Sickness, medical welfare and the English poor, 1750–1834

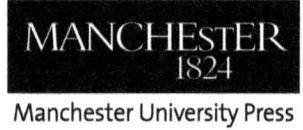

Manchester University Press

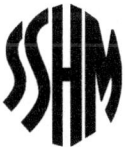

SOCIAL HISTORIES OF MEDICINE

Series editors: David Cantor and Keir Waddington

Social Histories of Medicine is concerned with all aspects of health, illness and medicine, from prehistory to the present, in every part of the world. The series covers the circumstances that promote health or illness, the ways in which people experience and explain such conditions, and what, practically, they do about them. Practitioners of all approaches to health and healing come within its scope, as do their ideas, beliefs, and practices, and the social, economic and cultural contexts in which they operate. Methodologically, the series welcomes relevant studies in social, economic, cultural, and intellectual history, as well as approaches derived from other disciplines in the arts, sciences, social sciences and humanities. The series is a collaboration between Manchester University Press and the Society for the Social History of Medicine.

Previously published

The metamorphosis of autism: A history of child development in Britain *Bonnie Evans*

Payment and philanthropy in British healthcare, 1918–48 *George Campbell Gosling*

The politics of vaccination: A global history *Edited by Christine Holmberg, Stuart Blume and Paul Greenough*

Leprosy and colonialism: Suriname under Dutch rule, 1750–1950 *Stephen Snelders*

Medical misadventure in an age of professionalization, 1780–1890 *Alannah Tomkins*

Conserving health in early modern culture: Bodies and environments in Italy and England *Edited by Sandra Cavallo and Tessa Storey*

Migrant architects of the NHS: South Asian doctors and the reinvention of British general practice (1940s–1980s) *Julian M. Simpson*

Mediterranean quarantines, 1750–1914: Space, identity and power *Edited by John Chircop and Francisco Javier Martínez*

Sickness, medical welfare and the English poor, 1750–1834

Steven King

Manchester University Press

The right of Steven King to be identified as the author of this work has been asserted by him in accordance with the Copyright, Designs and Patents Act 1988.

Published by Manchester University Press
Altrincham Street, Manchester M1 7JA

www.manchesteruniversitypress.co.uk

British Library Cataloguing-in-Publication Data
A catalogue record for this book is available from the British Library

ISBN 978 1 5261 2900 0   hardback

First published 2018

The publisher has no responsibility for the persistence or accuracy of URLs for any external or third-party internet websites referred to in this book, and does not guarantee that any content on such websites is, or will remain, accurate or appropriate.

Typeset by
Servis Filmsetting Ltd, Stockport, Cheshire
Printed in Great Britain by
TJ International Ltd, Padstow

*For Elizabeth, His Majesty King Bear, Lyddington-the-Mouse
and the Lord Tetbury*

Contents

Figures

Figures

Tables

Acknowledgements

This book has been long in the making: on one count at least thirty years. It brings together archival material from many projects, and I am grateful to those who have contributed to those projects. Richard Biddle, Margaret Hanly, Alison Stringer, Richard Gilbert, Ben Harvey, Alan Weaver and above all Peter Jones have all been instrumental in garnering the data used here. My co-authors over the years – especially Andreas Gestrich, Elizabeth Hurren, Alannah Tomkins and Peter Jones – have made me focus my ideas and perspectives. It goes without saying that I owe a debt to all of the archives noted in the bibliography and to the numerous archival staff who have put up with rapid turn-over of material as I sought out fugitive pauper letters. My colleagues Peter King, Andreas Gestrich and Keith Snell have had, sometimes unwittingly, substantial influence on my thinking for this book, and I am grateful for their help and friendship. While the book is not a product of a particular grant, the material I draw on was collected under the auspices of awards from the Wellcome Trust, British Academy, Leverhulme Trust, AHRC, British Council and Pasold Trust. I am grateful for the funding at a time when such opportunities were to say the least scarce. At the other end of the research process, I am grateful to Keir Waddington and staff at Manchester University Press for their careful steerage of this book. Keir engaged perspectives from two referees. Their acute observations and suggestions on the draft of the original manuscript highlighted plenty of areas where substance, style and presentation could be improved. I am grateful to them, and this volume is certainly better than it might otherwise have been. Above all I need to thank Elizabeth Hurren: You are a natural book writer, I am not. My shouting at the computer and exasperated opening of

wine bottles may well have been entertaining, but the long nights, early mornings, lack of holidays and pressure of writing were, I am sure, less welcome. But here we come to an end. Just as you must leave the dead, so I must leave the poor. No doubt we will remain at elbows with the world, but it will at least be together and in the company of His Maj.

Steve King, Lyddington, 2017

Abbreviations

BALS:	Bolton Archives and Local Studies
BRO:	Berkshire Record Office
BURO:	Buckinghamshire Record Office
COWAC:	City of Westminster Record Office
CPL:	Chorley Public Library
CRO:	Cheshire Record Office
CURO:	Cumbria Record Office
DHC:	Doncaster History Centre
DRO:	Dorset Record Office
EYRO:	East Yorkshire Record Office
GRO:	Gloucestershire Record Office
HALS:	Hertfordshire Archives and Local Studies
LCRO:	Leicestershire County Record Office
LRO:	Lancashire Record Office
MCL:	Manchester Central Library
NORO:	Norfolk County Record Office
NRO:	Northamptonshire Record Office
ORO:	Oxfordshire Record Office
RCSE:	Royal College of Surgeons, England
RL:	Rawtenstall Library and Local Studies
RPC:	Rothersthorpe Parish Church
SRC:	Surrey Record Centre
SRO:	Somerset Record Office
STRO:	Staffordshire Record Office
SURO:	Sussex Record Office
WRO:	Wiltshire Record Office
WYRO:	West Yorkshire Record Office

Note

This study focuses on seven counties. For the purposes of data organisation it works on the basis of pre-1972 boundaries and joins together the different Ridings of Yorkshire into one referential unit.

Part I

Locating sickness and medical welfare

1

The ecology of poor relief

Overview

On 18 July 1821 the overseer of Kingswood parish (Gloucestershire) received a letter from George Lewis of Bristol. Asking for 'Some preas-ant relife', Lewis claimed that he was sick and 'allmost intirely from my Worck'. He was

> in a verrey Weacke State my self i have a verrrey Soare throat as i am afraide as i am getting the Same Disorder as my family we am harekening Every moment to be the Last of one Chyld the Lords best to put is end to its Breath the biges bot was tacken ill Later day Last which i have five that is very bad ... which have not one to give aney assistance with the family for there is great Danger in Cathing the Disorder as i have no body as a friend to come to do aney thing for us ...[1]

This wonderfully orthographic letter, dripping with the desperation that might be occasioned by individual and familial illness, lays bare the core questions that frame the current study. What was wrong with Lewis and how does his sickness elide with a wider picture of the frequency and intensity of illness among the poor? Where did this particular episode fit into a life-cycle of ill-health? If he or his children did die, as Lewis prefigured, what would have happened to the body and the family left behind? Why did Lewis use the rhetorical vehicles that we see in his letter and why did he ask for present relief rather than the services of a doctor? How important as an element of expenditure was relieving sickness under the Old Poor Law? And how would local officials have viewed the letter and the predicament it encompassed?

Answering the latter question in particular is problematic. The English and Welsh Old Poor Law provided the legal basis for the

provision of welfare at parish level until the advent of the New Poor Law in 1834.[2] While the 1601 Act is more complex than is often allowed, its essence was to require parishes to punish vagrants and the undeserving poor, put the unemployed to work and relieve the 'impotent' (later 'deserving') poor using the proceeds of a local property tax.[3] Yet at no point did the 1601 legislation definitively establish which people should be seen as deserving and at what level and with what regularity their poverty should be relieved by the elected or selected, and for most of the Old Poor Law period amateur, parochial overseers of the poor.[4] The decisions of such men and the vestries which sometimes (and increasingly from the 1800s) stood above them were not, however, completely unconstrained. The Act also enshrined for the poor a right of appeal to a supra-local body (the Quarter Sessions and from 1691 individual magistrates) where they felt that their legitimate requests had been unfairly denied. This right of appeal became a more powerful commodity once the settlement laws of the 1660s and 1690s established that every English and Welsh person had a 'place' in which they were settled – to which they 'belonged'.[5] The settlement laws did nothing to clarify who was to be regarded as 'deserving', but they did establish a right for paupers to apply for poor relief in, at or to their parish of settlement, and thus grounds for contesting local decisions. Against this backdrop, it has been argued that we should read the combination of a right to apply and an avenue of appeal as conveying rights to receive relief on the part of paupers and an obligation on parishes to provide it.[6] Other commentators have not seen rights to relief, but have suggested that uncertainty over how magistrates would react to local decisions shaped, or rather constrained, the actions of officials.[7] For Peter King the individual decisions of magistrates coalesced into a powerful body of justice-made, 'local', law which constituted a remaking of justice from the margins.[8]

Yet empirical evidence on either perceptions of rights or the attitudinal impact of magistrate decisions is surprisingly slim. Paupers certainly had rights of appeal, but it is unclear how many used them.[9] Even where they did appeal, some studies have questioned how far magistrates were willing to go in supporting the poor.[10] More widely, it is striking that the language of 'rights' to receive, or obligations to give, relief is almost completely absent from pauper letters, vestry minutes and overseers' correspondence. While the poor might use yardsticks

of dignity as a way of asserting parochial obligations, these and other claims-making strategies were clearly conceived of by paupers as part of a *negotiation* of their eligibility for relief as well as its level, form and longevity. In fact, it could be argued that by the early 1800s the 'law of the Old Poor Law' had become such a complex constellation of oblig-atory legislation (much of it involving only partial re-interpretation or repeal of previous laws), enabling Acts and case law, that no one really understood it.[11] The ultimate impact of these multiple levels of 'the law' was a very considerable grey area in the minds of both officials and pau-pers over eligibility. In this space it was possible for custom rather than law to shape relief practice and for officials to vary their practice from year to year irrespective of continuity or change in the underpinning conditions of poverty.[12] Some of these issues are revisited in Chapter 3.

It was also possible for parishes and officials to construct relief mech-anisms – the Speenhamland system or the out-parish relief network – for which the legal basis was either questionable or non-existent.[13] In the end, much of the day-to-day practice of the English and Welsh Old Poor Law was underpinned by actual, perceived or claimed discretion on the part of officials.[14] Dorothy Marshall suggests that there 'was an enormous gulf between theory and practice … the latter was a misera-ble travesty of the former'.[15] While this view is heavily value-laden, the fact of the 'gulf' is reflected in work by Joanna Innes and others sug-gesting that national legislation frequently had to catch up with what was already happening at local level.[16] Against this backdrop, detailed empirical consideration of relief practice has suggested considerable intra-regional and local variation over both short and long terms.[17] This state of affairs began to break down in the early 1800s under the dual impetus of the statisticalisation of the poor law by central government and an increasing appetite on the part of vestries for knowledge about comparable practice elsewhere.[18] By this time, however, historians have conventionally come to trace a loss of official, public and rate-payer confidence in the Old Poor Law – a so-called 'crisis' – and a rapid waning of humanitarian sentiment towards the poor.[19] Indeed, Lynn Hollen Lees suggests that by the early nineteenth century 'the destitute had lost much of the legitimacy that they had earlier enjoyed in communal eyes'. The poor, she argues, 'were pushed to the margins of their communities well before' the New Poor Law, and there were persistent attempts to tighten eligibility to relief.[20] Whether one in fact

sees such a draining of sentiment by the early 1800s is a matter to which this study returns on a number of occasions.[21]

Reflecting and driven by diversity in local practice, the historiographical literature on the Old Poor Law has become increasingly rich. Administrative and institutional histories have dwindled in favour of attempts to reconstruct the world of poor people like George Lewis. Top-down approaches have been superseded by studies, such as that of Innes, which put a dynamic interaction between state and locality at their heart.[22] London has been transformed from a backwater of the Old Poor Law literature as large-scale studies have portrayed it as a microcosm of policy and practice across the country.[23] More widely, sustained work on the economy of makeshifts has begun to unpick the key issue of the extent to which local poor law practice was contingent – on the scale of informal and endowed charity, the presence or absence of self-help initiatives, the depth of petty earning and the degree of familial support networks – or self-contained.[24] Further research is needed on these important issues, not least to observe the shifting role of the poor law over the life-cycle of paupers and families.[25] Such work would usefully feed through to the wider question of how one should think about the geography of the Old Poor Law in its later phases. For some commentators practice was so situational – inexorably conditioned by the scale of local poverty and resources, as well as the personalities of overseers, paupers and vestrymen, and therefore fluid – that intra-regional and local variation defies any attempt to discern patterns of experience, practice and sentiment.[26] By contrast, I have argued that if one works within broad limits of tolerance for local (often short-term) variation it is possible to see regional patterns of expenditure and practice, themselves underpinned by distinct regional sentiments towards paupers on the part of officials and to the poor law by the poor.[27] More recently, I have refined and extended this argument, suggesting that it is possible to classify and organise local studies across Europe into 'welfare regimes' which span administrative, linguistic, religious and state boundaries.[28] Rather than focus on 'national' narratives of the character of welfare systems or the state of attitudes towards the poor, I argue, we must focus on the nature and longevity of local welfare practice as it was constructed and experienced. Such modelling is not uncontentious but it is informed by a sense that to understand a welfare system one must focus not on

the noise of everyday practice and short-term variation, two of the core rationales for individual micro-studies, but on the key yardsticks by which ingrained *local* sentiment can be judged.

The poor and the Poor Law

The need to make sense of diversity and to locate the individual stories of paupers like George Lewis has informed four trends in the historiography of the Old Poor Law that are central to this study. The first has been to place the pauper experience at the centre of an analytical agenda, fusing together issues of belonging and agency. Keith Snell, for instance, has sought to disentangle the issues of settlement and belonging for the dependent poor. While in practice settlement played a much larger part in defining the identity, 'place' and 'belonging' of the poor and potentially poorer than it did for other groups, even for paupers the question was more complicated than this.[29] Belonging was multi-layered – the legal status of belonging created by settlement law; the custom of belonging created by long residence; a belonging created by participation in local institutions, by paying taxes or receiving charity[30] – and could be bestowed, inherited and earned. It might be fragile or contested, stronger at some life-cycle points or in some socio-economic contexts than others. For groups like married women belonging could be very complex.[31] In turn, work on pauper letters or other ordinary writing reveals that the dependent poor had a keen appreciation of how belonging was claimed, maintained and lost.[32] And while the fact that some paupers were treated appallingly under the Old Poor Law is ever present,[33] this must be balanced with evidence of compassion, humanity and recognition of 'belonging' by parochial officials, neighbourhoods and communities.[34] This complex patchwork suggests the limitations of focusing on national narratives of sentiment towards the poor.

Of course, asserting, claiming and maintaining an acknowledgement of belonging was no easy matter for those at the sharp end of the relief system. One of the most powerful developments in recent historiography, however, has been a rethinking of the matter of pauper agency. The voices of paupers like George Lewis have been increasingly rediscovered, reproduced and re-interpreted. Early work by James Taylor and Thomas Sokoll revealed intriguing caches of letters from or about

paupers in Westmorland and Essex.[35] We now know that these represent a small sample of those available across England and Wales, and an even smaller sample of those written but which have not subsequently survived.[36] Such documents explode the complex world of pauperism. We are faced with paupers who varied in literacy terms from word-perfect to those like Lewis who employed basic orthographic spelling. These writers adopted complex rhetorical modes and systematically exploited the grey areas of the law over entitlement and parochial obligation by melding together arguments about respectability, gender,[37] fatherhood and motherhood,[38] familial duty, contribution, honesty, custom, duty, humanity and belonging. In contrast to deferential petitions, such narratives reveal paupers who by and large felt that they had a right to try and shape their relief.[39] Sometimes their 'familiar letters' were supplemented or substituted with appearances at the door of the overseer or the correspondence of epistolary advocates, or, as Steve Hindle has shown for an earlier period, by literally occupying liminal spaces within the parish community such as the church porch.[40] Questions over the limits of pauper agency and whether it translated into better relief outcomes for the poor remain to be fully answered.[41] Nonetheless, a new focus on the words and lives of the poor has suggested the existence of an alternative Old Poor Law: one in which paupers like George Lewis were not simply subject to the unconstrained will of parochial officials and vestries. It seems unlikely in this context that positive sentiment towards the poor ebbed in any uniform way across time and space.

Meanwhile, a second broad trend in the historiographical literature has been to juxtapose questions of agency with attempts to understand the nature of the power relationships into which poor law structure and practice was inscribed and which the poor law itself partly embodied. For the middling sorts who might dominate vestry politics, the relief system was about more than simply reconciling the demand for and supply of welfare. It provided an opportunity to weigh oneself against other people in the parish, to establish a collective identity and to construct and impose behavioural and attitudinal norms upon the poor. In this sense, the issue of what was dispensed to whom and for how long was anything other than a mechanistic decision. Rather, it was tied up with the micro-politics of poor relief and wider questions of social order and stability. During the early modern period such power relations seem to have given the initiative to officials. French and Barry,

for instance, suggest that the poor had to continually work to 'establish their honesty, or their social and moral autonomy' and that there was an inherent bias on the part of parish officials against 'claims of truthfulness and honesty' by the poor.[42] Hindle has argued persuasively that dependence in this period came to be associated with the loss of dignity and submission to a relationship in which ongoing entitlement was closely linked to obedience of moral codes, the rhetorical and behavioural norms of deference and gratitude and subjection to the will of the donor.[43] Such perspectives resonate with some of the writing on the crisis decades of the Old Poor Law. The Webbs, for instance, saw the central purpose of the Old Poor Law as 'repressing the freedom and regulating the conduct' of the poor.[44] John Broad suggests that the gentry regarded the poor law as 'a personal fiefdom', while Tomkins portrays female paupers as 'not just short of money; they were also short of influence'.[45] For Lees 'The welfare bargain was a local one between givers and receivers in a particular political context. Negotiated among unequals, it defined the limits of social obligation and of communal membership in a hierarchical society.'[46] In their turn, parochial officials 'had little hesitation in intervening in the lives of parishioners … across a positively kaleidoscopic range'.[47]

How far the Old Poor Law and its decision-making structures *actually* institutionalised expectations of deference and certain, moral, forms of behaviour is unclear for the post-1750 period. Poor law administration may have been a forum for the creation of middling identity, but the personalities of parochial officers and splits within vestries on policy matters periodically compromised exercise of the power that such social identity might confer.[48] On the other side of the welfare bargain, pauper letter writers often used the rhetoric of deference in their initial claims-making. We see this in the example of George Lewis. Yet over a sequence of letters from the same pauper such rhetoric usually slipped, and with no great impact on the outcome of the negotiation. The poor did not behave in workhouses, and readily (often successfully) contested decisions which vestries saw as final.[49] This picture, developed at length in Chapter 3, should not perhaps surprise us; the period from the 1780s to the 1830s was one in which ordinary people increasingly sought to engage with and confront the local and national state through rioting, rural unrest, petitions to Parliament, rallies, machine-breaking and innumerable acts of everyday resistance. Whether as expressions

of class, popular radicalism, a sense that the powerful ought to adhere to customary norms or wider attempts to establish what Isaac Land has called 'street citizenship', these very visible acts changed the landscape in which power might be exercised.[50] As we will see, sick paupers like George Lewis posed acute moral problems for ratepayers, hedging their notional power and undermining the sorts of structures of deference to which other groups might have been subject. Their plight also generated advocacy on the part of friends, neighbours, clerics, doctors, magistrates and even the gentry, bringing multiple understandings of power, obligation and the malleability of the local state into confrontation at parochial level.

A third and related development in the recent historiography has been the tendency to move away from analysis of the simple mechanics of poor relief (broadly, who got what, and with what regularity and longevity) towards a deeper understanding of the relief process. If we concentrate on the character and scope of relief as evidenced by overseers' accounts, the mainstay of most early studies of the Old Poor Law, a suite of problems emerge. These include the absence for most places of age-related data that would facilitate an analytical link between allowances and life-cycle stage, and the fact that the operation of the out-parish relief system from the 1780s means that one cannot be sure that all of those named in overseers' accounts were resident in, or paid for by, the community concerned. More importantly, recorded payments represent the final step of a process during which demands might be modified, amalgamated or dropped and claims accepted or rejected. These matters are discussed at greater length in Chapters 2 and 3. In part reacting to such complexities, there has been a tendency to rethink the scale of analysis – particularly the investigation of contiguous or proximate parishes as opposed to single parochial or township units[51] – and to link poor law data more systematically with other local sources. Thus, Richard Smith, Barry Reay, Pam Sharpe, Henry French, Samantha Williams, Barry Stapleton, Susannah Ottaway and myself have all linked overseers' accounts to family reconstitutions.[52] Such exercises collectively reveal a different kind of poor law from that seen by early commentators such as Dorothy Marshall,[53] one in which *inter alia* women tended to dominate the relief landscape measured by value for much of the eighteenth century;[54] officers were sometimes acutely sensitive to need; parishes sought partnerships with families;

small groups of paupers proved extraordinarily expensive; attitudes towards regular pensions (size, duration, etc.) might vary markedly; inter-generational poverty was growing; and parochial officials were often finely attuned to the local economy of makeshifts. It is doubtless this alternative structure that Lees saw when noting that while 'The price of relief was acknowledged dependence and a submissive air', the poor law tied claimant and parish into a 'morris dance of interlocking obligation'.[55] Focusing on the process of poor relief, then, refigures our understanding of parochial administration. It suggests that rather than practising a reactive parsimony or a deep adherence to the remedies emanating from national debates over Malthusianism and individual versus societal causes of destitution, vestries and overseers were sensitive to the situational needs of the poor, flexible in their relief strategies and less able to exercise discretion in cases such as that of George Lewis than has often been supposed.

Following from this observation, a final, and fundamental, trend in the recent historiography of the Old Poor Law has been to dissect the lumpen category of 'the poor'.[56] The elderly (however defined) have been foremost in this development. We now know that the aged poor were often seen as having definitive moral and customary claims on parochial poor relief, such that they could absorb a considerable proportion of local welfare resources. Ottaway's study of Terling in Essex and Tollpuddle in Dorset, for instance, reveals a long-term and remarkably robust focus of poor law resources on the aged poor.[57] Smith's analysis of the number and proportion of 'pension weeks' devoted to the aged poor in fourteen parishes adds a further dimension, suggesting that parochial administrations came to systematically support older men excluded from the labour force.[58] More widely, both Pat Thane and Lees have suggested that the elderly poor maintained their legitimacy in the eyes of ratepayers for much longer than other groups in the closing decades of the Old Poor Law.[59] Sokoll is more circumspect, arguing from the letters of Essex paupers that age alone was not a basis for poor relief. Entitlement in advancing years was often linked in the minds of both officials and paupers with sickness, decay, kinship deficit and the changing capacities for work.[60] In turn the moral dilemma that old age imposed on officials and communities allowed the aged poor to employ particular rhetorical strategies in their letters that were not available to other life-cycle paupers, and their success rates were high.[61]

Similarly, the problem of what to do with orphaned or abandoned children or the large families of poor parents created a thorny dilemma for parish officers. Sending them to an institution like the foundling hospital or workhouse could quickly curtail the problem given the high death rates.[62] Yet most dependent children did not end up in such places.[63] Meanwhile, this 'anatomisation' of the poor has also extended to those with mental and physical impairments, and recent commentators have questioned an ingrained view from new disability histories that communal support for such groups was threadbare and episodic.[64] Such experiences speak to a widespread local assumption that some groups of the dependent poor could not be held responsible for their own poverty and to the long-term survival of paternalistic attitudes towards certain groups of the poor, notwithstanding a national narrative which, as we have seen, might suggest a narrowing of eligibility and a renewed focus on constraining allowances given the spiralling costs of welfare from the 1790s.[65]

To weigh up the broad thrust of the recent historiography of the Old Poor Law is a heroic task. Signs of parsimony, inconsistent policy and a tendency to engage in periodic slashing of the relief lists are regular features of empirical studies. Scandals, though not as well documented as they would be under the New Poor Law, were common.[66] Such experiences play powerfully to wider contemporary commentary which called into question the moral status, deservingness and even humanity of the poor. On the other hand accumulating evidence of pauper agency and the fact that some groups garnered widely understood and acknowledged customary rights to relief offers a more optimistic sense of the final decades of the Old Poor Law. Paul Slack's reading of 'signs that English society's threshold of tolerance of deprivation was always low' might easily be applied to many of the parishes whose archives underpin this study.[67] The way in which parishes treated sick paupers like George Lewis is one such sign.

The sick poor

The character, scope and scale of medical welfare under the Old Poor Law are issues that have attracted relatively little historiographical attention in comparison to the post-1834 period.[68] In some ways this is surprising. The period encompassed by this volume was one in which

older diseases (such as smallpox) retained a hold on the population while new ones (such as cholera) were emerging and others (typhus, strokes and tuberculosis) were being reinvigorated. At the same time the rise of institutional medicine and a more frequent engagement of patients with doctors of various stripes were driving in the general population an increased medicalisation of conditions that might previously just have been 'lived with'. While increases in the range and effectiveness of surgery were at best incremental and the curative potential of drugs remained limited, there is a clear sense by the 1800s that conditions could be and were remediable. Against this backdrop of rapid change in understandings of health and ill-health for the wider population, it would be very unusual not to see percolation of language, demands and ideas down to the expectations and actions of the poor law.

In other ways, however, the lack of work on medical welfare is less surprising. The 1601 Act imposed no absolute obligation on parishes to recognise the sick poor as 'deserving' and to care for them.[69] Since the state did little to either monitor or regulate local practice, definitions of sickness and the resources devoted to combating it could vary substantially even between adjacent parishes. For historians the very process of defining medical welfare, let alone tracing it in sources such as overseers' accounts, is a complicated process. We return to these matters in Chapter 2. Meanwhile, much of the secondary literature on the Old Poor Law has followed the lead of the Webbs,[70] assuming that sickness was such a 'normal' part of the poverty life-cycle that there is little point in trying to disentangle medical from other forms of relief.[71] Many studies thus dwell only briefly on the question of the sick poor and their particular experiences or place in the poor law system. Of those medical and welfare historians who have moved further, Martin Gorsky and Sally Sheard suggest that the poor law tended to 'differentiate its health care from its relief duties', a view echoed by Tomkins in her study of Northampton, Shrewsbury and York.[72] E. G. Thomas similarly concludes that sick paupers in Berkshire, Essex and Oxfordshire received 'sympathetic and humane consideration'.[73] More widely, the scale and scope of medical welfare under the Old Poor Law appear to have been somewhat better than that to be had in the initial decades of the New Poor Law. Anne Digby, for instance, concludes that 'Both the comprehensive nature and the overall quality of the medical help given under the Old Poor Law were impressive.' She concurs with Loudon

that before 1834 paupers had access to medical care of equal quality to other parishioners.[74] Likewise Tomkins contrasts medical relief under the New Poor Law – 'at best undesirable and at worst …. repellent' – unfavourably with that available in the final decades of the Old Poor Law.[75]

The questions of what Thomas's 'consideration' meant in terms of the range and depth of medical care, whether it was uniformly offered across the country, how medical relief was negotiated and the mechanisms for its delivery have prompted a series of important but contradictory studies. Hilary Marland, for instance, argues that medical relief for the northern poor was 'limited', comprising in most places less than 5 per cent of total outdoor relief. Indeed 'poor law medical relief was the least important form of medical provision in existence for the poor throughout the nineteenth century'. French concludes for Terling that medical welfare in the form of *ad hoc* allowances absorbed 8.6 per cent relief resources over the period 1762–1834.[76] By contrast, Joan Lane suggests that the Old Poor Law provided a 'comprehensive welfare service' for the sick poor and identifies an upward spiral in medical expectations of the parish from the later eighteenth century. In fact there was 'no area of medical or welfare provision that the … authorities did not undertake'.[77] Crowther's characterisation of the 'chaotic and overlapping medical services' of the eighteenth and nineteenth centuries similarly reserves a key place for the Old Poor Law.[78] As Dorothy and Roy Porter remind us, vestries in even the most parsimonious communities recognised that small sums spent on treating sickness or alleviating its knock-on effects could save substantial bills in the long term.[79] Within this general context, medical and welfare historians have seen an increasingly central role for doctors. Samantha Williams, for instance, traces a late eighteenth-century upsurge in the practice of parishes contracting doctors as opposed to using them on an *ad hoc* basis.[80] Doctors themselves appear to have embraced such contracts,[81] and Roy Porter is in no doubt that for the poor 'being treated by the doctor became a way of life'.[82] Even in the notionally harshest of poor law counties, as we shall see, there is evidence of doctors extending their sway over the medical lives of poor people.[83] The intertwining issues of the changing nature of the engagement between parishes and medical people (doctors, fringe practitioners, nurses) and of the quality of the care they provided are revisited in Chapter 5.

In the meantime, the range of benefits encompassed by 'medical welfare' expanded from the late eighteenth century.[84] As well as employing doctors on contracts, paying extra cash allowances to families and buying food and drink for the sick, some parishes began to send their poor to specialist medical men.[85] Indeed, Lane suggests that the Old Poor Law provided '[medical] services from the cradle to the grave'.[86] Local studies suggest a willingness on the part of parochial officers to invest considerable sums in restoring individual and familial health, paying for midwives, rent arrears occasioned by sickness, false limbs, fuel, nursing care and sojourns in a wide variety of medical institutions.[87] Moreover, the range of what was recognised as 'sickness' also appears to have expanded, with Tomkins for instance arguing that parishes recognised melancholy by the early nineteenth century.[88] In the case of groups such as the insane (revisited in Chapter 8) or those with physical impairments, officers often proved particularly sensitive to their moral and practical obligations.[89] Indeed, Dorothy Porter even claims that it is possible to see the evolution in the nineteenth century of a definitive 'health citizenship'.[90] Whether range and variety in medical welfare were matched by depth is taken up from Chapter 4 onwards.[91] In the meantime, the question of how to interpret increased parochial engagement with sickness relief is complex. Such patterning may reflect a tightening of the definition of who was properly eligible for relief in the last decades of the Old Poor Law. Paupers as a group may have been losing their legitimacy in the eyes of ratepayers, as welfare historians focusing on national commentaries have often argued, such that parochial officers sought to increasingly focus resources on those traditionally seen as deserving. On the other hand, we may be witnessing responses to an increasing tide of sickness, a vibrant pauper agency or a positive sense that the sick poor had valid and substantial claims on parochial resources.[92]

However we interpret the broad picture, it is important to acknowledge that these perspectives arise out of a mere handful of empirical studies covering individual communities or (much more rarely) county samples. They remain to be tested against a large-scale database of evidence on medical relief drawn from parishes across the typological, chronological and geographical spectrum. There is also much that we do *not* know. While the literature on voluntary hospitals has become ever richer, our understanding of the medical aspects of the

institutional infrastructure of the Old Poor Law itself – workhouses, fever hospitals, nursing homes – is to say the least threadbare. Nor do we have a firm grasp on the medical economy of makeshifts. The voluntary hospital system, allied with increasing self-help provision through the growth of friendly societies and burial clubs, gave some paupers real alternatives to the poor law. So did the fact that, as Porter notes, medical practitioners themselves increasingly treated poor people free of charge, or at reduced cost, from charitable or other imperatives.[93] And, of course, irregular practitioners, dispensing druggists and quacks could increasingly claim the poor and very poor among their customers.[94] The question of how – or given the work of Tomkins on the discrete constituencies of infirmaries and workhouses, whether[95] – the sick poor like George Lewis assembled a medical economy of makeshifts at fixed points in time and over the life-cycle requires much further work.

Addressing these lacunae for such an important sub-group of the poor is a vital task. Yet the sick poor also matter for another reason. People like George Lewis posed, as we will go on to see, the most acute moral dilemma for the parochial officials. Sickness could be faked, and the unemployed and morally suspect could build a legitimate case for relief by appropriating the rhetoric of sickness, something which, if widely adopted, ought to influence our reading of quantitative trends in medical welfare spending. We return to this issue in Chapters 2 and 3. Even if genuine, sickness might be caused and exacerbated by moral failings such as heavy drinking. In this sense, parochial intervention invited sustained moral hazard. More generally, treating sickness could be extremely expensive, but not doing so might reduce individuals and families to long-term penury and lead to much higher relief costs than an engagement with the illness would have incurred. Failing to treat sick children or to throw enough resources at problems such as epidemics or accidents could foster both lifelong pauperism and its inter-generational transmission. Genuine, sickness placed ratepayers and their officials firmly in the territory of what we now understand as the moral economy, and studies of pauper letters have begun to point to an ingrained belief among the epistolary advocates of the sick poor that parishes had an absolute duty to act at times of sickness.[96] A bedrock of custom, intertwining by the late eighteenth century with the inexorable subjection of the labour market to exogenous shocks (trade

depression, war or harvest failure), demographic instability,[97] and evidence of rising background medical standards, proved a challenging framework for officials. Yet recognising sickness as a moral basis for relief would give the poor a fixed reference point in navigating the rules of relief systems where the actions of officials were underpinned by discretion and individual case analysis. It was in these grey areas over entitlement that the sick poor and their advocates could potentially apply an agency greater by far than for any other paupers. To reject claims meant accepting prolonged negotiation, repeated application, public discussion inside and outside the parish and potential damage to reputations where officials were seen or characterised as uncaring, inhumane, unchristian and penny-pinching. This is not to say that officials were immune from reacting summarily, slowly or negatively to the claims of the sick poor. It *is* to observe, however, that such actions were, and were often seen to be, contentious. Thus, while studying the sick poor and medical welfare in their own right is important, these matters also offer a wider lens onto bigger issues about the nature, purpose and sentiment of the Old Poor Law and the traction of 'national' debates about eligibility and deservingness at local level. In this sense, one of the central arguments of this study is that those who became poor because they were sick or became sick when or because they were poor constitute *the* iconic sub-group of 'the poor'. Their treatment at the individual and collective level can and should be used as a key yardstick by which one might judge the sentiment of the Old Poor Law in its final 'crisis' period.

Looking forward

In this context the current study has five interweaving aims. The first is to construct a broad comparative picture of the scale of medical welfare in England across the period 1750–1834. A second is to analyse the range, depth and constellation of medical welfare in different parochial, regional and typological settings, and through such an analysis to explore the everyday experiences of the sick poor. A related and third aim is to locate poor law support within the wider medical economy of makeshifts. Fourthly, the study aims to come to a better understanding of the agency of sick paupers like George Lewis in shaping the incidence, character and duration of medical welfare. Finally, the study will

question the sense that the poor – or at least the sick poor – lost their legitimacy in the eyes of ratepayers and officials, seeking to rethink the sentimental architecture of the Old Poor Law in its final decades.

Exploring these issues in a meaningful way requires a large-scale comparative dataset, and my study draws on four sets of sources. Firstly, I use operational data (overseers' accounts, vestry minutes, correspondence, bills, vouchers, correspondence) from 117 parishes across the counties of Berkshire, Norfolk, Wiltshire, Northamptonshire, Leicestershire, Lancashire and West Yorkshire. The Appendix provides further analysis of the reasons for choosing these counties and the socio-economic and demographic complexion of the sample. Meanwhile, Chapter 4 focuses on the methodological and practical issues involved in constructing a chronological, typological and spatial overview of medical welfare from this empirical core. Secondly, I draw episodically (and particularly from Chapter 5 onwards) on material from a second tranche of communities where operational data is more fractured. Comprising 146 parishes both within the core county envelopes and much more widely in England, these places provide a window onto the experiences of medical welfare across a wider spectrum. Once again, the Appendix provides more detail on this sample. Thirdly, the study draws (particularly in Chapters 2 and 5–10) on a set of miscellaneous sources collected and analysed as part of prior projects. These include the records of coronial courts for Lincolnshire, Midland and Wiltshire circuits, printed diaries and memorandum books, contemporary pamphlets, advertising material for irregular practitioners, notes on patient cases kept by voluntary hospitals and workhouse medical staff, newspaper articles, friendly society certificates, pre-1841 census material and parochial registers. Finally, I use in most chapters data from the tri-partite epistolary world of the parish: letters from poor claimants, their advocates and officials. Covering every county in England, the dataset comprises 12,904 narratives by or about the poor, and Chapters 2 and 3 deal at greater length with the sickness component of this material and also its wider methodological and substantive complexities.[98] Collectively, these datasets represent the most extensive and intensive corpus ever brought to bear on the Old Poor Law.

An important prior step in using this data is to understand the scale and character of sickness that the parochial welfare system had to

cope with and to construct a working definition of medical welfare. Chapter 2 takes up these matters. It argues that the frequency and duration of sickness among the poor increased even as the impact of epidemic disease fell away from the later eighteenth century. The chapter also argues that our definition of medical welfare should be driven by the practice of contemporary overseers and vestries. They often did not confine themselves to narrow definitions centred on the provision of doctors and medicines. Rather, they funded (and recorded as a coherent whole) a range of needs when confronted by sickness episodes, including rent payments, funerals, institutional sojourns, cash, and consequential relief for bereaved families. This evidently raises problems of measurement, record linkage, source coverage and official recording policy. Chapters 2 and 4 take up these questions and the practical application of a wide definition of medical welfare. Chapter 3 completes Part I. At its core lie questions about the scope for and effectiveness of the agency of the sick poor on the one hand and the receptiveness of officials on the other. While the sick poor rarely claimed definitive rights to relief, the chapter will suggest that there was an accepted ground of contestation which points ultimately to the fluidity and flexibility of local policy even in the crisis years of the Old Poor Law. Chapter 4 opens Part II of the study, which is centrally concerned with the complexion of medical welfare and everyday experiences for the sick poor. It reviews the methodological and procedural issues involved in using and interpreting analysis of the data, ultimately arguing that medical welfare became a more and more important part of overall relief spending during the last decades of the Old Poor Law. There were important spatial nuances to this picture, but typological variation will be seen to be muted. Chapters 5–7 (focusing respectively on medical people, wider forms of parochial medical welfare, and last illnesses and pauper funerals) offer a dissection of the broad quantitative picture. Combining summative analysis and more detailed perspectives on emblematic parishes or paupers, the chapters reconstruct an Old Poor Law that was willing and able to respond inventively to the needs of the sick

Part III of the study moves our focus away from issues of complexion, place, community typology and chronological change and to wider questions about the place of parochial support in the life-cycles of paupers and the wider medical market in which they engaged.

Chapter 8 focuses on the particular role of institutional care. Perhaps not unexpectedly given the proliferation of voluntary institutions, private asylums and workhouses in the later decades of the Old Poor Law, it argues that institutional sojourns became a more common part of the parochial response to sickness, albeit with marked differences of emphasis in certain counties. Chapter 9 sets the resources offered by the parish into the wider infrastructure of medical care available to the poor at points in time and over the life-cycle. Painting a rich picture of the medical economy of makeshifts, it argues that paupers individually and collectively navigated a complex assemblage of shadow, supplementary and substitute sources of medical care. Finally, Chapter 10 turns to the questions of how we make sense of spatial chronological and typological diversity and what such a synthesis can offer to our understanding of the character and role of the Old Poor Law in its final years.

A starting point

Jack Langton has suggested that welfare historians must recover the overarching 'human ecology' of poor relief. This includes, *inter alia*, the subjective experiences of being poor; pauper agency; the words and sentiments of the poor and their advocates; the micro-politics, personal enmities, jealousies, hopes and fears that drove both sides of the interaction between officials and paupers in the process of poor relief; and above all the impact of underlying socio-economic, topographical and cultural systems on policy.[99] It is particularly important to undertake such an exercise for the sick poor. This group inspired local sentiments on a spectrum from absolute loathing to a sensitive acknowledgement of Christian duty. Treating the 'plight' of paupers like George Lewis brought parochial officials into sustained contact with the stories of the desperate, the hopeless and hopeful, the honest, the crafty, the skilled and clumsy narrator, the mean and the generous, and the out-and-out charlatan. To build the human ecology of poor relief involves starting with this group rather than seeing them as part of the historiographical wallpaper.

That said, my study has not set out to engage with every sub-group of the sick poor. The Irish, Welsh and Scottish, black seafarers and ex-slaves, the Dutch and the Spanish all appear in the underlying

data, but I have not been centrally concerned with ethnicity, not least because parishes themselves often appear to have been blind to origin or colour.[100] And while issues of life-cycle are considered throughout, my study does not have individual chapters on particular life-cycle groups. In practice the sickness of one person often enmeshed whole families, neighbourhoods and kinship groups, and it makes more sense to talk about the sick poor collectively. Even so, sick children were ubiquitous in the underlying sources and they thus make frequent appearances. The study also has spatial and chronological limitations. It focuses, and was intended to focus, on England. This is not to say that Scotland is unimportant, but to acknowledge that the sources for studying medical welfare are radically different for the country, as they are for Ireland.[101] While Wales notionally shared the same laws as England, the character of its Old Poor Law was so distinctive as to demand a study in its own right. Within this broad spatial context, the parochial sample is substantial and (see the Appendix) designed to cover the typological spectrum from tiny rural parishes, town hinterlands, industrial and proto-industrial communities and coastal parishes to larger towns, both growing and decaying. I do not, however, claim that this is a systematic sample. London is under-represented though not absent; many pauper letters were written from the metropolis. The very largest towns are also under-represented, a reflection of both the scale of the task and associated problems of source coverage and depth. This is not, however, a study of rural England. Some twenty-three of my 117 base communities are 'urban' on conventional definitions of the term. Meanwhile, the chronological focus is firmly on the final decades of the Old Poor Law. This is partly for pragmatic reasons of source creation, preservation and depth. It also reflects, however, a desire to engage with wider questions of 'national' sentiment towards the poor and the poor law, which, as we have seen above, is constructed as waning at any time across the period from the 1750s. In this sense, my study will offer a more favourable reading of the relief system than has often been given, suggesting that the substantial tide of illness confronted by parishes in this period generated an essentially humanitarian response. We should thus construct the 'crisis of the Old Poor Law' as a rhetorical and strategic exercise that had limited impact on the lives of key groups such as the sick poor.

Notes

1 GRO, P193 OV/7–1, letter.
2 The Old Poor Law represents the only *constant* legally enshrined and national European welfare system before 1800: J. Innes, 'State, church and volunterism in European welfare 1690–1850', in A. Cunningham and J. Innes (eds), *Charity, Philanthropy and Reform from the 1690s to 1850* (Basingstoke: Macmillan, 1998), pp. 15–65; and J. Innes, S. King and A. Winter, 'Settlement and belonging in Europe, 1500–1930s: Structures, negotiations and experiences', in S. King and A. Winter (eds), *Migration, Settlement and Belonging in Europe, 1500s–1930s* (Oxford: Berghahn, 2013), pp. 1–28.
3 43 Eliz. I c. 2 (1601). On the need to read this statute alongside the Statute of Charitable Uses, see S. Hindle, '"Good, godly and charitable uses": Endowed charity and the relief of poverty in rural England, c.1555–1750', in A. Goldgar and R. Frost (eds), *Institutional Culture in Early Modern Society* (Leiden: Brill, 2004), p. 164.
4 S. Webb and B. Webb, *English Poor Law History Part I: The Old Poor Law* (London: Cass, 1963), p. 406.
5 For a case study in the Lancashire context see J. Healey, 'The development of poor relief in Lancashire, c.1598–1680', *Historical Journal*, 53 (2010), 567–72.
6 L. Charlesworth, *Welfare's Forgotten Past: A Socio-Legal History of the Poor Law* (London: Routledge, 2009). This works echoes similar claims by R. Mitchison, *Coping with Destitution: Poverty and Relief in Western Europe* (Toronto: University of Toronto Press, 1991), pp. 45–8, and L. H. Lees, *The Solidarities of Strangers: The English Poor Laws and the People 1700–1948* (Cambridge: Cambridge University Press, 1998), p. 39, who argues that 'citizens with parish settlements had a right to relief, and they knew it'. Dorothy Marshall in *The English Poor in the Eighteenth Century* (London: Longman, 1926), p. 252, has argued that 'The poorer sort took relief as their right whilst the ratepayers despised them for their indolence and insolence, and even for their very misery.'
7 P. Dunkley, *The Crisis of the Old Poor Law in England 1795–1834: An Interpretive Essay* (New York: Garland, 1982), pp. 54–6 and 78.
8 P. King, *Crime and Law in England 1750–1840: Remaking Justice from the Margins* (Cambridge: Cambridge University Press, 2006) and P. King, 'The rights of the poor and the role of the law: The impact of pauper appeals to the summary courts 1750–1834', in P. Jones and S. King (eds), *Obligation, Entitlement and Dispute under the English Poor Laws* (Newcastle: Cambridge Scholars Press, 2015), pp. 235–62. See also

D. Eastwood, *Governing Rural England: Tradition and Transformation in Local Government 1780–1840* (Oxford: Clarendon Press, 1994), pp. 44, 106, 112 and 133.

9 S. King, 'Negotiating the law of poor relief in England 1800–1840', *History*, 96 (2011), 410–35. Officials found ways of preventing appeals. See S. Broadbridge, 'The Old Poor Law in the parish of Stone', *North Staffordshire Journal of Field Studies*, 13 (1973), 11–25, at p. 12.

10 P. King, 'Social inequality, identity and the labouring poor in eighteenth century England', in H. French and J. Barry (eds), *Identity and Agency in England, 1500–1800* (Basingstoke: Macmillan, 2004), pp. 60–87; G. Morgan and P. Rushton, 'The magistrate, the community and the maintenance of an orderly society in eighteenth century England', *Historical Research*, 76 (2003), 54–77.

11 S. King, '"In these you may trust": Numerical information, accounting practices and the poor law, c.1790 to 1840', in T. Crook and G. O'Hara (eds), *Statistics and the Public Sphere: Numbers and the People in Modern Britain, c.1750–2000* (London: Routledge, 2011), pp. 51–66.

12 See S. Shave, 'The dependent poor? (Re)constructing individual lives "on the parish" in rural Dorset 1800–1832', *Rural History*, 20 (2009), 67–98; S. Ottaway, *The Decline of Life: Old Age in Eighteenth-Century England* (Cambridge: Cambridge University Press, 2004), pp. 42–86.

13 M. Neuman, *The Speenhamland County: Poverty and the Poor Laws in Berkshire 1782–1834* (New York: Garland, 1982), pp. 76 and 164. The out-parish relief system comprised bi-lateral and multi-lateral deals between settlement parishes and host communities whereby the poor 'out of their place' at the time they applied for relief were relieved in host communities, obviating the need for removal: S. King, '"It is impossible for our vestry to judge his case into perfection from here": Managing the distance dimensions of poor relief, 1800–40', *Rural History*, 16 (2005), 161–89. S. Hindle, 'Power, poor relief and social relations in Holland Fen c.1600–1800', *Historical Journal*, 41 (1998), 67–96, at p. 87, argues that there was considerable hostility on the part of host parishes to the non-settled poor. For a contrary view see Broadbridge, 'The Old Poor Law', p. 16, who notes that Stone (Staffordshire) had relief arrangements with more than sixty parishes by 1820.

14 Webb and Webb, *English Poor Law History*, p. 149.

15 Marshall, *The English Poor*, p. 250.

16 J. Innes, 'The local acts of a national parliament: Parliament's role in sanctioning local action in eighteenth-century Britain', *Parliamentary History*, 17 (1998), 23–47; J. Innes, *Inferior Politics: Social Problems and Social Policies in Eighteenth-Century Britain* (Oxford: Oxford University Press,

2009); R. Connors, 'Parliament and poverty in mid-eighteenth century England', *Parliamentary History*, 21 (2002), 207–31.

17 J. Langton, 'The geography of poor relief in rural Oxfordshire, 1775–1832', in Jones and King (eds), *Obligation, Entitlement and Dispute*, pp. 193–234.

18 D. Eastwood, 'Rethinking the debates on the poor law in early nineteenth-century England', *Utilitas*, 6 (1994), 97–116.

19 Historians differ considerably over the timing of this waning sentiment. For D. Valenze, 'Charity, custom and humanity: Changing attitudes to the poor in eighteenth century England', in J. Garnett and C. Matthew (eds), *Revival and Religion since 1700: Essays for John Walsh* (London: Hambledon, 1993), p. 78, the poor lost their legitimacy in the later eighteenth century; Eastwood, *Governing Rural England*, pp. 101 2 and 118, sees a softening of attitudes from 1750 systematically reversed in the 1790s; A. Tomkins, 'Women and poverty', in H. Barker and E. Chalus (eds), *Women's History: Britain 1700–1850* (London: Routledge, 2005), p. 166, suggests that favourable sentiment towards female paupers had disappeared by 1810. For a wider discussion, see A. Tomkins, *The Experience of Urban Poverty, 1723–82: Parish, Charity and Credit* (Manchester: Manchester University Press, 2006), pp. 7–8.

20 Lees, *Solidarities of Strangers*, pp. 20 and 82.

21 For more positive views see J. Taylor, *Poverty, Migration and Settlement in the Industrial Revolution: Sojourners' Narratives* (Palo Alto: Stanford University Press, 1989), pp. 4, 9, 105 and 173; Mitchison, *Coping with Destitution*, p. 33; P. Thane, *Old Age in English History: Past Experiences, Present Issues* (Oxford: Oxford University Press, 2000), pp. 107–8, 112–13; M. Daunton, *Progress and Poverty: An Economic and Social History of Britain 1700–1850* (Oxford: Oxford University Press, 1995), p. 452; D. Eastwood, 'The republic in the village: Parish and poor at Bampton 1780–1834', *Journal of Regional and Local Studies*, 12 (1992), 17–28, at p. 25. J. Broad, 'Parish economies of welfare 1650–1834', *Historical Journal*, 42 (1999), 985–1006, at p. 989, suggests that 'parish histories profoundly influenced the dynamism of local provision for the poor'. Contemporaries likewise held very divergent views. See, for instance, the plan for a national, government-funded, network of asylums for the aged and sick outlined in Common Sense, 'Rights of the poor asserted', *Monthly Magazine*, 34 (1812), 231, pp. 123–7.

22 Innes, *Inferior Politics*.

23 D. Green, *Pauper Capital: London and the Poor Law, 1790–1870* (Farnham: Ashgate, 2010); J. Boulton and L. Schwarz, '"The comforts of a private fireside": The workhouse, the elderly and the poor law

in Georgian Westminster. St Martin-in-the-Fields, 1725–1824', in J. McEwan and P. Sharpe (eds), *Accommodating Poverty: The Housing and Living Arrangements of the English Poor, c.1600–1850* (Basingstoke: Palgrave, 2011), pp. 221–45; J. Boulton, '"The charity of our life and healthful years"? Approaches to inter-vivos giving to the poor in the Metropolis 1600–1720', in Jones and King (eds), *Obligation, Entitlement and Dispute*, pp. 20–52; E. Murphy, 'The metropolitan pauper farms 1722–1834', *London Journal*, 27 (2002), 1–18.

24 S. King and A. Tomkins (eds), *The Poor in England 1700–1850: An Economy of Makeshifts* (Manchester: Manchester University Press, 2003); Tomkins, *The Experience of Urban Poverty*, pp. 204–29; and S. Lloyd, *Charity and Poverty in England, c.1680–1820: Wild and Visionary Schemes* (Manchester: Manchester University Press, 2009).

25 For an excellent example see H. French, 'How dependent were the "dependent poor"? Poor relief and the life-course in Terling, Essex, 1762–1834', *Continuity and Change*, 30 (2015), 193–222, at pp. 215–16.

26 S. Hindle, *On the Parish? The Micro Politics of Poor Relief in Rural England 1550–1750* (Oxford: Clarendon Press, 2004), pp. 282–99.

27 S. King, *Poverty and Welfare in England 1700–1850: A Regional Perspective* (Manchester: Manchester University Press, 2000). For different regional models see M. Lyle, 'Regionality in the late Old Poor Law: The treatment of chargeable bastards from Rural Queries', *Agricultural History Review*, 53 (2013), 141–57, and K. Price, *Medical Negligence in Victorian Britain: The Crisis of Care under the English Poor Law 1834–1900* (Basingstoke: Palgrave, 2015).

28 S. King, 'Welfare regimes and welfare regions in Britain and Europe, c.1750–1860', *Journal of Modern European History*, 9 (2011), 42–66.

29 K. Snell, *Parish and Belonging: Community, Identity and Welfare in England and Wales 1700–1950* (Cambridge: Cambridge University Press, 2006).

30 Lloyd, *Charity and Poverty*.

31 P. Sharpe, 'Parish women: Maternity and the limitations of Maiden Settlement in England 1662–1834', in Jones and King (eds), *Obligation, Entitlement and Dispute*, pp. 168–92.

32 See contributions to A. Gestrich, E. Hurren and S. King (eds), *Poverty and Sickness in Modern Europe: Narratives of the Sick Poor* (London: Continuum, 2012).

33 D. Feldman, 'Migrants, immigrants and welfare from the Old Poor Law to the welfare state', *Transactions of the Royal Historical Society*, 13 (2003), 79–104, at p. 102, suggests that parochial officials had a 'moral disdain' for paupers. For other negative commentary see E. Murphy, 'The metropolitan pauper farms', p. 4.

34 K. Snell, *Annals of the Labouring Poor: Social Change and Agrarian England, 1660–1900* (Cambridge: Cambridge University Press, 1985), pp. 105–7, argues that for those with settlement in southern England the Old Poor Law was 'flexible and humane'; D. Thomson, 'Welfare and the historians', in L. Bonfield, R. Smith and K. Wrightson (eds), *The World We Have Gained: Histories of Population and Social Structure* (Oxford: Basil Blackwell, 1986), p. 370, likewise argues that the poor law did not simply provide minimal and miserly relief. See also Daunton, *Progress and Poverty*, pp. 450–2, and J. Taylor, *Poverty, Migration and Settlement*, p. 51.

35 T. Sokoll, *Essex Pauper Letters 1731–1837* (Oxford: Oxford University Press, 2001); J. Taylor, 'Voices in the crowd: The Kirkby Lonsdale township letters, 1809–1836', in T. Hitchcock, P. King and P. Sharpe (eds), *Chronicling Poverty: The Voices and Strategies of the English Poor, 1640–1840* (Basingstoke: Macmillan, 1997), pp. 109–26. Such work should lead us to doubt that the voices of ordinary people were 'increasingly less audible' by the end of the early modern period. See R. Esser, '"They obey all magistrates and all good lawes … and we thinke our cittie happie to enjoye them": Migrants and urban stability in early modern English towns', *Urban History*, 34 (2007), 75.

36 S. King, T. Nutt and A. Tomkins, *Narratives of the Poor in Eighteenth Century Britain* (London: Pickering and Chatto, 2006).

37 P. Sharpe, 'Survival strategies and stories: Poor widows and widowers in early industrial England', in S. Cavallo and L. Warner (eds), *Widowhood in Medieval and Early Modern Europe* (London: Longman, 1999), pp. 220–39; S. King, '"The particular claims of a woman and a mother": Gender, belonging and rights to medical relief in England 1800–1840s', in A. Andresen, T. Grønle, W. Hubbard, T. Rymin and S. Skålevåg (eds), *Citizens, Courtrooms, Crossings* (Bergen: Bergen University Press, 2008), pp. 21–38.

38 J. Bailey, '"Think Wot a Mother Must Feel": Parenting in English pauper letters c.1760–1834', *Family and Community History*, 13 (2010), 5–19.

39 L.-H. van Voss (ed.), *Petitions in Social History* (Cambridge: Cambridge University Press, 2001). On the transition from early modern petitions to different sorts of narratives, see P. Jones and S. King, 'From petition to pauper letter: The development of an epistolary form', in Jones and King (eds), *Obligation, Entitlement and Dispute*, pp. 53–77.

40 S. King and P. Jones, 'Testifying for the poor: Epistolary advocates and the negotiation of parochial relief in England, 1800–1834', *Journal of Social History*, 49 (2016), 351–82; S. Hindle, 'Destitution, liminality and belonging: The church porch and the politics of settlement in English

rural communities, c.1590–1660', in C. Dyer (ed.), *The Self-Contained Village? The Social History of Rural Communities, 1250–1900* (Hatfield: Hertfordshire University Press, 2006), pp. 46–71.

41 For sceptical voices see P. King, 'Social inequality', pp. 66–74, and Tomkins, 'Women and poverty', p. 169.

42 H. French and J. Barry, 'Identity and agency in English society, 1500–1800: An introduction', in French and Barry (eds), *Identity and Agency*, pp. 1–37, at pp. 26 and 31.

43 S. Hindle, 'Civility, honesty and the identification of the deserving poor in seventeenth century England', in French and Barry (eds), *Identity and Agency*, pp. 38–59, at pp. 40, 47 and 52.

44 Webb and Webb, *English Poor Law History*, p. vi. In the North Riding such sentiments seem to have become ingrained after 1815. See R. Hastings, *Poverty and the Poor Law in the North Riding of Yorkshire 1780–1837* (York: Borthwick Institute, 1982), p. 32.

45 Broad, 'Parish economies of welfare', p. 989; Tomkins, 'Women and poverty', p. 169.

46 Lees, *Solidarities of Strangers*, pp. 7, 22 and 36.

47 D. Eastwood, *Government and Community in the English Provinces 1700–1870* (Basingstoke: Macmillan, 1997), p. 48.

48 On the importance of overseer personality, see Eastwood, *Governing Rural England*, p. 40. See also A. Kidd, *State, Society and the Poor in Nineteenth Century England* (Basingstoke: Macmillan, 1999), p. 4, who argues that the Old Poor Law demonstrated 'paternalistic and comparatively generous philanthropy'.

49 D. Green, 'Pauper protests: Power and resistance in early nineteenth-century London workhouses', *Social History*, 31 (2006), 137–59.

50 I. Land, 'Bread and arsenic: Citizenship from the bottom up in Georgian London', *Journal of Social History*, 45 (2005), 89–110, at p. 90.

51 Building on older works such as E. Neuman, 'The Old Poor Law in Kent 1606–1834' (unpublished PhD thesis, University of Kent, 1979); N. Hopkin, 'The Old and New Poor Law in East Yorkshire, 1760–1850' (unpublished MPhil thesis, University of Leeds, 1968); V. Walsh, 'Poor Law administration in Shropshire, 1820–1855' (unpublished PhD thesis, University of Pennsylvania, 1970). More recent comparative surveys include J. Hill, 'Poverty, unrest and response in Surrey, 1815–1834' (unpublished PhD thesis, University of Roehampton, 2006).

52 B. Stapleton, 'Inherited poverty and life-cycle poverty: Odiham, Hampshire, 1650–1850', *Social History*, 18 (1993), 339–55; B. Reay, *Micro-Histories: Demography, Society, and Culture in Rural England, 1800–1930* (Cambridge: Cambridge University Press, 1996); R. Smith, 'Ageing

and well-being in early modern England: Pension trends and gender preference under the English Old Poor Law 1650–1800', in P. Johnson and P. Thane (eds), *Old Age from Antiquity to Postmodernity* (London: Routledge, 1998), pp. 64–95; S. Williams, *Poverty, Gender and Life-Cycle under the English Poor Law 1760–1834* (Woodbridge: Boydell, 2011); P. Sharpe, *Population and Society in an East Devon Parish: Reproducing Colyton, 1540–1840* (Exeter: Exeter University Press, 2002); S. King, 'Reconstructing lives: The poor, the poor law and welfare in rural industrial communities', *Social History*, 22 (1997), 318–38; S. King, 'Pauvreté et assistance: La politique locale de la mortalité dans l'Angleterre des XVIII et XIX siècles', *Annales*, 61 (2006), 31–62; H. French, 'An irrevocable shift: Detailing the dynamics of rural poverty in southern England, 1762–1834. A case study', *Economic History Review*, 68 (2015), 769–805.

53 Marshall, *The English Poor*, p. 11, argues that parishes had 'blindness to all interests but their own'.

54 See S. Williams, 'Malthus, marriage and poor law allowances revisited: A Bedfordshire case study, 1770–1834', *Agricultural History Review*, 52 (2004), 56–82, at pp. 64–7.

55 Lees, *Solidarities of Strangers*, p. 36.

56 S. Williams, 'The experience of pregnancy and childbirth for unmarried mothers in London, 1760–1866', *Women's History Review*, 20 (2011), 67–86; T. Evans, 'Unfortunate objects': *Lone Mothers in Eighteenth-Century London* (Basingstoke: Palgrave, 2005).

57 Ottaway, *The Decline of Life*. More recently, Henry French, 'An irrevocable shift', pp. 784–6, has argued that the thrust of relief in Terling moved firmly towards men of working age in the early nineteenth century as the importance of short-term allowances to supplement income grew exponentially.

58 R. Smith, 'Ageing and well-being', pp. 90–5.

59 Thane, *Old Age in English History*; Lees, *Solidarities of Strangers*, pp. 58–60.

60 T. Sokoll, 'Old age in poverty: The record of Essex pauper letters, 1780–1834', in Hitchcock, King and Sharpe (eds), *Chronicling Poverty*, pp. 127–54.

61 T. Sokoll, 'Negotiating a living: Essex pauper letters from London, 1800–1834', *International Review of Social History Supplement*, 8 (2000), 19–46.

62 A. Levene, *Childcare, Health, and Mortality at the London Foundling Hospital, 1741–1800: 'Left to the mercy of the world'* (Manchester: Manchester University Press, 2007).

63 A. Levene, *The Childhood of the Poor: Welfare in Eighteenth Century London* (Basingstoke: Palgrave, 2012).

64 A. Borsay, *Disability and Social Policy in Britain since 1750: A History
    of Exclusion* (Basingstoke: Palgrave, 2005); D. Turner, *Disability in
    Eighteenth-Century England: Imagining Physical Impairment* (London:
    Routledge, 2012); S. King, 'Constructing the disabled child in England,
    1800–1860', *Family and Community History*, 18 (2015), 56–89.

65 On these debates see J. Poynter, *Society and Pauperism: English Ideas on
    Poor Relief, 1795–1834* (Toronto: University of Toronto Press, 1969);
    G. Himmelfarb, *The Idea of Poverty: England in the Early Industrial Age*
    (London: Knopf, 1983); and Innes, *Inferior Politics*.

66 On later scandals, see contributions to J. Reinarz and L. Schwarz (eds),
    Medicine and the Workhouse (Rochester: University of Rochester Press,
    2013).

67 P. Slack, *Poverty and Policy in Tudor and Stuart England* (London:
    Longman 1988), p. 207.

68 For a summary see S. King, 'Poverty, medicine and the workhouse in
    the eighteenth and nineteenth centuries: An afterword', in Reinarz
    and Schwarz (eds), *Medicine and the Workhouse*, pp. 228–52. See also
    R. Hodgkinson, *The Origins of the National Health Service: The Medical
    Services of the New Poor Law 1834–1871* (London: Croom Helm, 1967);
    M. Flinn, 'Medical services under the new poor law', in D. Fraser (ed.),
    The New Poor Law in the Nineteenth Century (Basingstoke: Macmillan,
    1976), and M. Crowther, *The Workhouse System 1834–1929* (London:
    Batsford, 1981). Nor did the matter attract sustained contemporary
    attention through the Royal Commission into the Operation of the Poor
    Laws of 1832 or in F. M. Eden's *The State of the Poor: Or, an History of
    the Labouring Classes in England, from the Conquest to the Present*, 3 vols
    (Cambridge: Cambridge University Press, 2011). The latter frequently
    notes, however, that a short illness was enough to bring dependency on
    the parish.

69 See M. Gorsky and S. Sheard, 'Introduction', in M. Gorsky and S. Sheard
    (eds), *Financing Medicine: The British Experience since 1750* (London:
    Routledge, 2006), pp. 1–20, at p. 3.

70 Webb and Webb, *English Poor Law History*, p. 170.

71 See A. Tomkins, '"Labouring on a bed of sickness": The material and
    rhetorical deployment of ill-health in male pauper letters', in Gestrich,
    Hurren and King (eds), *Poverty and Sickness*, pp. 51–68, pp. 51–2.

72 Gorsky and Sheard, 'Introduction', p. 2; Tomkins, *The Experience of
    Urban Poverty*, pp. 120–62.

73 E. Thomas, 'The Old Poor Law and medicine', *Medical History*, 24 (1980),
    1–19, at p. 1; A. Tomkins, '"The excellent example of the working class":
    Medical welfare, contributory funding and the North Staffordshire

Infirmary from 1815', *Social History of Medicine*, 21 (2008), 13–30, at p. 14.

74 A. Digby, *Making a Medical Living: Doctors and Patients in the English Market for Medicine* (Cambridge: Cambridge University Press, 1994), p. 230; I. Loudon, *Medical Care and the General Practitioner 1750–1850* (Oxford: Clarendon Press, 1986), pp. 231–5.

75 Tomkins, 'Women and poverty', p. 164.

76 H. Marland, *Medicine and Society in Wakefield and Huddersfield 1780–1870* (Cambridge: Cambridge University Press, 1987), pp. 53, 56–7, 58 and 66; French, 'An irrevocable shift', pp. 797–805.

77 J. Lane, *A Social History of Medicine: Health, Healing and Disease in England 1750–1950* (London: Routledge, 2001), pp. 49, 51 and 54.

78 M. Crowther, 'Health care and poor relief in provincial England', in O. Grell, A. Cunningham and R. Jütte (eds), *Health Care and Poor Relief in 18th and 19th Century Northern Europe* (London: Routledge, 2002), p. 206.

79 D. Porter and R. Porter, *Patient's Progress: Doctors and Doctoring in EighteenthCentury England* (Cambridge: Polity, 1989), p. 8. For similar points see A. Brundage, *The English Poor Laws 1700–1930* (Basingstoke: Macmillan, 2002), pp. 17–18, and A. Borsay, *Medicine and Charity in Georgian Bath: A Social History of the General Infirmary* (Aldershot: Ashgate, 1999), p. 212.

80 S. Williams, 'Practitioners' income and provision for the poor: Parish doctors in the late eighteenth and early nineteenth centuries', *Social History of Medicine*, 18 (2005), 159–86.

81 I. Loudon, 'Medical practitioners 1750–1850 and the period of medical reform in Britain', in A. Wear (ed.), *Medicine in Society: Historical Essays* (Cambridge: Cambridge University Press, 1992), p. 242; Digby, *Making a Medical Living*, p. 119, notes that by the early nineteenth century at least one doctor in five held poor law office, while two out of five may have held such office at some point in their careers. See also S. Cherry, 'General practitioners, hospitals and medical services in rural England: The East Anglian region, 1800–1948', in J. Barona and S. Cherry (eds), *Health and Medicine in Rural Europe (1850–1945)* (Valencia: Seminari d'Estudis sobre la Ciència, 2005), pp. 17–41.

82 R. Porter, 'The patient in England 1660–1800', in Wear (ed.), *Medicine in Society*, pp. 91–118, at p. 100.

83 Crowther, 'Health care and poor relief', p. 209. See also M. Fissell, 'The disappearance of the patient narrative and the invention of hospital medicine', in R. French and A. Wear (eds), *British Medicine in an Age of Reform* (London: Routledge, 1991), p. 106.

84 This was recognised in early historiography. See G. Oxley, *Poor Relief in England and Wales 1601–1834* (London: David and Charles, 1974), pp. 72–3.

85 Borsay, *Medicine and Charity*.

86 Lane, *A Social History of Medicine*, p. 54.

87 Marland, *Medicine and Society*, pp. 53–67.

88 Tomkins, '"Labouring on a bed of sickness"'.

89 Borsay, *Disability and Social Policy*, p. 148, suggests that benefits granted to the disabled were 'parsimonious in the extreme'. This view is revisited in later chapters of this study, but for some groups of the physically impaired at least the picture is opaque. See G. Phillips, *The Blind in British Society: Charity, State and Community, c.1780–1930* (Aldershot: Ashgate, 2004).

90 D. Porter, 'Health care and the construction of citizenship in civil societies in the era of the Enlightenment and industrialisation', in Grell, Cunningham and Jütte (eds), *Health Care and Poor Relief*, pp. 15–37, at p. 26.

91 Tomkins, *The Experience of Urban Poverty*, pp. 121, 135, 141–55, suggests that while range was impressive, the chance of individual paupers accessing the full spectrum of potential treatments was slim.

92 Thomas, 'The Old Poor Law', pp. 14–17; Digby, *Making a Medical Living*, p. 225.

93 R. Porter, 'The patient in England', pp. 94 and 100.

94 I. Loudon, 'The vile race of quacks with which this country is infested', in W. Bynum and R. Porter (eds), *Medical Fringe and Medical Orthodoxy, 1750–1850* (London: Wellcome Trust, 1987), pp. 116–17.

95 A. Tomkins, 'Paupers and the infirmary in mid-eighteenth century Shrewsbury', *Medical History*, 43 (1999), 208–27; Tomkins, *The Experience of Urban Poverty*, pp. 135–55.

96 S. King, '"Stop this overwhelming torment of destiny": Negotiating financial aid at times of sickness under the English Old Poor Law, 1800–1840', *Bulletin of the History of Medicine*, 79 (2005), 228–60.

97 R. Smith, 'Charity, self-interest and welfare: Reflections from demographic and family history', in M. Daunton (ed.), *Charity, Self-Interest and Welfare in the English Past* (London: UCL Press, 1996), pp. 36–41.

98 This material was variously collected as part of a Wellcome Trust Project Grant, a Wellcome Trust Strategic Award, a British Academy Project Grant and an AHRC Standard Project Grant (jointly with Professor Andreas Gestrich of the German Historical Institute, London). I am grateful to those who worked on these projects as research officers (RO): Alison Stringer, Alan Weaver, Peter Foster and Margaret Hanly

were ROs for the Wellcome Grants; Richard Biddle and John Glennie were ROs for the British Academy project; Peter Jones, Steven Taylor, Richard Gilbert, Richard Dyson and Jane Rowling were ROs on the AHRC–Deutsche Forschungsgemeinschaft project.

99 Langton, 'The geography of poor relief'. Steve Hindle, *On the Parish?*, pp. 282–94, also refers to the ecology of poor relief as a vehicle for linking variation in poor law practice to intensely local conditions. Langton's understanding of ecology is rather wider, even running to a call for us to relate practice to underlying soil structures.

100 Though see also N. Myers, 'Servant, sailor, soldier, tailor, beggarman: Black survival in white society 1780–1830', *Immigrants and Minorities*, 12 (1993), 47–74, and S. Braidwood, *Black Poor and White Philanthropists: London's Black and the Foundation of the Sierra Leone Settlement 1786–1791* (Liverpool: Liverpool University Press, 1994).

101 Irish welfare has received comprehensive consideration. See V. Crossman and P. Gray (eds), *Poverty and Welfare in Ireland, 1838–1948* (Dublin: Irish Academic Press, 2011); M. Cousins, *Poor Relief in Ireland, 1851–1914* (Bern: Peter Lang, 2011); V. Crossman, *Poverty and the Poor Law in Ireland 1850–1914* (Liverpool: Liverpool University Press, 2013).

2

Defining and measuring

Introduction

In an undated letter John Brooker addressed 'the Churchwardens, Overseers, and Others, the Gaurdians [sic], and Directors, of the Poor' of Tilehurst (Berkshire). He contended that his:

> business *you well know* is very pernicious to most Men that follow it after they have been a few years in the employ. But there is no doing without Painters, for Paint not only preserves but ornaments a Building without which the best of Structures would soon look mean, and filthy, as well as come to decay. But it is a Misfortune to them who are brought up to such a Trade that in the prime of life, lose the Use of Limbs by a relaxation of their Nerves, attended with Violent Coughs, Asthmas, &c. And have only to *linger out a few miserable Months, or years*, in Anguish, and Pain of Body, which Renders the miserable Objects, unable to get that Relief whereby they might be able to get their bread.

During his illness Brooker had sought to improve his own health through 'a little time in the Country'. But

> finding myself better I came to London last May twelve months, in hopes I might be able to follow my business again, having no other way of getting my living. But I had not long tried to work, when my Complaints returned worse than ever, and I have been above twelvemonths, and only done Seven days work put it altogether. As often as I have tried to work for two, or three hours, I have been so ill as to be obliged to leaved my work, and take to my Bed, where I am confined most of my time, and am now so Bad, I do not expect ever to be any better in this Life, as no Physition can administer to me the least Relief.

Tilehurst had previously afforded support during the worst episodes of ill-health and the parish was now asked to renew its 'kindness'.[1]

Brooker's letter encapsulates the problems that welfare and medical historians have faced in trying to understand and reconstruct both the scale of sickness and the nature of parochial responses. Six are particularly relevant to the basic framework of this study and require consideration at length. Firstly, was the claim of illness 'true'? For some early nineteenth-century commentators sickness and mendacity were linked firmly together, with the unworthy seeking to 'hire a few sprigs of poverty' in the form of feigned disability or ill-health in order to enhance their chances of obtaining welfare.[2] Chapter 3 takes up this theme at length. Secondly, there are issues about when an illness was recognised or crystallised and thus comes into the visible ambit of the historian. Brooker claimed chronic sickness. He gave up his job and went to the countryside to relieve his trembles and chest complaints. When ill-health returned he took to his bed, without apparently having recourse to any doctors. He felt his condition was beyond their cure, a 'natural' consequence of his work. Only late in the illness did he ask for a renewal of welfare payments. This tendency for paupers to suffer in silence before coming to the poor law,[3] or to experience continued ill-health between engagements with officials, was common. George Tull wrote to Oxford St Martin from Clewer (Berkshire) on 24 August 1760 to 'Let you know that I am very ill and *have Been for nine weeks'*.[4] Meanwhile, the advocate who wrote to St Martin on behalf of 'Silvester's wife' noted that her husband had struggled for a considerable period before coming to the parish, having 'been obliged to sell most of his goods' to pay a doctoring bill.[5] Sometimes this 'disguised' ill-health could last literally years.[6] The same narrative of suffering in silence can be found in all the vestry books used for this study. It does not therefore simply reflect the fact that paupers outside their parish of settlement needed to justify their honesty and suffering as a precursor to relief. At best, then (and a matter revisited in Chapter 9), even the highest-quality poor law records encompass only a subset of the sick poor and their sickness. This observation is important for my study in two ways: because it would seem likely that medical cases with a definitive timescale or well-understood symptoms – midwifery or smallpox for instance – were crystallised in the records more regularly, earlier and more clearly than chronic cases such as Brooker's; and because

changes in perceived medical welfare expenditure might reflect earlier or later engagement with the parish rather than a change in underlying sickness patterns themselves. These issues are ultimately unresolvable, but they mean that we must approach the quantification of both sickness and medical welfare with caution.

A third question, meanwhile, is that of the recording of sickness when it did become visible to parochial officers. John Brooker's rent was paid by Tilehurst. We might not have guessed the transaction to be sickness-related had his letter not survived. At least there was a record of the payment. As a young male pauper on outdoor relief, Brooker was always likely to be visible in the parochial sources given the moral hazards he posed. Payments to other subsets of the sick poor – married women, children and the mentally or physically impaired[7] – appear in all sources less often than perhaps they should because applications for relief were frequently made by husbands, carers or epistolary advocates. The patchy survival of workhouse records also represents a potential problem. Between 1776 and 1803 the number of workhouses recorded nationally climbed by 22 per cent such that they numbered 3,765 by the latter date.[8] Their distribution was not, however, uniform, and Taylor argues that Norfolk, Suffolk, Sussex, Essex, Middlesex, Wiltshire, Kent and Surrey collectively accounted for one half of all inmates.[9] More widely, where workhouses were, and were intended to be, homes for the very sick, decrepit or impaired, then overseers' accounts provide only a partial rendering of the nature, purpose and cost of medical welfare in a community unless the workhouse accounts are available and differentiate reasons for payment.[10] And Brooker applied to a parish with a long history of efficient administration such as was not always duplicated elsewhere. Medical relief, often given at short notice and frequently upon inspection at the houses of the poor with all that this entailed in terms of noise, bustle and fear of infection, may have been particularly prone to being recorded on slips of paper or in the memory and then lost or miscounted.[11] Sometimes parochial policy militated against the efficient recording of welfare transactions.[12] There are also, of course, questions as to the sensitivity of the records. John Brooker, along with almost all other in- and out-parish paupers, experienced periods of health or relative health, partial ill-health and chronic illness across even short life-cycle periods. In some communities such varying circumstances were reflected in periodic changes to

the scale or composition of allowances. Elsewhere – and particularly in relation to groups such as the very aged in long-term physical or mental decline[13] – static or long-term allowances make it potentially difficult to understand and locate the difference between 'medical' and 'normal' relief. Rectifying these recording problems, as we will see below and in Chapter 4, requires a synthesis of local sources to detect different aspects of the experiences of sickness and medical welfare.

Meanwhile, John Brooker's case also raises an important fourth question, about how illness was understood both by paupers and officials. The state of being ill was a fluid one, with bodily symptoms and mental constructions of them moving from day to day.[14] It is for this reason that people in their correspondence kept up a running commentary of the progress of their diseases or injuries and the timing of recuperation. If illness was genuine, overseers and paupers had to deal with and understand a disease landscape which might include the well-known, the unexplained, the newly discovered (cholera, for instance) and the re-labelled (particularly mental illnesses).[15] They also had to conceptualise occupational diseases. A reasoned diagnosis of John Brooker's case would almost certainly identify the debilitating effects of lead poisoning. For him ill-health was an inevitable consequence of his trade, something well known to those engaged in it and (he explicitly assumed) the officials who might be expected to pick up the pieces. Brooker is unusual (but not unique) in the sample of pauper letters and vestry minutes used here in the sense that paupers often constructed their claims around the fact that sickness prevented work rather than that work caused sickness.[16]

In short, understanding and rhetoricising illness was demanding for both officials and the poor, the more so given the changes in understanding of health, ill-health and curative potential briefly outlined for this period in Chapter 1. In this they can be seen to have struggled. Brooker was precise about his symptoms: a 'relaxation' of his nerves had given him the trembles and he suffered from periodic violent coughs and asthma. He occupies a place on a rhetorical spectrum which runs across my letter sample between the detailed, not to say gruesome, explications of some of those writing to Essex parishes through to the vague rhetoric of being ill or very ill which are typical of some of the English border counties. The majority of writers, however, tended towards the vaguer end of the spectrum across the whole period from the 1750s to

the 1830s. A consideration of the 540 surviving letters by or about the sick poor from the contiguous counties of Berkshire, Oxfordshire and Northamptonshire reveals occasional mentions of specific illnesses (rheumatism, smallpox, cholera, 'Anxiety, Fatigue & Distress', fever, blindness, stroke, palsy[17]), but almost all rhetoricised more general indicators of sickness. People were 'distressed'; 'Afflicted'; 'Lying veary ill'; 'deranged in his Intellect'; 'sick' (and variants thereof); in a 'State of Distraction', a 'sullen State' or a 'disabled state'; confined to bed; lacking the use of limbs; 'reduced by illness'; 'unwell sometime'; 'unwell and not fit to be mov'd'; 'so very ill' (and variants thereof); 'in no ways likely to do for herself'; in a 'very poor condition'; 'bad for some time'; in a 'state of pain & infirmity'; 'very weak'; 'helpless'; and 'in extreem pain'.[18] This sort of rhetorical focus on descriptions of the intensity and broad impact of illness rather than detailed symptoms and causation was duplicated in the correspondence of the epistolary advocates of the sick poor, and it is arguably much more orientated towards recognition than it is towards definition. While it would be tempting to see vagueness as a function of imperfect medical knowledge – a reflection of the fact that people did not know what was wrong – such conclusions would sit uneasily with the increasingly sophisticated knowledge of patients, the reach of medical advertising and the fact that doctors extended their influence over familial ill-health across the social spectrum during the early nineteenth-century.[19] In other work I have argued that to be precise or not about sickness was a rhetorical choice for paupers linked to the perceived sentiment of the officials who received their letters.[20] However we interpret these narratives, the imprecision extends to overseers' accounts, vestry minutes and even the bills of doctors. These sources tend to offer minute detail on the nature of accidental ill-health (burns, workplace accidents, etc.) but to be much less specific about chronic or infectious illnesses outside of smallpox. The label 'fever' is as endemic as the suite of conditions that caused it, for instance.[21] Such fuzziness in labelling has important consequences for our ability to offer precision on the scale and chronological or life-cycle patterning of the illnesses that feed into medical welfare spending because in terms of traceability these two variables are often co-dependent. I revisit this question throughout this chapter.

In turn, a fifth and related issue centres on the definition of parochial medical welfare. John Brooker claimed to be chronically sick but his

letter did not ask for the attendance of doctors, provision of drugs or even extra nourishment, the core of medical welfare in other studies.[22] Rather, he wanted help with his rent and the renewal of a cash allowance. Such demands are repeated across the diverse data underpinning this study and extended to requests for payment of friendly society dues, funeral costs, clothing, visiting relatives, nursing care, allowances for family members when the breadwinner or wife was ill, caution money for voluntary hospitals, temporary childcare, costs of transport, family allowances in the event of death and apprenticeship fees for impaired children. On the opposite side of the negotiating relationship, medical welfare might be culturally, socially and, above all, administratively constructed. It was after all parochial officials, not doctors, who decided whether claims of ill-health were valid and mapped benefits onto perceived intensity of sickness. Where the limits of a definition of 'medical welfare' sit is thus an issue thrown into sharp relief by the Brooker case.

The discretionary nature of the Old Poor Law system frames a final question about the process of recognising and treating sickness. John Brooker received exactly what was asked for. Yet, as Chapter 1 reminds us, overseers' accounts record payment level, form and regularity at the end of a process of negotiation, exclusion and modification. Thus, John Lines applied by letter to the vestry of Oundle (Northamptonshire) on 3 April 1833 'for extra relief for the Doctor's bill for the eldest Stanion's head'. Mr Lines was the grandfather of the child concerned and had taken him in when his daughter died. The vestry ordered 'That it be refused'. At the same time 'A letter was laid before this vestry from John Glithero of Paddington [London]' asking that his daughter Arabella be placed in an asylum. The vestry resolved that 'no attention be paid to it'. Three months later on 19 June 1833, an 'Application was made by George White for a Pair of shoes for Samuel George White.' The vestry 'taking into consideration the accident Geo. White has been labouring under' gave him 5s 'with the understanding that in future he shall maintain him according to his first agreement viz to receive 2/- a week from the parish to maintain & clothe him'.[23] In Oundle, then, the forms and scale of medical welfare recorded in the overseers' accounts render only a subset of what was asked for and felt to be needed by the poor themselves.

Confronting these issues requires us to synthesise as many poor law sources as possible and to regard both sickness and medical welfare as

processes rather than events. We also need to recognise that medical welfare in particular is a construct arising out of the subtle interplay of local power relationships (doctors versus overseers; overseers versus vestries; vestries versus ratepayers), negotiation (between officials themselves, officials and paupers, and officials and other advocates), spatial differences in ingrained sentiment towards the poor, economic constraints, the richness of the wider medical economy of makeshifts in any locality, scale of underlying sickness and the strengths and weaknesses of the recording process. The rest of this chapter must be read against this backdrop. It will focus on two questions. What were the broad scale, causation, intensity and duration of illness across the chronological period covered by this study? And what definition of medical welfare should be employed so as to encapsulate both parochial responses to sickness and wider pauper understandings of the role of the poor law in alleviating their suffering? Operationalisation of this definition is taken up in Chapter 4 and the Appendix.

Sickness

The scale and trajectory of infant, childhood and (to a lesser extent) adult *mortality* are relatively well-understood for the period from the 1750s to 1830s.[24] Urban death rates in particular were muted in comparison to those on the Continent. Wider risks of mortality were uneven across variables such as gender, region and family size, but the weight of evidence would point to a resurgence of infant mortality rates in particular by the early nineteenth-century.[25] Epidemics remained common, but with the exception of cholera in the 1830s the mortality associated with them moderated at the aggregate level.[26] Parish registers, bills of mortality and reports of the General Register Office and medical officers of health point to an increasingly varied complexion in causes of death and even the beginnings of a demographic transition.[27]

Less systematically addressed, at least for our period, has been the question of ill-health short of death. A general sense that poor and ordinary people experienced an intense palette of illnesses is compelling. Using aggregate data for the Ancient Order of Foresters Friendly Society, James Riley has argued that for the later nineteenth century there was an inverse relationship between mortality and morbidity rates: as people lived longer so they experienced more ill-health.[28]

How far the 'sickness' recorded in friendly society accounts reflected
the total experience of ill-health for the individual as opposed to the
financial capacity of the organisation is a moot point. Nonetheless,
subsequent sampling of friendly society data in rural Hampshire has
also highlighted a tendency for sickness episodes to increase in duration, if not frequency.[29] Friendly society data for the eighteenth and
early nineteenth centuries, by contrast, is relatively sparse.[30] This is
true even if we allow for substantial differences between the number of
friendly societies recorded by central government and those actually
in existence.[31] In my sample of overseers' accounts and vestry minutes,
instances where communities paid benefits to sick paupers and then
reclaimed the money from local societies provide evidence for frequent
and sometimes elongated claims.[32] Across my entire dataset there is a
steady increase in references to the collection of friendly society certificates, payment of dues, the collapse of organisations as a reason for
relief and (in pauper letters, for instance) the receipt or non-receipt
of society benefits. Given that friendly societies were increasing in
number, size and gender balance across our period, such observations
do not invariably signal an increase in underlying sickness, but the
material is suggestive.

Other sources also point to frequent sickness among the poor and
labouring populations during the last decades of the Old Poor Law.
The 9,000 cases of the Lincolnshire Coronial Circuit between 1773
and 1851 throw light on unexplained deaths. They additionally contain
information on background conditions of illness via the testimonies
of witnesses or the life histories of the deceased. Chronic ill-health –
resulting variously in suicides, incorrectly administered medicines and
sudden deaths – was commonplace. Thus, Susannah Dean, 'upwards
of 60 years of age' and afflicted with an unknown long-term illness,
went to an apothecary's shop in South Kyme on 17 February 1814
and 'purchased a pennyworth of white mercury', which she consumed
'in a dry state immediately after leaving the shop, as she complained
of being very thirsty on reaching home' and promptly died.[33] Jane
Worsdale hanged herself from a beam on 30 October 1816 having previously suffered a stroke and 'of late been very incoherent'.[34] Coronial
records also show us that while domestic and work accidents killed
prodigiously, they often left many more maimed and injured than died.
While some indicators of the scale of illness – spending on doctors by

parishes for instance, trends which can be variously explained by better, earlier or later recording of illness – might be constructed as unreliable, the thick description explicit in coronial records gives substance to a Riley-esque sense of significant background levels of illness.

Similar perspectives emerge from contemporary diaries and memorandum books, which often reported (albeit unsystematically) the melancholy effects of explosions or pit collapses, and which at their most detailed also confirm the pervasiveness of ill-health in the ordinary population. The Rev. Richard Cobbold's collection of life histories for the Suffolk parish of Wortham between 1824 and 1877 is considered at length in Chapter 9 but is also helpful here. While epidemic diseases other than smallpox were rarely mentioned, chronic illness and temporary sickness, often with long-term effects on capacity and ability, were common. Indeed, mental and physical impairment on a spectrum from dangerous insanity or elephantitis on the one hand to idiocy and disease-related amputations on the other were so common that all young residents of Wortham would have been alive to the scale of chronic ill-health.[35] At the other side of the country, William Rowbottom's diary of events in Oldham (Lancashire) between 1787 and 1799, demonstrates a deep fascination with public and personal health. He confirms the ubiquity of tuberculosis, fever, typhus and childhood epidemics which stride across the work of historical demographers, both as killing diseases and as originators of chronic long-term sickness. In August 1788, for instance, he noted that:

> the disorder called the influenza prevailed very much all over England and there died some few. They were affected by a great pain in their limbs, a sore throat, and in recovering they were subject to sweat prodigiously, and the flesh wasted astonishingly and left them very weak and low.[36]

This was one of more than forty national, regional or local epidemics recorded by Rowbottom. More widely, medical historians have done much to trace a rising tide of insanity over the course of the nineteenth-century. Whether this reflects a 'real' upsurge in mental conditions as opposed to new labels, the breakdown of family care structures propelling more people with mental conditions into the public domain or a wider socio-medical drive to pathologise certain types of behaviour is unclear.[37] Contemporaries certainly thought

that mental impairments of various stripes were increasing; the exasperated overseer of Rothersthorpe (Northamptonshire) replied to a
letter from his Birmingham counterpart asking him to relieve Mary
Smith, who had been declared insane, and noted that 'we are caught
in an endless tide of lunatics and idiots for which our rates are quite
insufficient'.[38]

Against this general backdrop, three intertwining issues – causation,
the frequency of sickness among those who became sick when on poor
relief or whose sickness drove them to dependence, and its duration
and intensity – are fundamental to the conduct of my study. After all,
one of the potential explanations for any variation in the volume and
character of medical welfare may be the scale, duration and character of sickness generated in different spatial or typological contexts.
Alternatively, such variation could reflect differences in the nature of
recording processes or in the age focus of relief. These issues must
be addressed through a multi-source approach. To turn first to
causation, some ailments are relatively easy to both locate and quantify. Charles Creighton's view that late eighteenth-century and early
nineteenth-century English communities were periodically ravaged by
regional or national epidemics finds support across the data employed
in this study.[39] Smallpox remained a common problem for the poor,[40]
as evidenced in persistent attempts by doctors to exclude it and other
infectious diseases from their parochial contracts or the proliferation
of schemes to inoculate and vaccinate the dependent and labouring
poor as a precaution.[41] The Dorset parish of Swanage was by no means
unusual when its vestry agreed on 15 April 1796 'that to prevent any
danger of contracting an infection of the Small Pox in the natural way
the Benefit of Inoculation be offered at the Parish expense to the well
disposed who being through poverty unable to pay it themselves'.
Authorising the broadcasting of this time-limited opportunity around
the parish, it was noted that:

> A committee will meet every day during the seven days in the Vestry
> Room from twelve to one o'clock to receive applications of such as are
> necessitated to apply for this assistance. As Messrs. Staines and Dolland
> are agreed with by the Parish to avoid further expense it is expected that
> no other person will be employed as the Parish will have nothing to do
> with any future charges which may be incurred through negligence or
> for want of judgment.[42]

Across my whole dataset (see Chapter 1) we can trace 594 specific small-pox epidemics. Cholera was equally recognisable. John Collingwood, assistant overseer of Spotland (Lancashire), noted in a letter of 14 August 1831 that Richard Farmer was 'Sick, and likely to continue' but then added a wider community context: 'We have many [of our own] Sick at this time, with a lax of Blood and throwing up also.'[43] John Gunnell was more specific when he wrote from Manchester to Oxendon (Leicestershire) on 19 August 1832 to say that

> Cholera it is this day stated that there has been 100 deaths this last week (God knows how soon it may be our lot) and it seems everyday to gain strength. A Neighbour 6 Doors below us was seized last Wednesday about 4 o'clock in the morning – Visited in the forenoon took to the Cholera Hospital about 2 in the Afternoon and died before 4 the same afternoon.[44]

Cholera is traceable in twenty-six of the 117 base communities encom-passed by this analysis. Many others were like Oundle, where on 9 May 1832 'Notice was given that application would be made at the next Select Vestry that the parish may provide a building for the reception of Cholera patients *in the event* of that disease appearing in this town.'[45]

Vestry minutes, overseers' accounts, correspondence and news-paper reporting also point to periodic outbreaks of measles, whoop-ing cough and other epidemic childhood diseases, mirroring the experiences of the wider population traced by Creighton.[46] At rural Brimpton (Berkshire), for instance, measles visited the parish in 1763 and 1773 and then at regular intervals until the final recorded out-break in 1821. Whooping cough and scarlet fever made appearances in 1777, 1786, 1795, 1801, 1814 and 1820.[47] Above all, unspecified epidemics were common. The overseer of Clewer (Berkshire) wrote to his counterpart in Oxford on 3 November 1754 to warn that several of the paupers from Oxford living in Clewer were 'very bad now of a Sickness which Rages very much where the[y] be'.[48] In Woodford Halse (Northamptonshire), unspecified epidemics changed both spending levels and policy. That of 1783, for instance saw an upsurge in fuel payments and funeral costs. Further unspecified epidemics in 1785, 1794, 1800, 1807, 1814, 1818 and 1824 generated temporary spikes in spending and innovative responses on the part of officials.[49] On average the communities considered here experienced broadly

defined demographic 'crisis periods' in one year out of every nine, with greater frequency after 1800 than before.[50] It is difficult to discern precisely whether the latter trend is merely an artefact of better data and better recording after 1800. The sense from my collected sources that the frequency of 'real' epidemics did increase is consistent with the observations of Creighton and with the logic of increased population size and density by the early nineteenth century. In these instances, the ranks of the long-term and casual poor (sick and otherwise) were significantly swelled by those propelled into poverty by sickness and for whom dependence was a temporary condition. Indeed, during the unspecified epidemic of 1783, the overseer of Woodford Halse deliberately changed his recording policy to distinguish the two groups, labelling those who were longer-term or chronically sick as 'ill' while those whose need was temporary, usually for no more than two weeks, were labelled 'not well'. Uneven recording of the sort that we have already encountered prevents the drawing of definitive conclusions but there is little evidence of systematic spatial or typological variations in the frequency of crisis years. Communities with census populations of 2,500 or more seem to have experienced slightly more crises than their rural counterparts. Of course, the absence of the very largest urban areas from this analysis introduces bias, but the sample contains, as can be seen in the Appendix, much evidence from unhealthy town hinterlands by way of balance.

The picture of the causation of ill-health is more problematic for 'normal' years. Mental impairments were recognised and treated in every parish considered here, and there is no evidence of the sorts of systematic variation in insanity levels across space, time or community typology that we see by the later nineteenth century.[51] This is not to deny that for some places the burden was intense and long-term. In Oundle, for example, ten different individuals were identified as lunatics in vestry minutes stretching between 1828 and 1836, with a further eighteen people placed in lunatic asylums in London at earlier dates and some thirty-three people identified as 'idiots' in other sources. With an 1831 census population of just 2,308, this level of mental impairment (at least 11 per cent of all families hosted an individual with such conditions) represented a significant burden on the parish rates. Vestrymen struggled with whether to place the insane in London asylums, return them to families and subsidise care, board them or find space in the

workhouse.[52] Oundle's experience was shared by the nearby town of Wellingborough, but both constituted outliers to a normative experience for other Northamptonshire parishes in which insanity and idiocy in its various forms was episodic rather than sustained.[53] This picture is repeated in all of the county samples employed here. In terms of explanatory variables there is no obvious relation to the existence in outlier communities of workhouses which might have led to more people being defined as 'insane' simply because there was somewhere to put them. We return to this question in Chapters 8 and 9.

Meanwhile, 'normal' years also saw a regular litany of accidents to those who were already poor, while others were thrown into dependence by the accident itself. Of course, such accidents were more common in industrial centres or communities with extensive transport hubs than they were elsewhere. In Doncaster (South Yorkshire) between 1794 and 1795, for instance, accidents included 'lame of an arm from the bite of a pig', 'harmed his hand at mill', 'some ribs broken', 'hurt by a misfortune at the brickyards', 'blind of an eye', and limbs lost to splinters, explosions and collapsing coal and clay pits.[54] Yet even in relatively rural Northamptonshire a consideration of vestry minutes, overseers' accounts and correspondence reveals 406 accident cases for the period between the 1790s and 1830s. These included being mangled in a paper mill, frequent burns and scalds, cuts, accidents connected to fits, crushing by falling buildings, road accidents, drownings, entombment in marl pits, bones broken by kicks from animals, falls and slips, and gruesome injuries occasioned by bad weather or use of farm implements. It was no doubt the ubiquity of everyday accidents and their potential for long-term poverty that led vestries throughout the Midlands to try and ensure that accidental injuries were included in the fixed price of a doctoring contract. The formula for Crick (Northamptonshire) in March 1820 is typical:

> it was agreed that Mr Tho Walker has engaged to attend upon the paupers of this place together with the outpoor within 5 miles for the sum of 20 Pounds per annum including surgery, midwifery and medicine together with fractured limbs, dislocations and all kinds of Wounds excluding only the small pox.[55]

We return to the issue of doctoring contracts in Chapter 5, but the sense from a simple quantitative reading of my sources that the number

of accidents increased over time finds resonance with the emerging historiographical literature on this issue.[56]

Outside easily recognisable or sudden conditions, the spectrum of ill-health causation for the dependent poor becomes more difficult to reconstruct. Figure 2.1 attempts to take the widest view of causation over the period considered here. The underlying methodology is admittedly crude. I take all of the sources available to this study (see Chapter 1) and identify 674 discrete sickness labels which were applied to the poor or self-applied by them. Many are recognisable (dropsy, stroke, epilepsy, amputation, asthma, etc.) and appear uniformly across the typological and spatial dimensions of the sample.[57] Others are more situational. These include 'dreake' (meaning 'melancholic' or 'depressed', found only in Yorkshire), 'clamsing' ('asthmatic', found only in Somerset), 'groaning' (in childbirth, found almost entirely in Northamptonshire and Oxfordshire), 'horming' (broadly equating to 'decline' in children and found only in Northumberland) and 'selag' ('incontinent', found largely in the Welsh borders). I then count for each year of the study the number of times each of these labels were applied or self-applied. This is an imprecise exercise in several respects: a letter might mention several conditions all applying to a single individual at the same point in time. At the opposite extreme an overseer might mention a smallpox outbreak in his accounts (which would count as a single case) without then defining which people in those accounts were suffering, so that we miss multiple cases of that disease. As has been suggested above and in Chapter 1, there is often little specificity to the conditions detailed when illness was claimed or welfare granted. The single most common label was 'ill' or 'very ill' and its variants. Because I am not concerned at this stage with discrete relief and sickness histories, a single individual can appear with the same or multiple illness labels in rapid succession. And there is an inevitable inter-correlation between the later decades of the graph and the tendency for improving medical and diagnostic knowledge in this period to generate more focus in labelling even if the nature of the underlying diseases did not change. It is important, then, that we do not ascribe more precision to Figure 2.1 than it warrants, though the 25,486 illness references generated by this process perhaps suggest that the sheer sample size may obviate some of the concerns noted above.

A third stage of the methodology involves collapsing the 674 labels into the manageable set of larger categories that we see in Figure 2.1.

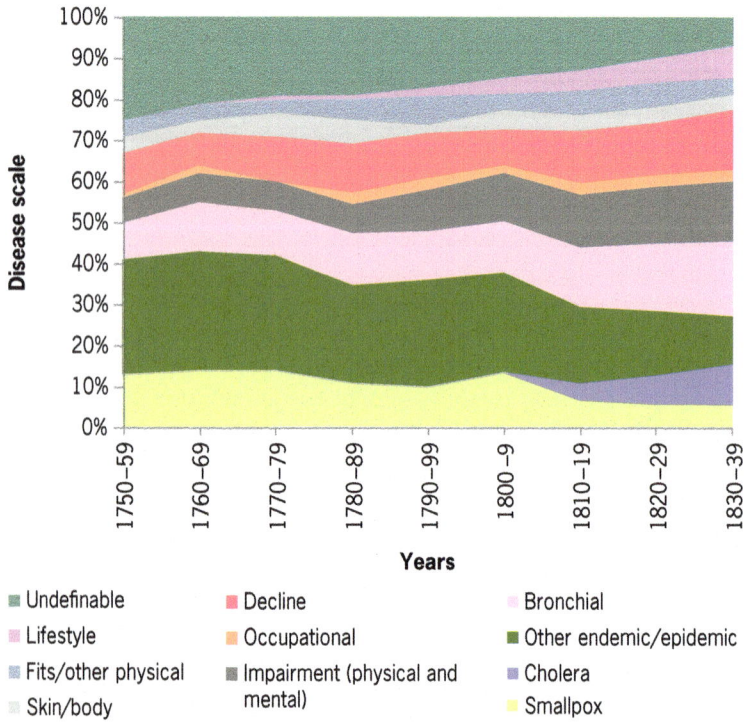

2.1 Chronological trends in identifiable illnesses

This process is informed by debates among historical demographers over how to classify cause of death, but also by the categories used for patients admitted to the early nineteenth-century Westminster Hospital, which was used as a control sample for this strand of analysis.[58] Finally, I remove the catch-all category 'Ill' from the count, so that Figure 2.1 focuses only on the 13,476 named conditions even if (in the 'undefinable' category) I do not know what they were. This strategy will, of course, skew the analysis if certain conditions (perhaps 'decline' among the aged, for instance) are disproportionately masked by the labels 'ill' and 'sick'. Notwithstanding these sorts of caveat, Figure 2.1 has important synergies with the work of James Riley (see above) and other historical demographers: epidemics were common but their presence in the illness landscape declined over time, to be

replaced by a significant surge in bronchial conditions, the 'decline' associated with an absolute increase in the number of old people in the early nineteenth century, lifestyle conditions such as gout and strokes, accidents, and a suite of chronic illnesses on a spectrum from 'the itch' to various macular issues short of blindness. The health experiences to which these labels point do not look very different from those found in the account books of contemporary doctors, suggesting that the range of illnesses borne by paupers was distinctly 'ordinary'.

Quantifying the frequency of ill-health among the dependent poor is problematic, even where family reconstitutions exist for individual parishes. We have seen that episodes of sickness could easily be fully or partially under-reported. Alternatively, Chapter 1 has suggested that the poor were increasingly subject to the attention of doctors such that more of their ill-health experiences may have come within the recorded ambit of the poor law, creating an illusory sense of increasing sickness by the early nineteenth century. More generally, using over-seers' accounts as a base source for sickness frequency would focus on the end of a process of determining relief, which might of itself lead to the under- or over-recording of sickness. Attempts to constrain the eligibility of unemployed family men during the 1810s may, for instance, have resulted in the dismissal of illness-related claims that in the 1780s would have reached the written record. And of course by the 1830s the average parish archive is richer in terms of retained sources than was the case in the 1750s, such that the sick poor have a statistically greater chance of remaining visible and seeing multiple sickness episodes recorded by the end of our period.

The correlation between recorded medical welfare spending and underlying sickness is thus uncertain. It is partly for these reasons that the dataset generates conflicting pictures on frequency. Thus, the Wighton (Norfolk) workhouse account book records a considerable spectrum of illnesses and impairments, either carried into the building on admission or caught there in the 1790s and early 1800s: 'Bedrid, speechless and infirm', 'Ill 4 weeks', 'sickly and infirm', 'insane', 'only one arm', 'troubled with fits', 'so very infirm', 'in a Deplorable state', 'blind, pass'd home from Colchester in Essex', 'in a most Deplorable State, Ill'. Those of unsound mind appear to have been particularly likely to end up in this workhouse. On 17 April 1791, for instance, Mary Long was searched on her admission and 'Poison found in her

pocket with Intent to Destroy her self', while Eliza Wade was one of nine female paupers between 1791 and 1799 who were recorded as requiring restraint. Moreover, the Wighton workhouse was also a receptacle for venereal disease cases. Thus, the workhouse master wrote to the mayor of King's Lynn on 14 March 1791 with dire warning about Mary Barns, who:

> was sent to the Workhouse at Wighton established for the maintenance of the Poor belonging to the united Parishes of H[olkham], W[ighton] and W[arham] where she was treated with all possible kindness having every indulgence her disorder (the Venereal) would admit. A Cure just being found she has this morning left the House (without the smallest provocation whatever) and I suppose is gone to Lynn again. Mary Barns has been once publickly whipt and 6 months imprison'd in Walsingham Bridewell for thieving & other misdemeanours three times cured of the Venereal disease and this is the ninth time of her running away from the House. The saying thus much is sufficient as it's very easily prov'd that she is almost a bandon wretch. Sir, Permit me to assure you after what is said that there can't be any reason for me to wish the Return of so bad a Person, yet think it my duty to inform you of the above circumstance as such a woman residing in Lynn must be of bad consequence.[59]

Most of those entering or living in the workhouse were, then, sick. At the opposite extreme, Tim Philipson's finding that fourteen sets of Oxfordshire vestry minutes record only a minuscule 0.15 per cent of all payments being made to sick paupers is also repeated for elements of my sample.[60] In Cliviger and Colne (both Lancashire), for instance, vestry books running periodically from 1815 to 1838 and 1792 to 1797 respectively record less than 5 per cent of all decisions and 1.2 per cent of all payments being made to applicants who were sick.[61] Yet for other communities sickness was more often the core concern of the vestry. In Oundle, broadly defined sickness cases made up 36 per cent of the business between 1828 and 1836.

A more substantial picture of the frequency of sickness can be obtained through an analysis of letters written by, about, or on behalf of the poor. Chapter 1 noted that the underlying dataset contains 12,904 letters of this sort. Sickness broadly defined is an insistent theme in such material, with 81 per cent (10,452) of all letters referencing some aspect of ill-health directly or part of a series from or about the same person in which sickness was the core claims-making

vehicle. Regional, typological and gender differences within this broad framework are surprisingly muted, pointing to a generic experience among the dependent or potentially dependent poor. It is difficult to establish chronological trends in frequency but the fact that 89 per cent of all letters for the period 1825–35 reference some form of ill-health is suggestive of either more comprehensive recording or more sickness. This issue gains sharper relief if we move from letters to letter writers, and in particular to those who wrote multiple times to their parish of settlement. While this group comprises only 29 per cent of all 2,629 distinct claimants, the letters written by, for or about them dominate the corpus numerically. Two features of such series are important for my analysis: that sickness almost always makes an appearance at some point; and that sickness usually becomes more prominent as a reason for writing, a claim for relief and a basis for contestation as the narrative series progresses.[62] Thomas Burditt wrote from Leicester to Market Harborough on 27 April 1828. Claiming to have been ill since Christmas and calling attention to his track record of independent living, Burditt added ominously, 'Surgeon tells me that my complaint is more serious than I am aware of.' Thus began a series of letters in which illness became a reason for the payment of a weekly pension, rent and episodic supplementary relief.[63]

Walter Keeling, writing from Hull to Colwich (Staffordshire) between 1786 and 1811, is an even better example. His correspondence opened on 27 November 1786 with sickness, Keeling reporting the

> deplorable condition of my self and Family … you can easily conceive to what a condition I am reduced with a Lame Son who is not in a condition to earn the lest subsistance for some years, and now for the space of seven or eight weeks I and Family all laid sick of a Fever.[64]

By July 1787 Keeling was telling the overseer that the family had 'Beread [his] oldest Sun Which Was Laim for two years Which Dide the 5 Day of Febuary Last Which me and all Fameley was Verry Bad in the Fever the Same time for half a year'.[65] Rather than recovering from these calamities, however, Walter Keeling began a series of correspondence in which the recounting of past troubles allied with new, often health-related, problems accreted into a wider claim and case for permanent support. In January 1788 he was obliged 'to Lett

you Know that I am Verrey Lame and Lost my Helth Every Since I had the Fever a twelve Month ago'.[66] Keeling also reported being discharged from his barracks (Chatham Barracks) 'for being Lame of Legg'; having a 'Verrey Bad Youmer Fell in my eyes as I have Been Sumtimes all most blind for this 2 months'; a wife 'Not able to help hir Self'; and 'getting Old and Lame in my Leg and side Where my bowels was Lett out … Which is Verry Trobelsom To me Now I am old Sir'.[67] By 1798 the situation had worsened and he was 'in grate Distress as my Wife Has Been Verry Bad In a fever for this Two monthes and me an old man Verry much Trobled With a pain in my Side'.[68] The final letter in the sequence (1811) was from Mr Osbourne, a magistrate in Hull who had refused to facilitate Keeling's return to Colwich on the basis that his settlement parish could not wish to upend an old couple. Osbourne reveals that Keeling and his wife were aged seventy-two and seventy-three respectively, suggesting (allowing for waiting times and the fact that he was ill when the correspondence began) that they had experienced episodic but related ill-health for a quarter of a century.[69] Keeling himself was subject to repeated bouts of fever, had impaired sight, experienced bowel problems and was lame throughout his later life. His wife was chronically sick, and his son, clearly lame before the correspondence begins, died during the period. Letters were dressed up in the rhetoric of hoping to be better and to clamber back to independence, but cumulatively these illnesses constituted a strong case, at least in the mind of Keeling and the magistrate who wrote on his behalf, for sustained relief.

Of course, Keeling and other serial writers, as well as those who corresponded only once or infrequently with parishes, could have been manufacturing or embellishing their sickness, fully aware of the moral and entitlement dilemmas that were embodied by sickness as opposed to other causes of poverty such as unemployment. In Chapter 3, however, I argue that such claims were almost invariably genuine. I also suggest that the concerns, rhetoric and experiences of these writers find reflection in the approaches that in-parish paupers made to vestries, reflecting a ubiquitous experience of sickness as the major cause of welfare claims. Accepting these arguments, we can also go further. Focusing on those with three or more letters to their name – that is those engaged in a genuine process of co-respondence – we can see that the average number of discrete sickness episodes encompassed

by a series rose inexorably in every decade to a peak of six in 1820–29. This does not, of course, prove that there was a rising tide of ill-health, especially given the lessons that we should draw from the case of John Brooker. Nonetheless, in the sense that letters of this sort represent the start of the process of poor relief rather than its end, we can point to the strategic importance of sickness for the operation of the poor law in its last decades.

Building on this material about frequency to consider issues of intensity and duration is a considerable task, not least because contemporaries themselves had only the most tenuous grasp on such matters. James Seed, long-time overseer of the poor of Billington in Lancashire during the 1810s and 1820s, offered a very precise demarcation of individual sickness episodes among the poor.[70] He was one of just a handful of officials in the underlying data that made such distinctions. More representative were Richard Tilburn and John Daniell, who surveyed the regular and casual poor of Doncaster, noting their general health conditions and allowances but giving little sense of how long illnesses had already lasted.[71] Imprecision extended to paupers themselves. William King of Bethnal Green was thus common among aged paupers in framing his claim not in terms of precise timing but as a broad phase of life that one would usually associate with declining health and capacity. He wrote to the overseer of Braintree (Essex) on 20 November 1828 to say that he was 'Subyect to an asthma and other Commmplaints in My Boddy'. Having 'yust Bore Up Under My Gret affliction of Mind', he asked the parish for an ongoing allowance.[72] King's letter marks the start of a sustained period of correspondence about his own and his wife's illnesses in which he claims variously to be 'Very Bad in My Breath and other Complaits', mired in the 'Gloom wich So often Bows Down the Spirits of Sach a Poor Man as My Self', in 'Unbeerble Trubble and Want and Great affliction', suffering 'Very Hevey inward Complaints', 'Under a Mind Sometimes Bent down with Sadness and Distress' and 'Very ill with the affliction wich has Carried off So Meny of our fellow Creatures of Late'. By late 1834 King found the 'failings of Nature to Be Very alarming Not only in Boddy But in Mind also Long Years of Trubble have Bowed Me down as it wheare'. Then in September 1834 he noted: 'I am Not able to Do as formerly – I feel a Great weakness and Sinking Such as I am perswaded all People feel who are told 60 years.' This skilful rhetoric generalised his particular

sickness, well known in its detail to the vestry, to all people over the age of sixty. He continued it in his final letter when acknowledging the risk of being confined to the workhouse in the crossover to the 1834 legislation. King suggested that he wished to see out his 'epointd Days wich are Now on the decline Tis October with me'.[73]

That intense bouts of individual and familial illness followed by prolonged and often partial or episodic recuperation were the lot of a significant subset of all paupers is not in doubt. Elizabeth Wilson wrote to her father in Market Harborough under the pseudonym of her husband John on 4 January 1824 to say that John had been very ill with rheumatic fever and 'had only one penny left last night till relieved by a Neighbour'. His 'shattered constitution' meant that 'it is very doubtful how it [the illness] will end'. Asking for aid from the family, Wilson revealed herself as the writer who was 'sorry to give so much sorrow to worthy parents but it is unavoidable and *she* hopes an immediate answer will be sent'.[74] Some relief was presumably afforded because the correspondence was taken up again eight weeks later. Noting in her own voice that she herself had been ill, Elizabeth was still

> very lame, my hips, thighs, & legs being much in pain, have not been out of Doors month yesterday, keep upstairs because it is warmer, afraid I shall not get over it for some time, although I am better my legs, thighs, waste very much, hard striating [straightening] then which makes me go almost double … it is impossible to get all up – it's a great pull for me with such a family as I have, have brought on this complaint with hard work heats & colds … the children are better have a good appetite but are like shadows.[75]

Taking these and subsequent letters (to both the parents and overseer) at face value suggests that illness raged through the family from late 1823 to early 1826, with hopes for recuperation consistently dashed by the onset of further illness.

While it is impossible to devise, from letters or any other source, intensity indices for sickness among the dependent poor, their correspondence suggests that intensity was an important matter for applicants. John Brooker applied for a renewal of relief only when his condition had reached a pitch which suggested long-term chronic ill-health. He assumed that this intensity and longevity of sickness would spark entitlement in the eyes of the parish. More widely, around 40 per cent of

those applying for relief and claiming sickness as a motivating factor did so when they perceived that the intensity of ill- health (variously measured in terms of the number of family members who were sick, the loss of residual working ability or the movement of an illness to a new and more ingrained stage) had increased. Thus, William Bardwell (or Barwell) applied for relief to the overseers of Market Harborough on 17 December 1823. Apologising for his application, he noted that he himself was ill but that he now had five of his six children 'ill at Home with the Small pox'. This level of familial illness meant that 'as for my wife I do not expect that she will be able to do for us much longer as she as being up with one of the children (the Eldest) almost Night and Day for 3 weeks'. The family had thus reached crisis point, and their coping mechanisms for 'normal' levels of illness had disintegrated.[76] This sense of the importance of threshold intensity was shared by epistolary advocates in their correspondence with overseers. Iorweth Lockwood, vicar of Croydon (Surrey), wrote on behalf of Mrs Tyrell, noting that he was contacting her settlement parish because 'of the continued illness of her Boy, about 10 years old, who has occasioned them very great expense by being off & on almost constantly under medical care', and asked the parish to send the family £1.[77] This and other writers, along with overseers themselves, assumed that the rules of the local state should be malleable in the face of evidence of intense and intensifying need. Whether at the level of the whole corpus of letters we see an increase in the intensity of illness will remain a moot point given the other source problems outlined in this chapter.

It is, however, clear from Table 2.1, that we see an increase in the duration of sickness episodes. This table takes the 13,476 illness references underpinning Figure 2.1 and uses all of those (7,994) for which we have or can imply a start or end date or duration. The figures must be regarded cautiously. As I have already observed above, we know from the work of medical historians that an increased availability of doctors and other providers of services in the medical market of eighteenth and nineteenth-century England saw more conditions defined as medical matters and a tendency for longer engagement with such providers. There is no doubt at all that paupers themselves increasingly understood and rhetoricised medical conditions as remediable, something that may have increased the perceived, recorded and claimed duration of individual sickness episodes even where the nature and

Table 2.1 The duration of sickness episodes

Years	Mean duration (days)	Standard deviation
1750–59	16	2.5
1760–69	15	2.2
1770–79	15	1.6
1780–89	17	1.4
1790–99	21	1.6
1800–9	24	1.2
1810–19	24	1.0
1820–29	26	1.2
1830–39	31	0.8

Sources: 7,994 illness references for which we can infer a start or end date or duration. See main text.

course of symptoms remained static. An institutional or medical stamp of legitimisation for those who were not cured, or needed a long recuperation, appears to have been particularly powerful in extending the duration of observed illness by the 1820s in a way that would not have been the case in the 1750s. Changes in the composition of the medical economy of makeshifts might also mean that more of the sickness of ordinary people over the life-cycle was captured by the poor law, rather than that the experienced duration of illness increased. And of course, poor law accounts and other records might simply be qualitatively better sources by the 1820s and 1830s.

Yet the lessons of Table 2.1 are unlikely to be generated by observational and classificatory artefact alone. Nor are they a function of very long-term chronic illnesses at individual and familial level skewing the mean figures. The consistency of standard deviation figures over time gives confidence that sickness episodes were genuinely lengthening, just as James Riley has claimed for the wider population. This observation sits neatly with many hundreds of discrete examples in the data which point, otherwise unsystematically, to the idea that chronic or at least repetitive illness became more common over the period 1750–1834 and across the regional and typological spectrum of communities. The level of chronic and serious sickness in Oundle reached such a pitch by the mid-1830s, for instance, that the master of the workhouse was obliged to approach the vestry 'for some more

persons to be put into the workhouse to do the work of the House he stating that the Inmates from Old age & disease are incapable of doing anymore and that the work they cause require some hands to assist himself & his wife to do the work of the House'.[78] Judged in the round then, sickness – and sickness potentially increasing in frequency and duration – was ubiquitous, and its amelioration via medical welfare was a core, perhaps increasingly the core, business of the Old Poor Law during its crisis years.

Defining medical welfare

Against this backdrop, deciding what counts as 'medical welfare' and measuring it in the sources available to us is a complex task.[79] The competing historiographical views of the nature and scale of parochial support for sickness outlined in Chapter 1 at least partly reflect the fact that it is possible and reasonable to define medical welfare across a wide spectrum. At one extreme we might consider it as encompassing costs associated with direct treatment of sickness (doctoring bills and contracts, drugs, dressings and institutional subscriptions), along with the extra cash relief and in-kind allowances accruing to people when they were noted as sick in vestry minutes or overseers' accounts. On the other hand, E. G. Thomas reminds us that while the direct costs of medical care were often modest, associated costs were invariably high, pointing to the possibility of a rather wider definition.[80] Something of the conundrum for welfare historians can be seen in the sources themselves. The vestry of Bispham-with-Norbreck (Lancashire) noted on 5 November 1833 that Mary Badger 'having had the misfortune to fall from the effects of a fit, into her yarn in her looms and so much damaged the same that it cannot be woven … [the vestry] do allow her 2s and agree to pay the damage caused by the misfortune'.[81] Badger never applied for, and the parish never offered, medical welfare related to the original fit. The cash payment of 2s and the costs of putting right the loom might, however, reasonably be regarded as consequential medical welfare. Instances such as this are common in the underlying dataset, and whether we include or exclude them from the definition of medical welfare has a significant impact on how we perceive the nature, scope, duration and importance of such spending at parochial level. Some accounting entries are intriguingly thorny, particularly where

an accident or sickness event was linked randomly or consequentially to another which was ostensibly not. William Clippard of Crowland (Northamptonshire) lost his cow in the winter of 1805–6. He would ordinarily have been able to pay the doctoring bill subsequently occasioned when 'his son received a bad fracture of the thigh' but in March 1806 found it impossible. In this case, payment of the doctoring bill would fall into all definitions of medical welfare. It is rather less clear how we should understand a regular allowance while his son recovered and a contribution to a new cow.[82] The link is even more complex in the case of the Jacob Curchin, resident in Wisbech (Cambridgeshire) but settled in Thrapston (Northamptonshire), who wrote to the overseer in 1828 seeking an allowance, being in a 'deplorable condition'. While himself fit and well, he noted that the cause of his distress was that 'no one comes to bring me any jobs since my children had the smallpox'.[83] Whether to understand a subsequent cash allowance as medical relief is thus an acutely fine decision, and one repeated across the subsets of data outlined in Chapter 1.

Adopting a wide perspective on medical welfare (and thus including all of the payments noted above) has significant resonance with the way in which some overseers recorded medically related spending. The account book of Alston (Lancashire), for instance, sees Richard Atherton relieved in cash and kind (and apparently healthy) between May and October 1820. In February 1821, however, a new relief cycle was begun with cash payments for Atherton, *ad hoc* support for his wife in childbed, the costs of burying the infant concerned, and nursing, coals and consequential cash payments as the family recuperated, all recorded as a single accounting item.[84] Overseers might, as Chapter 7 demonstrates, also record a final illness, burial costs and relief of all sorts (in cash or kind) for those left behind as one expenditure event, one seamless whole of medical welfare.[85] Drawing on the lessons of sources, like these it is possible to conceive of the wide definition of medical welfare represented in Table 2.2, which underpins the rest of the study.

Measuring spending thus defined is not unproblematic. We have already encountered generic source problems – missing accounts; some tendency to keep rough notes and update records only periodically;[86] failure to record reasons for relief; and chronological variations in source coverage – that impact the ability to measure any form of

Table 2.2 Potential components of a definition of medical welfare
expenditure

Expenditure category	Scope
Medical people	Fees/contracts for doctors, nurses, informal practitioners and all costs associated with employing and retaining such people including postage and legal advice
Material costs	Drugs, dressings, devices, food, drink, false limbs, and other services to the sick poor including shaving
Institutional care	Fees, subscriptions, caution money, costs of transport and correspondence, clothing, food and drink for those in institutions, allowances to families while members were in institutions, costs for washing and relatives visiting
Cash relief	Allowances to or on behalf of the sick poor, consequential cash payments, payments to families in bereavement, costs of transmitting cash and negotiating allowances including postage and conveyance, allowances to family members not afflicted by illness
Funerals	Payments in cash and kind, including costs of washing and laying out bodies, food and drink, coffins and associated material costs of burial, conveying relatives and bodies, and legal opinion
In-kind payments	Rents, house repairs, washing, coal and other fuel, conveyance of goods, costs associated with recuperation including clothing, etc.
Administering medical welfare	Postage costs, legal and medical opinions, examinations, journeys, entertainment, partial salaries of paid officials, costs of notices, settlement and examination costs for sick paupers
Workhouse	Share of spending on workhouse or costs of farming out the poor where quantifiable, spending on alternative institutional provision at parochial level including pest-houses, and alteration or building costs where associated with medical welfare
Other health	Vaccination costs, wage supplements for sick paupers or their families, parochial work opportunities for the sick and impaired poor or their relatives, boarding, the boarding of the children of the sick poor, apprenticeship fees for sick children or the children of the sick poor

relief. These are augmented by more specific problems. Understanding exactly when medical welfare begins, even where records are strong, can be problematic. William Rogers Pearce, the vestry clerk of Newbury (Berkshire), wrote to his counterpart at Marlborough (Wiltshire) on 2 March 1827 on the subject of Thomas Rymes, who 'is very ill, and stands in need of relief & medical attendance he appears indeed very ill'. Pearce noted that he had already advanced the family 10s in extremis and hoped that the settlement parish would now respond. Marlborough granted the request, but there is no evidence that the 10s was ever repaid, and the commencement of medical welfare may have been January, February or March 1827.[87] To overcome problems like these requires that we link information within and between the data types outlined in Chapter 1, in order to distinguish 'normal' from medically related relief at both aggregate and individual level. This task is taken up in Chapter 4.

Conclusion

Reflecting on a carting accident that claimed the life of a Benjamin Woolstoncroft on 13 August 1791, William Rowbottom recounted a poem:

The fortunate have years
And those they choose
The unfortunate have days
And those they loose[88]

For those who were driven to dependence because of sickness or who became sick when receiving relief, the losing of days was all too common, as Chapter 7 shows. Yet illness short of death was also ubiquitous. Some of it was transient or constituted a single event in the life-cycles of paupers and families. Much, however, was more serious, and recovery was episodic and non-linear. Mental and physical impairment were common, and there is evidence that sickness was increasing in both frequency and duration over the period covered by this study. While it is possible to identify particularly 'unlucky' communities – Kettering for instance experienced large-scale epidemics in 1750, 1751, 1755, 1759, 1763, 1764, 1768, 1773, 1775, 1777, 1780, 1782, 1786, 1787 and 1789[89] – the lack of evidence for intra- and inter-regional, or

indeed typological, differences in the incidence of sickness is striking. The complexities of how illness was constructed, accepted, defined and recorded (and by whom) mean that we detect only a subset of the sickness episodes experienced by communities and individuals. It necessarily follows that we detect only a fraction of the medical resources deployed to ameliorate illness. Nonetheless, by employing a wide definition of medical welfare, one that sits neatly with the way in which contemporaries appear to have thought about the package of benefits assembled to tackle individual and familial sickness, and by employing detailed data linkage and analysis stages, we can render a strong picture of the importance of medical welfare for poor law spending as a whole. Chapter 4 takes up this challenge. In the meantime, one set of important interpretative and contextual issues remain: while the sick poor appear to have accrued considerable moral, customary and philanthropic capital in the eyes of officials during the final decades of the Old Poor Law, it was still the case that paupers or their advocates had to claim and contest sickness, that officials or vestrymen had to recognise and accept such claims and that all parties had to agree a package of relief and to revisit that package over time. This bargain involved knowledge – of the poor people and their situations on the part of officials, of the potential position of magistrates when claims were ignored or not met,[90] and of officials and precedents in parish relief policy on the part of paupers – and the accumulation, interpretation and re-interpretation of that knowledge left many grey areas. These issues of entitlement and negotiation – the subjects of the next chapter – are a vital backdrop to the interpretation of quantitative data in Chapter 4.

Notes

1 BRO, D/P 132/18/15/40, letter (my italics). On the form, rhetorical structure and content of pauper letters, see S. King, 'English pauper letters, 1790s-1830s', *Groniek*, 204–5 (2015), 305–16.

2 Anon. (1822), 'Mendicants', *Literary Speculum*, March 1822, 299.

3 Stoicism was a more general phenomenon, particularly in the eighteenth-century. See D. Porter and R. Porter, *Patient's Progress*, pp. 1–52, and contributions to J. Hinnells and R. Porter (eds), *Religion, Health and Suffering* (London: Kegan Paul, 1999).

4 ORO, PAR 207/5/A7/7, letter (my italics).
5 ORO, PAR 207/5/A7/5, letter, 24 March 1754. This was also a ubiquitous claim.
6 See, for instance, ORO, Oxford St Martin PAR 211/5/C1/1/26 and 27,
letters.
7 Levene, *The Childhood of the Poor*. For the mentally and physically
impaired see Borsay, *Disability and Social Policy*, but also (and for the
argument that those with impairments were part of the parochial wallpaper) S. King, 'Constructing the disabled child'.
8 T. Hitchcock, 'The English workhouse: A study in institutional poor relief
in selected counties, 1696–1750' (unpublished DPhil thesis, University
of Oxford, 1985). For a discussion of definitional problems see S. King,
'Poverty, medicine and the workhouse', pp. 228–51.
9 J. Taylor, 'The unreformed workhouse 1776–1834', in E. Martin (ed.),
Comparative Developments in Social Welfare (London: George Allen and
Unwin, 1972), pp. 57–84, at pp. 62–4.
10 Walsh, 'Poor law administration in Shropshire', pp. 82–8, argues that
workhouse use was more sustained in rural industrial and coalfield areas
and that this would also have influenced detectable sickness patterns. On
the idea that workhouses were receptacles for the sick see G. Mooney,
'Diagnostic spaces: Workhouse, hospital, and home in mid-Victorian
London', *Social Science History*, 33 (2009), 357–90, and for an earlier
period J. Boulton and L. Schwarz, 'The medicalisation of a parish workhouse in Georgian Westminster: St Martin in the Fields, 1725–1824',
Family and Community History, 17 (2014), 122–40. J. Taylor, 'The
unreformed workhouse', p. 63, provides the clearest statement of this
hypothesis.
11 Some idea of how closely overseers were expected to engage with the
sick poor can be seen in the case of Doncaster, where the overseer noted
paupers who were 'evidently ill'. DHC, PLD1/1, memorandum book of
Richard Tilburn and John Daniell, 1794–95.
12 See, for instance, S. Peyton, *Kettering Vestry Minutes A.D. 1797–1853*
(Northampton: Northamptonshire Record Society, 1933), p. 2.
13 Thane, *Old Age in English History*.
14 The construction of disease and illness has attracted a considerable histo-
riography. See, for instance, C. Rosenberg and J. Golden (eds), *Framing
Disease: Studies in Cultural History* (New York: Rutgers University
Press, 1992); A. Frank, *The Wounded Storyteller: Body, Illness and Ethics*
(Chicago: Chicago University Press, 1995); and for an earlier period
M. Stolberg, *Experiencing Illness and the Sick Body in Early Modern Europe*
(Basingstoke: Palgrave, 2011).

15 See F. Bound-Alberti, 'Emotions in the early modern medical tradition', in F. Bound-Alberti (ed.), *Medicine, Emotion and Disease, 1700–1950* (Basingstoke: Palgrave, 2006), pp. 1–21. For the reinvention of childhood insanity linked to new therapeutics see A. Mathisen, 'Mineral waters, electricity, and hemlock: Devising therapeutics for children in eighteenth-century institutions', *Medical History*, 57 (2013), 28–44.

16 Though note Eastwood, 'The republic in the village', p. 18, who suggests that because vestries were not obliged to keep minutes until 1819, before this there is likely to be a bias in record-keeping towards large or faster-growing urban industrial parishes where accidents were more common.

17 The lack of extensive reference to communicable diseases other than cholera or smallpox is striking. K. Siena, 'Contagion, exclusion, and the unique medical world of the eighteenth-century workhouse: London infirmaries in their widest relief', in Reinarz and Schwarz (eds), *Medicine and the Workhouse*, pp. 19–39, argues that in London the workhouses siphoned off infectious cases, potentially making them less visible. Chapter 8 will suggest that the situation is rather less certain in the provinces, where workhouses often refused those with infectious disease.

18 Pain, as opposed to the rhetoric of 'suffering', is something that emerges in pauper letters only from the 1820s, suggesting that some of the wider discourse on the meaning and treatment of pain in this period was feeding through to pauper consciousness. See A. Hodgkiss, *From Lesion to Metaphor: Chronic Pain in British, French and German Medical Writings, 1800–1914* (Amsterdam: Rodopi, 2000), and J. Bourke, *The Story of Pain: From Prayer to Painkillers* (Oxford: Oxford University Press, 2014).

19 See R. Porter, 'Lay medical knowledge in the eighteenth century: The evidence of the *Gentleman's Magazine*', *Medical History*, 29 (1985), 138–68; W. Wild, *Medicine-by-Post: The Changing Voice of Illness in Eighteenth-Century British Consultation Letters and Literature* (Amsterdam: Rodopi, 2006); M. Brown, 'Medicine, quackery, and the free market: The "war" against Morison's pills and the construction of the medical profession, c.1830–c.1850', in M. Jenner and P. Wallis (eds), *Medicine and the Market in England and its Colonies, c.1450–1850* (Basingstoke: Palgrave, 2007), pp. 238–61; J. Lane, '"The doctor scolds me": The diaries and correspondence of patients in eighteenth century England', in R. Porter (ed.), *Patients and Practitioners: Lay Perceptions of Medicine in Pre-Industrial Society* (Cambridge: Polity Press, 1985), pp. 205–48; R. Porter and D. Porter, *In Sickness and in Health: The British Experience 1650–1850* (London: Fourth Estate, 1988), p. 193.

20 S. King, 'Regional patterns in the experiences and treatment of the sick poor, 1800–40: Rights, obligations and duties in the rhetoric of paupers', *Family and Community History*, 10 (2007), 61–75.

21 J. Pickstone, 'Dearth, dirt and fever epidemics: Rewriting the history of British "public health", 1780–1850', in T. Ranger and P. Slack (eds), *Epidemics and Ideas: Essays on the Historical Perception on Pestilence* (Cambridge: Cambridge University Press, 1992), pp. 125–48.

22 Marland, *Medicine and Society*, pp. 28–43.

23 NRO, 249p/166, vestry minutes.

24 The literature on this area is complex and large. For the foundation study see E. Wrigley, R. Davies, J. Oeppen and R. Schofield, *English Population History from Family Reconstitution, 1580–1837* (Cambridge: Cambridge University Press, 1997). See also P. Razzell and C. Spence, 'The history of infant, child and adult mortality in London, 1550–1850', *London Journal*, 32 (2007), 272–91; R. Woods, N. Williams and C. Galley, 'Differential mortality patterns among infants and other young children: The experience of England and Wales in the nineteenth century', in C. Corsini and P. Viazzo (eds), *The Decline of Infant and Childhood Mortality: The European Experience 1750–1990* (The Hague: Martinus Nijhoff, 1997), pp. 57–72; and R. Woods, *The Demography of Victorian England and Wales* (Cambridge: Cambridge University Press, 2000).

25 J. Landers, *Death and the Metropolis: Studies in the Demographic History of London, 1670–1830* (Cambridge: Cambridge University Press, 1993).

26 See F. Condrau and M. Worboys, 'Epidemics and infections in nineteenth-century Britain', *Social History of Medicine*, 22 (2007), 147–59; S. Duncan, S. Scott and C. Duncan, 'Smallpox epidemics in cities in Britain', *Journal of Interdisciplinary History*, 25 (1994), 255–71; S. Duncan, S. Scott and C. Duncan, 'The dynamics of smallpox epidemics in Britain, 1550–1800', *Demography*, 30 (1993), 405–23.

27 The demographic transition is contested. See M. Brown, 'From foetid air to filth: The cultural transformation of British epidemiological thought, ca. 1780–1848', *Bulletin of the History of Medicine*, 82 (2008), 515–44; G. Mooney, 'Shifting sex differentials in mortality during urban epidemiological transition: The case of Victorian London', *International Journal of Population Geography*, 8 (2002), 17–47; B. Harris, 'Morbidity and mortality during the health transition: A comment on James C. Riley, "Why sickness and death rates do not move parallel to one another over time"', *Social History of Medicine*, 12 (1999), 125–31; G. Mooney, 'Infectious diseases and epidemiologic transition in Victorian Britain? Definitely', *Social History of Medicine*, 20 (2007), 595–606.

28 J. Riley, *Sickness, Recovery and Death: A History and Forecast of Ill-Health* (Basingstoke: Macmillan, 1989); J. Riley, *Sick Not Dead: The Health of British Workingmen during the Mortality Decline* (Baltimore: Johns Hopkins University Press, 1997); J. Riley, 'Why sickness and death rates do not move parallel to one another over time', *Social History of Medicine*, 12 (1999), 101–24.

29 B. Harris, M. Gorsky, A.-M. Guntupalli and A. Hinde, 'Long-term changes in sickness and health: Further evidence from the Hampshire Friendly Society', *Economic History Review*, 65 (2012), 719–45 at pp. 719–21.

30 Though see M. Gorsky, 'Friendly society health insurance in nineteenth-century England', in M. Gorsky and S. Sheard (eds), *Financing Medicine: The British Experience since 1750* (London: Routledge, 2006), pp. 147–64; Marland, *Medicine and Society*, pp. 188–202; E. Lord, '"Weighed in the balance and found wanting": Female friendly societies, self-help and economic virtue in the east Midlands in the eighteenth and nineteenth centuries', *Midland History*, 22 (1997), 100–12; and A. Rusnock and V. Dietz, 'Defining women's sickness and work: Female friendly societies in England, 1780–1830', *Journal of Women's History*, 24 (2012), 60–85.

31 See S. Morley, *Oxfordshire Friendly Societies, 1750–1918* (Oxford: Oxfordshire Record Society, 2011), pp. 3–15 for discussion of this gap.

32 See for instance the policy of Cliviger. LRO, DDX 1822/1, Cliviger order book, particularly entries from 1819 onwards starting with payments to reimburse the parish for supporting Lawrence Clark at a substantial £2 7s 6d. Such claims were likely to reflect real sickness given that claimants had to be inspected by the society doctor.

33 *Lincolnshire, Rutland and Stamford Mercury*, 25 February 1814.

34 *Lincolnshire, Rutland and Stamford Mercury*, 8 November 1816.

35 D. Dymond (ed.), *Parson and People in a Suffolk Village: Richard Cobbold's Wortham 1824–77* (Ipswich: Wortham History Group, 2007).

36 A. Peat (ed.), *The Most Dismal Times: William Rowbottom's Diary 1787–1799* (Oldham: Oldham City Council, 1996), p. 23.

37 As well as Chapter 8 see L. Smith, *'Cure, Comfort and Safe Custody': Public Lunatic Asylums in Early Nineteenth-Century England* (Leicester: Leicester University Press, 1999) and C. Cox, H. Marland and S. York, 'Itineraries and experiences of insanity: Irish migration and the management of mental illness in nineteenth-century Lancashire', in C. Cox and H. Marland (eds), *Migration, Health and Ethnicity in the Modern World* (Basingstoke: Palgrave, 2013), pp. 36–60.

38 RPC, letter, 14 June 1811.

39 C. Creighton, *A History of Epidemics in Britain*, vol. 2: *From the Extinction of the Plague to the Present Time* (Cambridge: Cambridge University Press, 2014, repr.).

40 A. Rusnock, 'Catching cowpox: The early spread of smallpox vaccination, 1798–1810', *Bulletin of the History of Medicine*, 83 (2009), 17–36; D. Shuttleton, *Smallpox and the Literary Imagination 1660–1820* (Cambridge: Cambridge University Press, 2007); S. Williamson, *The Vaccination Controversy: The Rise, Reign and Fall of Compulsory Vaccination for Smallpox* (Liverpool: Liverpool University Press, 2007); P. Razzell, *The Conquest of Smallpox: The Impact of Inoculation on Smallpox Mortality in Eighteenth Century Britain* (Firle: Caliban Books, 1977). For a recent argument that the purpose of inoculation was not to eliminate smallpox but to ameliorate the symptoms of an inevitable disease see A. Eriksen, 'Cure or protection? The meaning of smallpox inoculation, ca.1750–1775', *Medical History*, 57 (2013), 516–36.

41 See M. South, 'Smallpox inoculation campaigns in eighteenth-century Southampton, Salisbury and Winchester', *Local Historian*, 43 (2013), 122–37; M. Bennett, 'Inoculation of the poor against smallpox in eighteenth-century England', in A. Scott (ed.), *Experiences of Poverty in Late Medieval and Early Modern England and France* (Farnham: Ashgate, 2012); and S. King, 'Nursing under the Old Poor Law in midland and eastern England 1780–1834', *Journal of the History of Medicine and Allied Sciences*, 69 (2014), 1–35.

42 Some 117 individuals were treated. DRO, PE/SW/VE1/1, vestry minutes.

43 STRO, D24/A/PO/3106, letter. On cholera more generally, see M. Holland, G. Gill and S. Burrell (eds), *Cholera and Conflict: 19th Century Cholera in Britain and its Social Consequences* (Leeds: Medical Museum Publishing, 2009).

44 NRO, 251p/98/3, letter.

45 NRO, 249p/166, vestry minutes (my italics).

46 See C. Duncan et al, 'Whooping cough epidemics in London, 1701–1812: Infection dynamics, seasonal forcing and the effects of malnutrition', *Proceedings of the Royal Society of London, Series B: Biological Sciences*, 263 (1996), 445–50; A. Cliff, P. Haggett and M. Smallman-Raynor, *Measles: An Historical Geography of a Major Human Viral Disease from Global Expansion to Local Retreat, 1840–1990* (Oxford: Blackwell, 1993); and C. Duncan, S. Duncan and S. Scott, 'The dynamics of scarlet fever epidemics in England and Wales in the 19th century', *Epidemiology and Infection*, 117 (1996), 493–9.

47 BRO, D/P 26/12, overseers' accounts.

48 ORO, Oxford St Martin PAR 207/5/C1/1/5, letter.

49 NRO, 372p/11/A/S, Woodford Halse overseers' accounts. For context see O. Davies, 'Cunning-folk in the medical market-place during the nineteenth century', *Medical History*, 43 (1999), 55–73.

50 I identify crisis years as those where between six and fifteen or more claim-
    ants mention an epidemic or endemic illness. This is not to suggest that
    the complexion of disease was uniform. Norfolk, for instance, recorded
    many more fevers across the collected sources than Northamptonshire,
    but rather less smallpox.
51 In particular there is no evidence that the building of new asylums led
    to an increasing identification of pauper lunacy. See C. Jones, 'Disability
    in Herefordshire, 1851–1911', *Local Population Studies*, 87 (2011),
    29–44; E. Miller, 'English pauper lunatics in the era of the Old Poor
    Law', *History of Psychiatry*, 23 (2012), 318–28; E. Miller, 'Variations in
    the official prevalence and disposal of the insane in England under the
    poor law, 1850–1900', *History of Psychiatry*, 18 (2007), 25–38. Nor were
    there typological differences between communities in levels of idiocy.
    See F. Hughes, 'Was lunacy and idiocy a rural or an urban condition? A
    comparison of two county asylum services 1845–1900', *Local Historian*,
    44 (2014), 301–11.
52 NRO, 249p/164 and 166, vestry minutes.
53 C. Smith, 'Living with insanity: Narratives of poverty, pauperism and sick-
    ness in asylum records 1840–1876', in Gestrich, Hurren and King (eds),
    Poverty and Sickness in Modern Europe, pp. 117–41; C. Smith, 'Parsimony,
    power, and prescriptive legislation: The politics of pauper lunacy in
    Northamptonshire, 1845–1876', *Bulletin of the History of Medicine*, 81
    (2007), 359–85.
54 DHC, PLD1/1, memorandum book of Richard Tilburn and John Daniell,
    1794–95.
55 NRO, 92p/117/3, memorandum book.
56 See contributions to T. Crook and M. Esbester (eds), *Governing Risks in
    Modern Britain: Danger, Safety and Accidents c.1800–2000* (Basingstoke:
    Palgrave, 2016).
57 It is not clear, of course, that those using the same terms in different places
    or at different times were actually describing the same illnesses.
58 A. Hardy, '"Death is the cure of all diseases": Using the General Register
    Office cause of death statistics for 1837–1920', *Social History of Medicine*,
    7 (1994), 472–92; N. Williams, 'The reporting and classification of causes
    of death in mid-nineteenth-century England: The example of Sheffield',
    Historical Methods, 29 (1996), 58–71; R. Woods and A. Hinde, 'Mortality
    in Victorian England: Models and patterns', *Journal of Interdisciplinary
    History*, 18 (1987), 27–54; L. Schweber, *Disciplining Statistics: Demography
    and Vital Statistics in France and England, 1830–1885* (Durham, NC:
    Duke University Press, 2006); RCSE, MS0162, 'Westminster Hospital
    Remarkable Cases' 1802–18.

59 NORO, PD 552/55–108, Wighton overseers' and workhouse papers. See also K. Siena, *Venereal Disease, Hospitals and the Urban Poor: London's 'Foul Wards' 1600–1800* (Rochester: University of Rochester Press, 2004).

60 T. Philipson, 'The sick poor and the quest for medical relief in Oxfordshire ca 1750–1834' (unpublished PhD thesis, Oxford Brookes University, 2009).

61 LRO, DDX 1822/1, vestry minutes; LRO, MBCo 7/1, vestry minutes.

62 Tomkins, '"Labouring on a bed of sickness"', pp. 51–68.

63 LCRO, DE 1587/156/16, letter.

64 STRO, D24/A/PO/2893, letter, 27 November 1786.

65 STRO, D24/A/PO/2894, letter, 29 July 1787.

66 STRO, D24/A/PO/2895, letter, 27 January 1788.

67 STRO, D24/A/PO/2898, letter, 5 February 1791; STRO, D24/A/PO/2902, letter, 10 November 1795.

68 STRO, D24/A/PO/2904, letter, 18 March 1798.

69 STRO, D24/A/PO/2919, letter, 30 October 1811.

70 LRO, PR 2387/12–15, PR 2386/1–18, PR 2397/37 and 41, overseers' accounts and pay sheets. See also PR 2391/2–16 and PR 2390/1–51, correspondence and pauper letters.

71 DHC, PLD1/1, memorandum book of Richard Tilburn and John Daniell, 1794795.

72 Sokoll, *Essex Pauper Letters*, pp. 111–12.

73 *Ibid.*, pp. 116, 118–19, 120–1, 130–39, 148, 149, 150.

74 LCRO, DE 1587/155/12, letter (my italics).

75 LCRO, DE 1587/155/18, letter, 4 March 1824.

76 LCRO, DE 1587/154/35, letter.

77 LCRO, DE 1587/156/43, letter, 25 February 1828.

78 NRO, 249p/166, vestry minutes, 1 July 1835.

79 There is of course an inevitable auto-correlation with the way in which illness was defined and recorded.

80 E. Thomas, 'The treatment of poverty in Berkshire, Essex and Oxfordshire 1723–1840' (unpublished PhD thesis, University of London, 1971), p. 65.

81 LRO, DDX 1/6, town book of Bispham with Norbreck.

82 NRO, 261p/242/38, letter from Matthew de Pear, surgeon of Crowland, 15 March 1806.

83 NRO, 325p/194/103, letter book, January 1828.

84 LRO, PR 1603, overseers' accounts. See also Marland, *Medicine and Society*, pp. 58–64 and 68–9.

85 Some charitable bodies also recorded multi-layered medical welfare as a single entity. See P. Morgan, 'Service of the truth: Quaker poor relief in

Staffordshire to the mid-eighteenth century', in P. Morgan and A. Phillips (eds), *Staffordshire Histories* (Keele: Staffordshire Record Society, 1999), pp. 157–76.

86 For a particularly good example, see SRO, D/P/She/13/2/30, Shepton Mallet daily receipts and expenditure 1831–36.

87 WRO, 871/185/10, Marlborough St Peter & St Paul correspondence.

88 Peat, *The Most Dismal Times*, p. 36.

89 NRO, 185p/94, vestry minutes.

90 See Dunkley, *The Crisis*, p. 78; P. King, 'The rights of the poor', pp. 235–62.

3

Negotiating medical welfare

Introduction

On an unspecified date the overseer of Pangbourne (Berkshire)
received a hand-delivered letter from Olive Barber. She wrote:

> these lines to say that I took it very hard and unkind as you would not
> send us so much as a shilling *yesterday* as we are greatly destresed or else
> believe me we would not trouble you but my husband has been very ill
> since He came home and is legs are very bad at this time his oblidged to
> keep hisself as still as he can or his legs swells and are in so much pain or
> else he would have come to you yesterday and I do asure you he is very
> weak for he has been nearly starved this month and how can one [?]
> get strong when they have nothing to surport them was he able to work
> and could get it to do believe me we would never trouble you again so
> sir I beg you will consider of it and send us something and I hope God
> will provide for us and send us a friend for we have not one on earth. I
> thought Mr Holmes you had a feeling for you know what affliction is
> as well as my self and how bad it is to be a cripple God grant you your
> health and may you never know the destress as we.[1]

A classic pauper letter in terms of its focus on illness, lack of punctuation, orthography, rhetorical range and the mixture of apology,
reporting and assertion,[2] it is underpinned by a belief that the pathos
of illness and incapacity should be met on the other side by empathy
and sympathy. Barber's previous engagement ('yesterday', presumably in person because no earlier letter survives) with the overseer had
been unsatisfactory. Now she wrote to portray the couple as totally
friendless, in the hands not of their parish but of God. She personal-
ised the negotiation, eliding the disabilities of the old couple with the
(presumed) impairment of the overseer himself.

Barber's letter gives form to the observation of Chapter 1 that no pauper under the Old Poor Law had a definitive right to relief. She wrote to request relief rather than demand it.[3] On the other hand, it also highlights the fact that entitlement to support – its form, duration and scale – was not something that officials could always or easily decide solely in their own right. Rather it was the subject of negotiation and contestation. We see this process most clearly played out in the letters of the poor living outside their parish of settlement because relief had largely (but not entirely, as Barber's prior engagement with officials shows) to be agreed at a distance. Nonetheless, the sense that poor relief in general and medical welfare in particular were negotiable is not confined to this group. The strategies employed when the in-parish poor applied for, or sought to maintain entitlement to, relief are often masked by bland decisions in overseers' accounts and vestry minutes. Yet we occasionally get much stronger evidence that they too both felt that parochial policy could be contested and actively contested it. Robert Sharp of South Cave (East Yorkshire) noted that a female pauper 'on Monday last threw a stone at me [who] had been stopped in her pay'.[4] Evidence for such direct and violent contestation of decisions is uncommon,[5] but the fact that the in-parish poor negotiated robustly is clearly apparent in vestry minutes. Thus, in Kettering (Northamptonshire) an April 1823 vestry meeting bore 'testimony to the general and good behaviour of the persons applying for relief' and noted that their 'deportment to the overseers and the Vestry' had seen 'very considerable improvement'.[6] Negotiation with overseers themselves was also commonplace. When John Daniell, the joint overseer of Doncaster (Yorkshire), considered the case of Ann Hill in October 1794 he wondered whether she 'should not be taken into the House, she wanting further relief'. After visiting, however he '*Agreed* to give her 2s a week instead of 1s', which is suggestive of an act of negotiation. Indeed, he frequently referred to payments being made 'according to agreement' with the paupers.[7]

The rest of this chapter will (after a discussion of the meaning of pauper letters) explore three aspects of the negotiation process: the nature of the legal, customary, agential and moral space within which the claims of the sick poor sat; the rhetorical and other strategies employed as they engaged with officials; and the way in which parochial officers understood the rights of the sick poor in particular.

It will suggest *inter alia* that, as we began to see in Chapter 1, claims of sickness represented a singular area of contestability for overseers; that sick paupers both appropriated rhetorical strategies used by other types of claimant and forged their own distinctive claims-making apparatus; that they were more successful than other groups, irrespective of parish typology or location, in securing parochial welfare; that officials demonstrated a complex but ultimately favourable attitude towards the customary and humanitarian claims of the sick poor; and that 'success' might be fragile or freighted with unintended consequences.

Writing and claiming

Reconstructing the negotiating spaces, strategies and rhetoric of the sick poor (in itself and in relation to other pauper groups) is complex. None of my sources are as potentially useful or problematic for this task as the 12,904 letters written by, for or about the poor that make up one strand of the evidence used here. As Chapter 2 noted, some 10,452 of these letters either directly reference or imply illness, or are part of a letter set where illness was the core of claims-making. Notionally covering the whole of our period, they increase exponentially in number and regularity from the early 1800s, a combined function of better postal services, increasing migration, which took people outside their places of settlement, and better mechanisms for transmitting money between places, which made it worthwhile to write.[8] All communities seem to have received such letters, but their subsequent survival is patchy. The single biggest community collection relates to Kirkby Lonsdale (Westmorland) and has 1,600 letters, dwarfing the 252 pieces retained for the whole of Devon, for instance. Some 29 per cent of the 2,629 distinct claimants wrote or had letters written for or about them multiple times, and the underlying corpus is dominated numerically by such people. Their letter series can be both large and long: Hannah Buckman wrote twenty-one times from Harwich (Suffolk) to Hurstpierpoint (Sussex) between 1826 and 1832, with a further thirteen letters concerning her also extant; Sophia and Jacob Curchin wrote forty-nine times from Wisbech (Cambridgeshire) to Thrapston (Northamptonshire) between 1812 and 1828; William Lloyd wrote thirty-seven times from Hulme (Lancashire) to Llanasa (North Wales) between 1808 and 1817.[9] If the core sample of operational data for

117 parishes is 'light' on coverage of the largest urban areas, the pauper letter data demonstrates no such bias. The letters were written extensively from the largest urban areas, and even collections for Cornwall and Cumberland contain material from the out-parish poor living in London parishes. Particularly where they can be synthesised with other parochial sources, then, such material provides an important perspective on the process of poor relief from its very beginning. In turn, welfare historians who have made extensive use of such letters have regarded them as embodying a – perhaps even the – voice of the poor. Others have been less sanguine, regarding pauper voices as 'muffled, audible only in relation to (and deeply shaped by) the highly strategic negotiations of formal poor relief'.[10] Clearly, pauper letters and associated correspondence raise a suite of interlinked questions about representativeness, authorship, authenticity and utility, and while these matters have been addressed by myself and others elsewhere, their centrality to understanding the negotiation process requires further engagement here.[11]

The representativeness of pauper letters and the rhetoric and strategies that they embody depend in part upon how many people were 'out of their place' and thus potentially tied into the out-parish relief system that largely generated such letters. Numbers could be considerable. In eighteenth-century Stratford-on-Avon at least 25 per cent of all households were resident without settlement, while a large number of Stratford residents had migrated outwards and created potential parochial liabilities elsewhere.[12] In the Yorkshire the figures are even more compelling. Between 50 and 100 per cent of all pensioners notionally recorded in the overseers' accounts of some parishes were actually either non-resident or physically present but the responsibility of parishes elsewhere.[13] For this study, bills and accounts for the out-parish poor in my Northamptonshire parishes suggests that 39 per cent of all paupers notionally receiving relief were either non-resident or non-settled. To this number one must add residents whose relief from settlement parishes was directed not through overseers (and hence potentially recordable in their accounts) but through tradesmen, carriers, vicars, neighbours or landlords.[14] Indeed, for some places it is possible to argue that the paupers who remained in their settlement parish were unrepresentative.[15] Other dimensions of the representativeness question perhaps have more purchase. Most collections, as I

have already observed, contain letters from London and plenty more from large urban areas, but such places in their turn appear to have retained relatively few of the letters that we know to have been sent to them.[16] The corpus contains very few narratives from the inmates of institutions, children,[17] the Scottish and Irish poor and the young unemployed. On the other hand, the aged, the impaired, widows and the Welsh are certainly over-represented in comparison to their likely share of the overall 'pauper host'.

The wider issue, however, is whether the stories, negotiating strategies and rhetoric that we find in pauper narratives are representative of the way sick 'in-parish' claimants engaged with parochial officials. There are good reasons to think that those who negotiated on paper might adopt different tactics from those who could approach the overseer in person. Margaret Crowther reminds us that for the out-parish poor 'the decision on where [and how] to seek relief was a delicate one'.[18] When they did apply, the visual signifiers of need, despair and hopelessness (and the matching responses of paternalistic humanism or Christian duty) implicit in face-to-face encounters with the sick were missing. Moreover, it might be that paupers writing from a distance (and often to parishes where they had not been seen for a while) would have to spend more time conveying their trustworthiness and deservingness than would a sick pauper applying in person who could be viewed easily by ratepayers and officials. Yet one can overstate, both in general and for the early nineteenth-century in particular, the discreteness of oral and literate cultures.[19] A surprising number of those who were sick when they applied or became sick while receiving relief both appeared before the vestry or overseer and wrote letters, either contiguously (out-parish paupers were often eager to emphasise their belonging by coming 'home' periodically as we saw above) or sequentially, as did Olive Barber. It seems unlikely that their rhetorical and strategic approaches would have been very different in either forum. By the same token, some of those applying to vestries did so by note or advocate, stressing that they were too ill to attend in person, a common enough claim among out-parish letter writers as well. Moreover, both in- and out-parish paupers faced two shared conundrums – how to navigate entitlement in a system where there were few fixed rules; and how to approach the different stages of the process of obtaining relief, ranging from the decision to ask for help, through making a case and

appeals to higher authorities where unsuccessful, to the decision to accept relief – which ought to have shaped their claims-making strategy in similar ways. This is particularly true of the aged sick, whose letters and appearances before the vestry share a basic rhetoric (outlined in Chapter 2) that a progressively decrepit old age equated to an absolute obligation for the parish to provide regular support.[20]

One can also argue that the claims-making strategies of both in- and out-parish paupers drew on a common heritage of storytelling. In part this was rooted in fairy stories, balladry and local memorials and languages of custom and obligation.[21] From the late eighteenth century, however, the poor were exposed to many more forums in which their 'stories' might be developed, told, demanded or recounted, in which their petitioning and rhetorical skills developed or where they might hear the stories of others. Coronial juries, case histories taken in voluntary hospitals, witness statements, petitions to charities, meetings and public petitions to parliament,[22] briefs, appeals for assistance via newspapers,[23] and migrant letters[24] all provided fora in which the poor could fashion themselves and their lives. It is hard to imagine that this storytelling heritage did not feed through to the ways in which the poor (in- or out-parish) represented themselves to parochial officials. In the particular context of the sick poor it is also important to note that from the later eighteenth century an ever larger corpus of scientific or medical knowledge and language appeared in the public domain. Advertisements, novels, poetry (particularly embodying the language of melancholy), popular medical texts, prescriptions, direct consultations with doctors and advice books coalesced to provide a common source of medical fact, rhetoric and authority with which paupers could engage officials.[25]

The question of authorship – of who originated the ideas embodied in a letter and wrote what appears on the page – also matters for our understanding of the meaning of medical welfare. It is ultimately impossible to prove that the person signing a letter was also the writer of it.[26] On the other hand, doubts over this matter can be, and have been, taken rather too far. In the pauper letter corpus used here the writing, grammar and punctuation were highly variable but tend strongly towards the more orthographic end of the spectrum (see Figure 3.1). Nonetheless, such letters point to a wide base of broadly functional literacy, and, as Martyn Lyons has argued, the English labouring poor

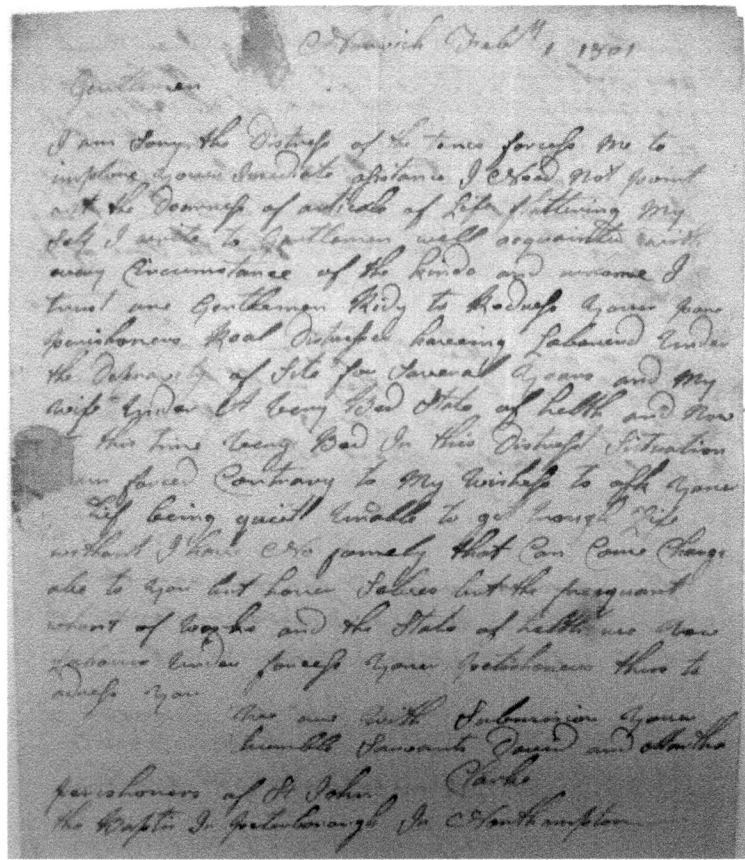

3.1 Sample pauper letter

were probably much more literate than has often been supposed or measured.[27] There are certainly cases where an amenuensis or close relative was used to write.[28] Yet, and in contrast to France, evidence for the operation of paid scribes is rare.[29] Moreover, we have already seen above that multiple letter writers and their letters are the core of the dataset, and the consistency of handwriting in these cases, often over long periods, suggests that author and signatory was usually the same person.

The internal evidence of the letters can tell us less about the problem of authenticity – the sense that paupers at a distance might embellish their stories or simply lie. The most cursory reflection on human nature would suggest that this must have been a problem. If, as seems likely, claims of sickness enhanced the likelihood of relief there was an incentive for both the out-parish poor and (though with more difficulty) the in-parish poor to dress their claims up in the rhetoric of sickness. The poor were more likely to adopt the rhetorical cloak of sickness when their ability to get relief for other causes of poverty (such as unemployment) was being closed down, as appears to have been the case in the last decades of the Old Poor Law. It is certainly possible, against this backdrop, to detect paupers such as Jacob and Sophia Curchin who told persistent and blatant lies. Piecing together their narratives reveals that Sophia Curchin was ostensibly pregnant in the 1820s and 1830s more often than is biologically possible, even allowing for miscarriages.[30] Other paupers were undone by particularly active officials. John Deaking, the overseer of Leicester, wrote to his counterpart in Market Harborough (Leicestershire) on 25 February 1823 to contradict the story of Widow Stringer. He wished to inform Market Harborough that 'no such Person has ever applied … for relief' and that 'the rest of her tale [of sickness] is a fabrication … and I take pleasure in exposing her, this is one of many impositions I have exposed of Paupers endeavouring to impose on Parishes to which they belong'.[31] Yet more were revealed as liars by people in host communities. Thomas Derwin thus wrote from Leicester to the overseers of Oxendon (Leicestershire) to 'Inform you of the conduct of a man named James Harmstead & his wife', who he claimed were 'living in Drunkenness, Riot and Debauchery' while receiving a parochial allowance for sickness. Worse, their house was a meeting point for 'men of Bad character at all hours of the Night, and at present they have 5 Lewd women in the house'.[32]

Though entertaining, however, these stories are also relatively unusual. If pauper letters 'share with other autobiographical sources a certain element of fiction',[33] it is possible to substantially overstate the degree to which writers were prone to embellishment, partial truths and downright lies. Thomas Sokoll has suggested that Essex pauper letter writers generally told the truth, not least because they could easily be inspected by their home parish, or officials could ask others (visiting tradesmen, fellow overseers) to drop in on them.[34] The corpus

used here is replete with such requests for inspection and subsequent replies, and almost none find that claimants were lying. Indeed, and as the overseer of Wellingborough (Northamptonshire) found in the 1790s, inspection sometimes revealed that paupers had understated the severity of their case.[35] The frequent claim in pauper letters that the writer had told officials only the half of their suffering thus seems to ring true. More widely significant numbers of writers got others to attest the truth of their letters by adding postscripts. And in so far as we can construct an 'average' set of correspondence relating to a single individual, it would certainly contain letters from officials, doctors, vicars and other advocates reflecting on the state of the individual, the cause of their poverty and the justice of the claims made. In short, I understand the corpus of pauper letters used here as broadly truthful; the unemployed or other groups who found their entitlements to apply for relief squeezed over time could not casually add sickness to their list of woes in order to enhance their standing.

A final problem centres round issues of utility. Pauper letters were strategic documents, simultaneously reporting fact, shaping the identity of the sender and embodying variable measures of appeal, silence, partial statement, anger, duty, gratitude, deference and the assumption of rights, in an effort to secure relief and influence its scale and duration. The very nature of the overseer–pauper relationship might influence their form and contents as Fitzmaurice and others have suggested.[36] Paupers may have shaped the 'facts' and omissions so as to best exploit the discretionary nature of poor relief. Silences (particularly on issues such as kinship) are important and frequent.[37] While there is little evidence in the underlying corpus of the use of letter-writing manuals, it seems unlikely that paupers would have been so far on the margins of society that they would be unaware of the epistolary conventions implicit in serialised novels and formal public petitions.[38] Moreover, the contents of the pauper letter were invariably situational: the aged had a wider rhetorical reach than the young and a wider set of claims-making apparatus simply because they had lived longer and moved more often. A man of forty could not use the rhetoric of decay to justify a claim (though he might use an equivalent such as chronic illness) any more than a married women writing to the settlement parish of her husband could claim attachment to a 'home' community. The content and form of letters were also shaped by the art of the possible. Urban paupers, for

instance, were more likely to co-opt or refer to the authority of doctors than their rural counterparts simply because there were more of them around when urgent letters required testimony. This core problem is insoluble, but counteracted in part by looking for broad patterns in a national database of pauper letters rather than focusing simply on individual rhetorical strategies. Triangulating pauper narratives with overseers' correspondence, letters by epistolary advocates and vestry minutes can also help to strip them back to the bare strategic essentials. Used sensitively and mediated via emblematic case studies, such narratives open an important window onto the lives, words and basic agency of the sick poor as they sought to influence relief decision.

Legal, customary and moral spaces

The discretionary nature of parochial decisions was briefly highlighted in Chapter 1. While overseers and vestries had duties to receive applications for relief, they had few obligations to approve such applications, to provide relief in the form or over the duration asked for or to respond promptly.[39] Indeed, pauper writers sometimes complained bitterly that their letters had not been attended to, pointing to the costs of sending mail and the mournful effects of waiting endlessly for a reply. Officials sometimes reacted angrily to such accusations: the overseer of Thrapston (Northamptonshire) added a postscript on his letter of 1 October 1829 to Elizabeth Brand, noting that 'I consider the parish of Thrapston very kind to your mother and hope you will in future treat them with respect and write in a civil and becoming manner as I assure you they never wish their paupers to lie out of their money.'[40] Within this discretionary system, and as suggested in Chapter 2, the applications of both in- and out-parish paupers could be turned down, deferred or commuted.[41] This is not to say that officials were careless about the poor and their applications. Indeed, the reality that parish officers frequently found themselves caught between a rock and a hard place is beautifully conveyed by a respondent to the *Cambridge Chronicle* in November 1800 who, pointing to families in 'inconceivable distress', suggested that 'Parish officers frequently know not what to do; the poor rates are already so high.'[42]

In this context it is clear that the capacity for agency across the pauper community was variable according to age, gender, place and, especially,

cause of poverty. Claims of sickness and associated conditions such as decline or troubled minds occupied a distinctive place. Parishes were legally obliged to care for their 'impotent' poor, and while there was scope on the margins for overseers to 'define away' sickness, conditions such as chronic illnesses, mental or physical impairment, recurrent sickness, accidents and sudden medical need occasioned by infectious diseases constituted the arena in which parish duties kicked in. Paupers thus afflicted – and there is little evidence that those claiming to be sick fabricated their conditions, as we have seen – posed particular moral hazards for overseers. Since sickness compromised the ability to work, the key test of deservingness in this period, and might have significant knock-on consequences for the viability of households, officials had a *de facto* case for responding favourably to appeals couched in these terms. On the other hand, to grant sickness relief as an automatic right might threaten unlimited future rate bills. It would also give the poor, as we have seen, a fixed reference point as they tried to navigate a system where the combination of opaque rules and the discretion of local administrators were crucial in balancing demand for and supply of welfare resources. Unsurprisingly, then, officials and vestries struggled with sickness, particularly where the claimant retained marginal capacity to work.

As the example of Olive Barber shows, the sick poor implicitly assumed a right to have their case heard favourably if not a right to relief itself. The underlying dataset is redolent with material which suggests that, notwithstanding some spectacular acts of pitiless parsimony, overseers themselves often agreed with this position. By way of example, Richard Palmer wrote from Hawick (North Yorkshire) to his counterpart in Billington (Lancashire) on 26 January 1829 to say that:

> James Ormerod's wife is very poorly indeed and the relief which they have had is thought by all who are acquainted with her situation to be quite insufficient: I have consulted Mr Hesmondhalgh on the subject and we have come to the following conclusion:
>
> 'That the overseer give a ticket to Richard Hesmondhalgh for 11s per week to furnish the old people with milk until such a time as they can provide for themselves.'
>
> James Seed had, therefore, better send a ticket to that effect with J. Ormerod to R. Hesmondhalgh.[43]

Palmer, then, was responding to a widely held community belief that severe sickness should be met with enhanced resources. Justice Hesmondhalgh codified the legitimacy of the claim with an implicit threat to take further action if the ticket was not issued. The irritation at the Billington overseer's breaching of normative standards is palpable. In turn, ingrained perceptions of the paternalistic and Christian duty of local elites, custom and correct behaviour, the tendency for magistrates to test the limits of deservingness, legal obligation and the activities of interest groups (such as doctors) and epistolary advocates for the poor coalesced to create a moral space within which the different sub-groups of 'the sick poor' could negotiate and contest their eligibility for welfare. And it was a short step from granting relief in one case to the assumption of local custom. As Thomas Wintle, the vicar of Brightwell-cum-Sotwell (Oxfordshire), noted in 1794, the poor were expert at translating discretionary payments into customary claims which 'are so soon establish'd, and with such difficulty broken thro'.[44] It is thus important to revisit suggestions that lopsided power relations meant the poor had to submit to obedience of moral codes, the rhetorical and behavioural norms of deference and gratitude and the broad will of ratepayers.[45]

Negotiating medical relief

The ways in which paupers (both in- and out-parish) rhetoricised their condition were partly shaped by wider developments in the 'narrative culture' of our period. A refashioning of the way in which the 'self' was constructed and understood yielded a new and more powerful interiority with a focus on the emotional condition, and one might expect to see this reflected in pauper writing.[46] Other aspects of this narrative culture – the increased accessibility of newspapers; development of the linguistic register and the mushrooming of a generalised epistolary culture, alongside the accumulating experience of medical storytelling outlined earlier – must also have influenced the scope, content and form of letters.[47] Moreover, this was a period of rising popular radicalism across a spectrum from local food riots through to organised large-scale unrest in both rural and industrial areas. There is little evidence from the corpus (though see below in relation to expressions of anger) that radical language made its way into the letters of the poor and no sense at all that there was a spatial patterning to rhetoric which might map

onto contemporary radical activity. Nonetheless, the unfolding of local unrest as well as the arrival of national movements such as Chartism may well have given claimants more confidence to make their case at the same time as the other developments noted above provided a wider linguistic register to frame it, and a more sophisticated rhetorical range with which to engage overseers.

How the sick poor sought to navigate the agential spaces open to them differed according to age and to some extent gender, location and causation of sickness. This said, we can identify a spectrum of strategies and rhetorical devices that were central to their claims-making.[48] Some claims were shared with other groups of paupers. Thus one of the obvious strategies was to invoke anger or threat. Henry Hunt wrote to the overseer of Tottington (Lancashire) in March 1826 stating,

> Sir, I got ure note of the last Munday and I say to u that u must releeve us family for we have nothing and no credit to get. It is now five weekes that I wrought the work to evn pay for our meat and my wife still sick and my children without clothes. U must show humannitie and if u do not then depend on it that I shall come to U and no thing will stop me from making apply to the justices for u propose.[49]

Hunt's wife was sick, and notwithstanding attempts to make do via work and credit, there was no prospect of independence. Without relief he would have to return to his 'home' parish and employ the full force of the law in order to ensure that relief was forthcoming. The assumption that sickness equalled entitlement is as clear here as in the case of Olive Barber, while the anger at initial refusal is palpable. As Sokoll has shown for Essex, this mixture of threat, appeal, abject despair and determination to return home is typical of many letters, though recognition of the extent to which paupers were able to operationalise the law has been a more recent historiographical theme.[50] In turn, the rhetoric of threat appears to have been a particular device for former ratepayers who fell sick, those turned down on first application and sick paupers who had their allowances withdrawn and modified.[51] Such was the case of William Arkwright, who wrote to the overseer of Manchester on 19 April 1830. He was

> sorry to inform you that I am unable to work at the present time in consequence of illness and the length of time that I have been unable to work the inclosed note will certify. I live in a house of £10 per year rent

I am now entered into the third quarter the second quarter was due on the 25 of the last month which is £2 10s. and the poor leys is also wanted and they will not excuse me anything but will they say force me to pay the utmost farthing so that all that I have is in danger of being sold for rent and leys for I am not able to pay either in consequence of sickness you know what family I have and how matters stand with regard the settlement for if I become a parishoner through rent all my children will belong Manchester likewise her. I have given you a true statement of the case and shall leave you to judge of it if my quarter rent is not paid immediately all my goods will be sold.[52]

This was a carefully crafted threat. Effectively, if the parishioners did not help Arkwright with the rent – as they should do because the situation and settlement of the family was well known and they were struggling to maintain themselves as respectable ratepayers – it would eventually cost them a lot more. And if the parish did not 'judge' fairly then presumably Arkwright would turn to a judge literally.

While both of these examples are drawn from Lancashire parishes, threat and anger appear in all the county letter collections. Charles and Hannah Sharman, writing from London to Market Harborough on 10 March 1828, accused the overseer of 'very great neglect'. James Richards, writing from Colleycroft (Bedfordshire) to Thrapston on 19 December 1829, complained that the 'one shilling a week you are pleased to allow me is not nearly sufficient ... you no doubt are quite aware of my privations in hearing and lameness'. John Frankish wrote from Louth (Lincolnshire) to Beverley (East Yorkshire) on 14 July 1816 to say, 'it is your Neglect that causes me to be so trubelsome'.[53] Threats were not confined to the out-parish poor, as the experience of Robert Sharp suggests. Indeed, since threatening letters accrued harsh punishment, direct action against officials, some of whom were themselves marginal characters, was most likely to occur in face-to-face relationships with the in-parish poor. The Garstang vestry, for instance, noted in May 1822 'the very improvident and insolent conduct of Jonathan Harrison and his wife'.[54] The fact that paupers used the rhetoric of threat is perhaps understandable given that parish relations under the poor law were themselves sometimes constructed within a linguistic register tending towards the threatening, conflictual or legalistic.[55] Nonetheless, what is surprising in the corpus of pauper letters is how infrequently the sick poor in particular resorted to the use of threats or

anger. Fewer than 2 per cent of their 10,452 letters were framed wholly or largely in these terms.

Sickness narratives also shared other rhetorical devices with the wider corpus of pauper letters, perhaps not unexpectedly given that sickness was only one of the causative factors making for a sustained relief history at the individual level. These devices, as the examples of Barber, Hunt and Arkwright above begin to suggest, included *inter alia* the respectability of the applicant; their desire to help themselves and not to be a long-term burden; the economic logic of 'relief now' to avoid larger bills in the future; the contribution of a family to host or settlement parishes; and the languages of custom (either that of the host or settlement parish) and humanity or fair treatment. These elements of a shared linguistic platform should not, however, lead us to downplay the sense that sickness added a twist to familiar claims-making vehicles. The appeals of the sick were different by moral degree from those made by, say, the unemployed. While there have been several attempts to create categorisations of pauper letters,[56] such an exercise for the sick poor stumbles on the fact that they were also inscribed with a number of distinctive rhetorical devices or embodied distinctive strategic approaches. These include the stark expression of a pauper's plight, melding seamlessly into hopelessness; requisitioning the voices and authority of others; speechlessness; the language of sudden and catastrophic need on the one hand versus that of chronic and inevitable decline on the other; invitations to inspect or seek accounts of familial plight; and the rhetoric of normative and customary standards of the sort assumed by Olive Barber.

Some emblematic examples can help us explore this rhetorical and strategic range. Thus the majority of sick paupers eventually centred claims-making round stark expressions of their plight. On 11 April 1764, Elizabeth Taylor wrote to James Daydde, the overseer of Shelton (Norfolk), to tell him that 'I have been so much afflictet since Michelmas with the St antinis Fire that I have had 5 holes in my thighs and I have had no health since March nor no my child.' She begged 'you to send me sumthing more to subsist me til I gett sumthing Better'.[57] This stark expression of her situation was folded into an acknowledgement of the discretion of the overseer ('send me sumthing') at the same time as the narrative was infused with a basic assumption that some relief would be forthcoming given the situation. John Salisbury, meanwhile, wrote

to the overseer of Barnacre-with-Bonds (Lancashire), on 27 April
1825 to:

> inform you that I cannot nor am not able using honest means to support
> my family so therefore I desire you will take it into consideration and
> give some assistance I have 3 children two little more than one year old
> and she in childbed at present and one child not likely to live so I pray
> consider my circumstances and for gods sake allow me something in
> this time of need. I Am John Salisbury, son of John Salisbury that served
> his prentiship under Edmund Salisbury Barnacre forge so you need not
> dispute me ... [58]

Salisbury sought to establish his respectability and (through settle
ment) his entitlement to apply. Yet it is the starkness of his case – death
and circumstance threatening to overwhelm them and an honest man
on the edge of having to use dishonest means – that is striking. A final
desperate appeal to the humanity of the ratepayers was couched in
terms of religious duty, a common addendum to the stark need presented in the letters of the sick poor, as we saw for Olive Barber. In
turn, statements on the severity of a situation were often enclosed in a
narrative of sudden need, as in the case of Isaac Curtis, who appended
a note intended for his family to a letter asking for medical relief when
he wrote to Longbridge Deverill (Wiltshire): 'I take the opertunity
of sending to you to inform you of the state of my wife at this time
for three days past I did not expect her life.'[59] For the in-parish poor,
vestry minutes usually record a considerable range of indicators of
'suddenness' – 'severe' injury or illness, 'dreadful' accidents, paupers
'seized' with illness – to account for the fact that an applicant had not
come in person, suggesting the universality of this approach.

The most powerful rhetorical vehicles were those which combined
a stark expression of plight with the threat of public knowledge of
the writer's suffering. James Wilson's letter to Hulme on 4 March
1831 said:

> I write to inform you that my famely lies in the most desperate state. I
> buried my son, not 4 years old, last Tuesday and because of my ill health
> have not been able to work this last month. Gentlemen, have a care
> and come to see our state with not the clothing we need and the hose
> [house] to live in. Our rent is now due and I have no means to pay. I beg
> you gentlemen not to dismiss our case for our friends know of the case

and will show you for what you are. But gentlemen I beg your support for my famely once more and I shall when in health hope never to be a pauper again if you look to us this once.[60]

Sickness, then, had dragged the family to a desperate state of nakedness of which the neighbours were well aware and which had already been on display at a public funeral. Wilson had nothing to hide, inviting the vestry to come and view the state of the family. But there was a sting in the tail. If relief was not forthcoming then his state and the part of the 'gentlemen' in continuing it by failing to pay the rent would become a local talking point. Other paupers were even more direct. William King, writing from Bethnal Green to Braintree (Essex), suggested that 'My Sean of wreachedness appeared in the News and in a Small track [tract] Likewise wich I Now Can Produce if Neads be …'.[61] Samuel Parker of Kidderminster (Staffordshire), writing to Uttoxeter (Staffordshire), said that he would go to the local newspapers and publicise his case if the vestry continued to ignore his claims,[62] and more widely there are 242 examples in the underlying letter corpus of paupers threatening publicity. In turn, paupers like Wilson, King and Parker were, at least in part, adopting a common rhetorical platform with officials themselves; overseers used the language of public knowledge and shame in their dealings with each other.

The rhetorical prospect of resuming an independent life if assisted was common to many paupers. But for the aged, as we saw in Chapter 2, stark representations of their situation were often accompanied by, or merged seamlessly into, rhetoric of hopelessness, decay, and chronic or inevitable decline which should attract regular support. The narratives of this group, as well as appeals by the in-parish poor recorded in vestry minutes, are redolent with phrases such as 'I am without hope'; 'I walk in the valley of death'; 'We are bowed low'; 'I am of the age at which I must have relief'; and 'I suffer from the afflictions of my age.' This rhetoric was, as we saw for William King in Chapter 2, developed over a series of correspondence in which pauper letters melded seamlessly with those of other advocates. Such cases are balanced by letters in which the writer sought to crystallise a lifetime of suffering in a single epistle, when all hope had been lost. Thus Anna Greenhalgh wrote from Manchester on 21 July 1825 to inform her husband's settlement parish that Samuel Greenhalgh was in 'a worse situation in respect of

his Bodily health then he was when last I wrote'. She would do everything she could for him: 'Under his afflictions and when it pleases prov-
idence to remove him from this transitory life may he meet with a kind
acceptance in heaven.' Present relief 'to sooth his present uncomforta-
ble misery' would, she assured the overseer, 'always be remembered'.[63]

At the other end of the age spectrum we encounter comparable
rhetoric as parents expressed their loss of hope for ailing children or
reflected pessimistically on their dark future if parishes would not help
to ameliorate sickness and impairment. Frances Soundy wrote to the
parish of Pangbourne (Berkshire) at an unknown date in 1823 asking
for an apprenticeship fee for her son John. Stressing that she had found
a good opportunity, Frances added a short postscript: 'Gentillmen this
poor boy John Soundy as got an empedement in his speach so that
he can not git his living by servitude.' Before Pangbourne could reply
Soundy wrote again, in October 1823, noting that the prospective
master required an answer forthwith. She warned that:

> My son his now turned 15 years so that he will soun be tou old to be
> boun prentise any ware and gentillmen I ham sorry to say if he his not
> bound I shall have him at home all the winter on my hands a gain as he
> as empediment in his speach so that he can not go Service as he can not
> vary wall be understud.

As if to reinforce the timeliness of intervention, James Soundy (John's
erstwhile estranged father) appended a further note to the effect that
John 'his quit incapable of giting his living other mens So gentillmen
we umblely pray you to assist this poor lad in giting his living'.[64] The
contention that John Soundy could not be well understood is, when set
against the remarkably orthographic communicative form of his parents, remarkable. Nonetheless, this and other follow-up letters convey
a sense of worry on the part of parents not to lose an opportunity which,
if relinquished, might lead to lifelong dependence upon both them and
the parish. The request was, in other words, proportionate, and the
parish responded in its stead, as a means of saving future costs but
also reflecting the wider humanitarian and paternalistic attitudes which
created the negotiating space for Soundy's letter in the first place.

For some claimants (in- and out-parish), the situation appeared so
hopeless or the suffering was so far beyond their capacity to describe
that they became actually or strategically speechless, transmitting

testimonials of their condition from others. Such external testimony simultaneously helped to establish the authenticity of the case and the respectability of the pauper. In July 1816 James Wilson, living at Appleby (Westmorland), attended the Garstang vestry 'wanting relief having buried his wife after her long sickness leaving him with 4 small children, oldest only about 9 years old and very infirm'. He 'brought an account [of his circumstances]' from the Appleby overseer.[65] Alternatively, both in- and out-parish paupers could simply requisition the language and authority of others, quoting their words or outlining their opinions to overseers in order to make up for their own speech-lessness. Thus Hannah Sutton's final letter in a sequence of five from Rugby (Warwickshire) to Rothersthorpe (Northamptonshire) did not seek to elaborate further on her illness, noting only that 'Doctor Barnes says that I have No Hopes now of Recovery from this Grave illness and you may Seek his testimoney as to the Truth of my words.'[66]

For both the speechless and those at other stages of the rhetorical construction of their sickness, it was common to draw on epistolary or personal advocates who did more than simply provide testimony of the sort noted above. In the case of multiple letters, as I have suggested above, the vast majority of narrative sequences contained material from an epistolary advocate. Indeed, the sick turned to advocates with persistent regularity in comparison to other subsets of the poor. In some cases the writers had obvious self-interest, as for instance with employers or landlords who joined paupers and overseers in a three-way negotiation for scarce resources. William Griffin, writing from Cheam (Surrey) to inform the parish of Shere (also Surrey) that his tenant, William Moore, owed him rent of £3, is a classic example of a demand for money supplemented by a case for the pauper: Moore, 'having a family of five Children, not one being able to work, [and] nor indeed is he scarcely able himself', was a deserving case for parish assistance.[67] Yet what strikes one about the corpus as a whole is how infrequently self-interest lay behind advocacy. We see this clearly in letters from overseers of the poor about or on behalf of individuals. On the face of it, such overseer advocacy can be read as a simple exten-sion of their day-to-day management of finite parish resources and the complexities of the laws of settlement. They wrote to establish whether a home parish wished to begin or continue a welfare arrangement; to request instructions on relief levels; to demand payment; to clarify

payment mechanisms; or to advise settlement parishes of changes in pauper circumstances. Yet officials did not just report facts or seek action. Rather, their letters often included personal appeals or information in support of a claimant's application for relief, and employed a rhetoric which implied a genuine concern for the poor. Overseer Bostock's letter to the home parish of Hannah Parkinson is a classic example. He wrote: 'I understand that she formerly received 1/6 per week from you, and that that the allowance was discontinued about seven weeks ago.'[68] Bostock continued:

> she is 50 years of age and consequently incapable of much bodily exertion – she used to go out washing, but has been obliged to give it up from inability ... Under these circumstances I hope you will consider to allow her the 1/6 as before, which *I really think is as little as you should do for her.*[69]

Of course, we can read this narrative as instrumental – a subtle attempt to avoid large future bills – but the personal last line suggests a different perspective, one much more attuned to the role of advocate.

For the settlement parish, the question of whether to turn down a strong recommendation from a fellow officer was a thorny one. Such concerns were magnified when sick paupers got people of higher social status or holding a clerical title to write on their behalf. In a series of eleven letters to Hulme (Lancashire) on behalf of the pauper Jane Higginson, William Hudswell, minister of George Street Chapel in Leeds, used sickness and impending death as a rhetorical vehicle. His letter of 21 May 1836 noted, 'I saw the old woman yesterday and found her very poorly she can scarcely do anything for herself ... now she is obliged chiefly to lie in bed from pain in her leg.' The reply of the overseer is telling, highlighting the way in which claims for medical relief could put intense strain on the poor law, something that we do not see in simple end-of-process expenditure statistics. It states, 'We cannot consistent with our duty either to receivers or payers increase the allowance. Our township is one almost entirely of cottages and we are at times as much pained at compelling payment of rates as we are in withholding in cases like this now before us.'[70] One could understand this letter as posturing, but an alternative reading would be that Hulme genuinely could not afford to pay medical welfare claims. Whatever the interpretation, faced with an annoyed reply from Hudswell, the

overseer promptly paid an allowance. The decision over how to react to an epistolary advocate was complicated further where that advocate was a medical man. The underlying corpus contains 479 letters from doctors. Some simply transmitted bills, reported that pauper X was sick and unable to work,[71] or were solicited by parochial officers in the host community. Yet we also find doctors going further. George Bottomley of Croydon (Surrey) affirmed that 'Hunt's Wife & three children are all very ill with Scarlet Fever [and] they stand in very great need of Medical attendance', adding that 'in fact they are in so very bad a state, that something must be *immediately* done for them'.[72] Such letters effectively changed the landscape of engagement with parish officers in comparison to other groups of the poor, for whom such professional advocacy was rarer. Indeed, it is striking how often the sick poor in even the smallest and most remote communities had access to medical men. We have less evidence of advocacy for the in-parish poor, but in communities where medical men were actually members of the select vestry, they were normally asked to inspect sick applicants and recommend a course of action. Few of those inspected were turned down, suggesting a spectrum of informal advocacy.

Within this broad framework, as I have already suggested, writers believed that officials would act. The rhetorical infrastructure of such assumptions is well displayed in the case of Jacob Curchin, the malingering resident of Wisbech encountered earlier. His letter of May 1825 on the occasion of his wife's impending childbirth claimed, 'you must know what an expensive time [this is]'. He went on to note that 'I can get my wife's attendance for 10/6. If I could pay the money before the Doctors leaves the room If not it will be £1–1–0.'[73] The assumption that his wife should have the attendance of a medical man is clear. Curchin took up this theme even more forcibly in a letter of 1 December 1826 in which he claimed, 'I have a place for them where I was born and depend upon it they shall come unless you deliver what is customary on these occasions.'[74] His other letters are rather less confrontational, though no less inscribed with notions of moral, paternalistic and customary duty. Sophia Curchin also periodically wrote to Thrapston and worked under the same basic assumptions. Her letter of 26 June 1826 asked for 'a Trifle more a week in my confinement as every one of feeling will allow it a shocking thing to want at such a time as I expect very shortly'.[75] The couple were periodically relieved, despite an observation from the

Thrapston overseer to his Wisbech counterpart in June 1824 that 'I beg to observe that he [Jacob Curchin] is a very troublesome and imposing man, and therefore shall be obliged by your being guarded against his crafty insinuations ...'.[76]

Of course, to consider pauper strategies in the abstract is misleading since multiple rhetorical vehicles could be combined within a single letter. P. N. Stewart wrote just such a narrative, worth quoting at length, to the overseer of Barnacre-with-Bonds on 3 April 1822. It was with

> regret and feelings that I cannot express that I send you these few lines to let you know our deplorable situation. It is now nine weeks since I wrought 3 weeks work and just as I was beginning to mend my wife took her trouble and was brought to bed on the 24 of last month and has brought on additional hardship such as must be seen to be believed. We were totally unprepared for any such thing and in my poor state of health and very neare in distraction tried every scheme in honesty to earn some money But to no purpose at last a neighbour advised me to go and sell one pair of our looms and not see my wife and children lost. I went and found a man to buy them and gave me 1 pound for them and he was so good as to give me 3 weeks to pay it back again and keep the looms. On Monday 15 the time will be expired and the money is not and more needed now. Gentlemen, I appeal to you as husbands and fathers to look to our deplorable conditions and prevent the breaking up of a house with 4 little ones under 6 years 2 months the oldest now. If you do not look to this last request that I shall ever make I shall have no other shift left but see what we have and keep my wife and children till she gets better and then she shall come to you Depend on what I say if I am live till she is well I will never starve both them and myself while the law of the land has made a place for her and them, if not for me. I am not fit to maintain myself at present But I shall not come to you I shall never undergo another brow beating by a fellow as fierce as if he had a brief to bleed my life away. I shall die in a ditch first if you think proper to stop this overwhelming torment of destiny. Send what you think good by the bearer of this and you will prove yourselves worthy the character of men with human feelings and forever oblige your humble servant.[77]

This letter is shot through with sophisticated rhetorical strategies: apology and deference, claims to respectability and future independence, threats, appeals to the humanity of the recipient, suggestions of the good value of acting immediately, the implication that his suffering was public knowledge, anger and hints that Stewart's very standing as a

man, father and husband had been compromised. He threatened them that the consequences of inaction would result in public scandal – he would 'die in a ditch' – and stated categorically that poverty was not his fault but the 'torment of destiny'. Above all the drama of his situation had been enhanced by the sheer suddenness of the medical situation for which the family 'were totally unprepared'.

Stewart's correspondence is particularly rich. It is balanced in the underlying corpus by a series of letters which often stretch to just a few lines and which simply stated that the pauper was very ill and in a desperate situation. Sudden sickness quite literally disabled the afflicted from making their case. On balance, however, the individual letters of the sick poor are certainly the most rhetorically varied and sophisticated sources in the underlying data. Whether this reflects claimant's understanding of the expectations of overseers, a sense that entitlements in general were fragile so that writers had to go the extra mile or a shared understanding between officials and applicants that potentially expensive and long-term medical relief required a certain rhetorical position is difficult to unpick. If, however, we switch our attention – from the writing of letters to the question of how overseers received them – it is possible to discern considerable shared under-standing between officials and paupers about the nature of negotiation, the malleability of the local state and the limits of parochial action.

Official responses

The question 'How were pauper appeals received?' is a deceptively simple one. Overseers' correspondence is one of the great remaining untapped resources for the study of poor law history and should in theory afford a clear answer. Comprising letters to and from other officials, suppliers, magistrates, ratepayers, bankers, lenders and vari-ous other parties, some collections even include draft or copy letters back to the poor themselves. And while largely externally facing, the corpora also includes material on the in-parish poor. It is precisely this abundance which begins to explain why overseers' correspondence has been so little exploited. To problems of volume, we might add the fact that the tone and content of material were tied up with the individual personality of the overseer. This, and the often rapid turnover of such officials,[78] makes uncovering detailed patterns of sentiment complex.

The patchy survival of select vestry records for much of the period means that it is no easier to discern how the appeals of the in-parish poor were met.

Nonetheless, we can discern core regularities that touch upon the issue of reception. In practice, and as I have already suggested, overseers appear to have been remarkably susceptible to the claims-making of the sick poor. James Taylor's observation that 'The cruelty and stupidity of the few [overseers] should not obscure the plodding competence of the many' applies particularly keenly where officials considered cases of sickness.[79] Moreover, there is much in the data to support Daunton's view of 'a broad identity between ratepayers and the recipients of relief ... overseers of the poor were not providing a system of relief for a distinct and despised class'.[80] We can trace the outcome of appeals by letter or epistolary or personal advocate for 8,224 of the 10,452 instances in which sickness formed the key claims-making vehicle. Some 82 per cent were 'successful' in the sense of not being immediately turned down. This observation applies across the county samples. It is by some distance the highest success rate of those applying for relief by letter: a comparable figure for those citing unemployment was just 32 per cent. The essential conundrum that parish officers faced with both in- and out-parish paupers who claimed sickness has already been explored, and perceived failure to act in such cases could generate extensive negative commentary and accusations of neglect. Even the most parsimonious overseer would have been wary.

Moreover, we should remember that the case for medical welfare was often constructed, delivered and dissected in public. Both the vestry and the overseer's parlour can be conceived of as public spaces.[81] By the time an application was made the fact of sickness would have been well established in the eyes of the host or settlement communities and even in the minds of overseers themselves, given often sustained interaction with sick paupers.[82] The consequences of a failure by officials to account for resulting public sentiment can be seen in other records, with coroners, for instance, regularly obliged to respond to rumours or formal complaints that a death had been occasioned through inaction by overseers. Hence on 2 November 1764, William Beasant of Canock (Wiltshire) died suddenly. In response to stories to the contrary, the coroner was forced to note, 'he had a sufficient allowance from the parish officers from the time of his being taken ill to the day of his

death'. On 3 April 1777 Betty Box of Broughton Gifford (Wiltshire) was 'reported to have died for want of necessaries and attendance in the smallpox and from neglect of the parish officers'. Similarly, on 28 August 1783 Ann Watts of Great Cheverell (Wiltshire) was 'said to be starved through neglect of the parish officers', while Thomas Caning's suicide in Bradford-on-Avon workhouse after he had been admitted in a melancholic state on 7 March 1787 led to widespread condemnation of the neglect of the officers.[83] At the other end of the period considered here, rumours of neglect pepper reporting of the Lincolnshire Coronial Circuit. Juries almost always found rumours to be false, but the very fact that they circulated at all testifies to an underlying seam of pressure to act constructively. They also suggest just how fragile the reputation of parochial officers might be.[84]

If there is little support in the data for the idea that the sick poor lost their legitimacy or were pushed to the margins of their communities, it is nonetheless clear some claims were more successful than others.[85] Appeals made on the basis of sudden or catastrophic medical need or accident usually received quicker and more favourable attention than those made on the basis of chronic ongoing illness. Where the pauper making such claims was living elsewhere overseers often asked their counterparts in the host parish to 'treat this pauper as your own', while the in-parish poor usually had an official or vestryman dispatched with authority to give whatever relief was needed. Claims that paupers were dying or in their final illness (explored in Chapter 7) and claims by women both in their own right and for sick children also attracted prompt and favourable responses. By contrast, the claims of sick men (unless they were made for sick wives and children), the young and the aged tended, even where ultimately successful, to be part of a more elongated decision-making process.

The term 'success' is, however, rather elastic. It certainly did not mean that paupers got what they asked for or that all people with similar circumstances were treated equally. Letter writers often complained that overseers had sent them less cash than they felt they needed, less than they had asked for or less than was customary. Out-parish recipients on long-term relief were particularly likely to express such resentment. For the in-parish poor, vestry minutes equally point to delay, the giving of less than was asked for or the translation of requests for cash payments into relief in kind. Those for Oundle and Garstang – in

Northamptonshire and Lancashire respectively, two highly contrast-
ing counties – are good exemplars: On 8 July 1829 the wife of John
Ives applied to the Oundle vestry for 'relief' on the occasion of her
husband's illness. At the same meeting her brother-in-law William Ives
applied for relief because his wife was ill. Faced with the two applications from people with similar family situations, the vestry awarded the
wife of John Ives 10s, while William Ives was 'granted meat and broth'.
In Garstang, the application of Jilly Stewart, 'she being very feeble and
unwell', was delayed pending further investigation, while that of Mary
Taylor resulted in authority for 'the overseer to make an agreement
with her as shall further the interests of the town'.[86] Both sets of vestry
minutes evidence repeated applications from paupers where overseers
were tardy in making their decisions, much as we see in the letters
of the out-parish poor. Moreover, some cases were simply granted,
while others involved requests for information from third parties such
as employers, vestrymen, doctors or even family members. If the sick
poor claimed and maintained a space in which their relief could be
negotiated and contested, it is clear that this space took considerable
navigating. Nor should we forget, in terms of reception, that relief
orders sometimes came with unforeseen consequences, including
ongoing surveillance. Vestries only reluctantly granted open-ended
commitments to paupers. They hedged responses to illness with caveats that allowances were temporary, would expire on a fixed date unless
ongoing need was proven, were dependent upon regular re-assessment
of the case or were simply given 'until XX gets well'. Chapter 6 explores
this issue in more depth, particularly in relation to cash allowances.
Officers might also seek to limit their ongoing liability for the sick poor
by discovering relatives and either forging a partnership with them or
simply requiring family support. Such was the case, for instance, with
the Colne (Lancashire) vestry, in June 1793 which ordered that 'Jas
Foulds is to be allowed 2s a week by his son for another month, he
being at present very sick'.[87] At the opposite extreme (and a theme
explored in Chapter 8) officials could eschew family care and simply
confine paupers in hospitals, asylums or other institutions as part of
recognising parochial liability.

The observation that officials were highly sensitive to the claims of
the sick poor, who themselves had considerable agency, must thus be
tempered with the sense that entitlement could be, or could be felt to

be, fragile. It had not just to be gained, but maintained, and negative consequences of accepting aid minimised. Hence both vestry minutes and the pauper letter corpus are littered with repeat applications, not just to ask for new allowances but to continue existing ones. While officials were clearly irritated by the steady flow of correspondence – there are twelve examples of copy letters from overseers asking paupers to desist writing – the fact of their sustained and detailed engagement with such letters points to acute problems of how to decide deservingness and to calibrate consequential benefits. Paupers often assumed that the overseer would remember their previous correspondence and might claim that basic rules of etiquette were not observed where the overseer failed to reply. Sustained correspondence could establish a customary right to be heard and to have allowances renewed, and it often allowed letter writers to claim friendship with or patronage from particular officials. Moreover, the fact of a prolonged epistolary relationship allowed paupers to mix up claims for themselves and their relatives and those on their behalf by others. Above all, a sequence of letters facilitated the development of rhetoric, such that paupers could move seamlessly from the need for trifling relief associated with individual instances of sickness, through claims to more substantial relief for family sickness, and finally to the need for permanent and ongoing relief linked to decline, the accumulated effects of sickness on the ability to work, melancholy or depression and chronic conditions. Of course, paupers had to temper the development of their rhetoric to fit the wider backdrop of knowledge of them in the 'home' parish, which gave subtle local and regional flavour to the rhetoric employed.[88]

Conclusion

Parochial spending represents the end of a process of application, decision-making and inclusion or exclusion. While for other groups of the poor this process could result in very large numbers of applications failing or being withdrawn, the sick poor had a privileged space in which to negotiate eligibility. Their original requests may sometimes have been modified; they might get less than they asked for and over a shorter duration than required; and certain groups of sick paupers may have had better chances than others. Nonetheless, the sick

poor did have real agency and could deploy sophisticated rhetorical devices – individually or in sequence – to press *de facto* rights onto the consciousness of the parish. In turn, there is no evidence to support a sense that other groups of the poor could casually add sickness to their list of ills in order to enhance their chances of relief. The medical welfare figures explored later in this study are, in short, a good reflection of the scale of initial applications driven by sickness. Considering the pauper letter corpus as a whole suggests definitively that poor people invested effort and care into their language and image even when, by definition if they were truly sick, the case was urgent. This reflected not just the fact that negotiating space had to be navigated, but that applying for and taking the parish shilling could occasion scrutiny of the most intrusive sort. Nowhere are such tensions better demonstrated than in the words of Walter Simcock, writing from Ashton-under-Lyne in Cheshire:

> to inform you that I have totally lost the use of my right leg and have to use a crutch to support me the few hours I'm able to go about during the day and consequently have not been able this last six months to hearn food sufficient for myself and family. From the repeated enquiries made after me and the impudence of the female Sarah Tolinson to my wife whilst I was absent at the doctors I'm inclined to think a false statement and rong impression may be given of my infirmity therefore beg to refer you to Dr Wood home I've been under three months without his being able to cure me or to dr Winsor of Manchr that I'm at present under for a corroboration of what I have stated – shan't do you of my severe affliction I will wait upon you at the office any time you may b pleased to appoint. With many thanks for the kindness you have shown me during so long a sickness.[89]

The poor were keenly aware of their vulnerability in a period of long sickness and the importance of having a good reputation if relief was to continue. 'Rights', if often assumed by both paupers and officials, had to be created, finessed, monitored, renewed and defended even in a situation where the poor 'were not a distinct underclass [but] a shifting population among whom almost any member of the community might fall' at time of sickness.[90] It is to the outcome of this process – spending on medical welfare and particularly the creation of normative standards of care – that subsequent chapters turn. In this context, David Eastwood's sense, framed in terms of family allowance systems, that

'the last years of the so-called unreformed parish system were years of vibrancy and experiment' will be seen as the key motif for parochial treatment of the sick poor.[91]

Notes

1 BRO, D/P 91/18, letter (my italics).

2 Sokoll, *Essex Pauper Letters*, pp. 1–72. See also Jones and King, 'From petition to pauper letter', pp. 53–77.

3 Eastwood, *Governing Rural England*, p. 121, who argues that by the mid-1790s near universal rights to minimal welfare payments existed.

4 J. Crowther and P. Crowther, *The Diary of Robert Sharp of South Cave: Life in a Yorkshire Village 1812–1837* (Oxford: Oxford University Press, 1997), p. 38. Hopkin, 'The Old and New Poor Law', p. 198, provides evidence of violence and intimidation in Yorkshire parishes during the 1830s.

5 J. Taylor, *Poverty, Migration and Settlement*, p. 47, argues that 'for every occasion a pauper spoke or acted badly, there were a hundred in which he spoke and acted humbly and hoped for a generous heart'.

6 Peyton, *Kettering Vestry Minutes*, p. 88.

7 B. Barber, *Memorandum Book of Richard Tilburn and John Daniell: Overseers of the Poor for the Township of Doncaster* (Doncaster: Doncaster and District Family History Society, 2009), pp. 24 and 26 (my italics). In Oundle (Northamptonshire) a proposal to cut the allowances of some widows and force others into the workhouse was revisited 'after hearing from each individual their remarks upon it'. NRO, 249p/166, Vestry Minutes, 1 July 1835.

8 S. King, '"It is impossible"'.

9 SURO, PAR.400/37/122; NRO, 325p/193 and 194, overseers' correspondence; MCL, M10/808–16, letter books.

10 A. Shepard, 'Poverty, labour and the language of social description in early modern England', *Past and Present*, 201 (2008), 51–95, at p. 53. By contrast Sokoll, 'Negotiating a living', p. 25, argues that pauper letters 'provide – literally – first hand evidence of the experiences and attitudes of the poor themselves'.

11 See Sokoll, *Essex Pauper Letters*; J. Taylor, *Poverty, Migration and Settlement*, pp. 149–64; S. King, 'Pauper letters as a source', *Family and Community History*, 10 (2007), 167–70; and A. Gestrich, E. Hurren and S. King, 'Narratives of poverty and sickness in Europe 1780–1938: Sources, methods and experiences', in Gestrich, Hurren and King (eds), *Poverty and Sickness*, pp. 1–34.

12 J. Martin, 'The rich, the poor and the migrant in eighteenth century Stratford-on-Avon', *Local Population Studies*, 20 (1978), 28–48.

13 Hastings, *Poverty and the Poor Law*, p. 28. See also J. Taylor, *Poverty, Migration and Settlement*, p. 142.

14 Note too Taylor's contention that in Devon paupers given casual relief were not considered chargeable and hence did not appear in the out-parish books. J. Taylor, *Poverty, Migration and Settlement*, p. 21.

15 The frequency of migratory moves across the average life-cycle provides an idea of how this situation emerged. See C. Pooley and J. Turnbull, *Migration and Mobility in Britain since the Eighteenth-Century* (London: UCL Press, 1998).

16 S. King, 'Friendship, kinship and belonging in the letters of urban paupers 1800–1840', *Historical Social Research*, 33 (2008), 249–77. With regard to B. Song, 'Parish typology and the operation of the poor laws in early nineteenth century Oxfordshire', *Agricultural History Review*, 50 (2002), 203–24, at pp. 205 and 208–12, there is no evidence in the corpus that open parishes systematically received more letters than closed parishes or vice versa. Langton's remarkable county study of Oxfordshire in any case suggests that much more complex typographical and topographical variables may have influenced both poor law sentiments and pauper agency. See Langton, 'The geography of poor relief', pp. 193–234.

17 Though see Barber, *Memorandum Book*, p. 23 for the application of a nine-year-old child.

18 Crowther, 'Health care and poor relief', pp. 211–12.

19 B. Bushaway, 'Things said or sung a thousand times: Customary society and oral culture in rural England, 1700–1900', in A. Fox and D. Woolf (eds), *The Spoken Word: Oral Culture in Britain 1500–1850* (Manchester: Manchester University Press, 2002), pp. 256–77.

20 See Sokoll, 'Old age in poverty', pp. 127–54.

21 D. Hopkin, 'Storytelling, fairytales and autobiography: Some observations on eighteenth and nineteenth century French soldiers' and sailors' memoirs', *Social History*, 29 (2004), 186–98, and contributions to M. Lyons (ed.), *Ordinary Writings, Personal Narratives: Writing Practice in 19th and early 20th Century Europe* (Frankfurt: Peter Lang, 2007). For a wider theoretical framework see R. Charon, *Narrative Medicine: Honoring the Stories of Illness* (Oxford: Oxford University Press, 2006).

22 C. Tilly, 'The rise of the public meeting in Great Britain, 1758–1834', *Social Science History*, 34 (2010), 291–9; J. Hanley, 'The public's reaction to public health: Petitions submitted to parliament, 1847–1848', *Social History of Medicine*, 15 (2002), 393–411, at pp. 394–95. See also

D. Lemmings, 'Introduction', in D. Lemmings (ed.), *The British and their Laws in the Eighteenth Century* (Woodbridge: Boydell, 2005), p. 18.

23 D. Andrew, 'To the charitable and humane: Appeals for assistance in the eighteenth-century press', in Cunningham and Innes (eds), *Charity, Philanthropy and Reform*, pp. 87–107; and Lloyd, *Charity and Poverty*, pp. 1–35.

24 D. Gerber, *Authors of their Lives: The Personal Correspondence of British Immigrants* (New York: New York University Press, 2006).

25 See, for instance, A. Ingram and L. Weatherall Dickson (eds), *Popular Culture*, vol. 4 of L. Weatherall Dickson and A. Ingram (eds), *Depression and Melancholy, 1660–1800* (London: Pickering and Chatto, 2012); A. Secord, 'Science in the pub: Artisan botanists in early nineteenth century Lancashire', *History of Science*, 32 (1994), 269–315; J. Topham, 'Publishing "popular science" in early nineteenth-century Britain', in A. Fyfe and B. Lightman (eds), *Science in the Marketplace* (Chicago: University of Chicago Press, 2007), pp. 135–68; G. Smith, 'Prescribing the rules of health: Self-help and advice in late eighteenth-century England', in R. Porter (ed.), *Patients and Practitioners*, pp. 249–82; R. Porter, 'Spreading medical enlightenment: The popularization of medicine in Georgian England, and its paradoxes', in R. Porter (ed.), *The Popularization of Medicine 1650–1850* (London: Routledge, 1992), pp. 215–31.

26 K. Snell, 'Belonging and community: Understandings of "home" and "friends" among the English poor, 1750–1850', *Economic History Review*, 65 (2011), 1–25.

27 M. Lyons, 'Writing upwards: How the weak wrote to the powerful', *Journal of Social History*, 48 (2015), 311–36. See also S. Whyman, *The Pen and the People: English Letter Writers 1660–1800* (Oxford: Oxford University Press, 2009).

28 For an excellent example see P. Jones, 'Widows, work and wantonness: Pauper letters and the boundaries of entitlement under the Old Poor Law', in Jones and King (eds), *Obligation, Entitlement and Dispute*, pp. 139–67.

29 C. Métayer, *Au tombeau des secrets: Les écrivains publics du Paris populaire, cimetière des Saints-Innocents XVIe–XVIIIe siècle* (Paris: Albin Michel, 2000). The stay maker Thomas Jeffries, charged with theft at the Old Bailey on 22 February 1786, is one of the few examples. A character witness said that Jeffries 'maintained himself by writing letters and petitions'. See Old Bailey Online, https://www.oldbaileyonline.org/browse. jsp?id=t17860222-104-defend1037&div=t17860222-104#highlight (last accessed 26 March 2017).

30 King, Nutt and Tomkins, *Narratives of the Poor*, pp. 75–125.

31 LCRO, DE 1587/154/1, letter.

32 NRO, 251p/99, letter.

33 L.-H. van Voss., 'Introduction', in van Voss (ed.), *Petitions in Social History*, pp. 1–10, at p. 9.

34 Sokoll, *Essex Pauper Letters*, p. 68. The best example in the underlying data is for Beverley (Yorkshire), which regularly asked George Lacey to inspect out-parish paupers in Hull. See in particular EYRO, PE1-702-48, letter of inspection, 20 June 1832.

35 NRO, 350p/166–9, overseers' accounts.

36 S. Fitzmaurice, 'Politeness and modal meaning in the construction of humiliative discourse in an early-eighteenth century network of patron-client relationships', *English Language and Linguistics*, 6 (2002), 239–65.

37 B. Poland and A. Pedersen, 'Reading between the lines: Interpreting silences in qualitative research', *Qualitative Enquiry*, 4 (1998), 293–312. On missing kinship references see A. Tomkins, 'Poverty, kinship support and the case of Ellen Parker, 1818–1827', in Jones and King (eds), *Obligation, Entitlement and Dispute*, pp. 107–38.

38 E. Bannet, *British and American Letter Manuals, 1680–1810* (London: Pickering and Chatto, 2008). For a wider culture of epistolarity on which the poor might draw see J. How, *Epistolary Spaces: English Letter Writing from the Foundation of the Post Office and Richardson's Clarissa* (Farnham: Ashgate, 2003).

39 On regional differences see King, *Poverty and Welfare*.

40 NRO, 325p/194, letter.

41 As one example, see M. Ramsbottom, 'Christopher Waddington's peers: A study of the workings of the poor law in the townships of the Fylde of Lancashire 1803 to 1865' (unpublished PhD thesis, Oxford Brookes University, 2011), pp. 114–17.

42 M. Murphy, *Cambridge Newspapers and Opinion 1780–1850* (Cambridge: Oleander Press, 1977), p. 50.

43 LRO, PR 2391/29, letter.

44 M. Spurrell (ed.), *The Brightwell Parish Diaries* (Oxford: Oxfordshire Record Society, 1998), p. 37.

45 French and Barry, 'Identity and agency', pp. 1–37, and Hindle, 'Civility, honesty', pp. 40, 47 and 52.

46 R. Porter, 'Introduction', in R. Porter (ed.), *Rewriting the Self: Histories from the Renaissance to the Present* (London: Routledge, 1997), p. 3.

47 On these matters see R. Dekker, *Autobiographical Writing in its Social Context since the Middle Ages* (Hilversum: Veloren, 2002); R. Gagnier, *Subjectivities: A History of Self-Representation in Britain, 1832–1920* (Oxford: Oxford University Press, 1991); R. Porter, 'Expressing yourself

ill: The language of sickness in Georgian England', in P. Burke and R. Porter (eds), *Language, Self and Society: A Social History of Language* (Cambridge: Polity, 1991), pp. 276–99.

48 On wider attempts to construct a tri-partite characterisation – restitution, chaos, quest – of sickness narratives, see Frank, *The Wounded Storyteller* and Shuttleton, *Smallpox*, pp. 43–9. The latter's discussion of the mythic quality of illness narratives is particularly important.

49 MCL, L82/8/3/14, letter, 3 March 1826.

50 Sokoll, *Essex Pauper Letters*, pp. 27–33. See also S. King, 'Negotiating the law'.

51 Anger was also prevalent where paupers sought to refuse medical treatment for diseases such as smallpox. See D. Brunton, *The Politics of Vaccination. Practice and Policy in England, Wales, Ireland and Scotland, 1800–1874* (Rochester: University of Rochester Press, 2008), and S. Burrell and G. Gill, 'The Liverpool cholera epidemic of 1832 and anatomical dissection – medical mistrust and civil unrest', *Journal of the History of Medicine and Allied Sciences*, 60 (2005), 478–98.

52 MCL, L82/8/3/30, letter.

53 LCRO, DE 1587/156/6, letter; NRO, 325p/194, letter; EYRO, PE1-702-19, letter, 14 July 1816, unsigned but identifiable as Frankish's from prior correspondence.

54 LRO, DDX 386/3, vestry minutes, 21 May 1822.

55 Some overseers' correspondence provides clear evidence that paupers had a hand in shaping the contents, as for instance when officials indicated they had been 'asked to write …'.

56 J. Taylor, 'Voices in the crowd', pp. 111–12, classifies letters into 'formal, informational, insistent and desperate'. This classification, however, has more to do with tone than content. See also T. Sokoll, 'Writing for relief: Rhetoric in English pauper letters 1800–1834', in A. Gestrich, S. King and L. Raphael (eds), *Being Poor in Modern Europe: Historical Perspectives 1800–1940* (Bern: Peter Lang, 2006), pp. 91–112.

57 NORO, PD 358/63, letter.

58 LRO, PR 2391/42, letter.

59 WRO, 1020/102, letter, 20 December 1817. For an even more insistent letter sent to Langho (Lancashire) see LRO, PR 2391/37, letter.

60 MCL, M10/808, letter.

61 Sokoll, *Essex Pauper Letters*, p. 116.

62 See STRO, B3891/6/100, letter. I am grateful to Alannah Tomkins for this reference.

63 MCL, L21/3/13/7, letter.

64 BRO, D/P 91/18/, letters.

65 LRO, DDX 386/3, vestry minutes, 19 July 1816.
66 RPC, letter, 23 July 1812.
67 SRC, SHER 28/8/2, William Griffin to Shere, 11 February 1828.
68 WYRO, WDP 20/9/3/15, J. Bostock to Asst. Overseer (name and parish unknown), 9 August 1827.
69 *Ibid.* (my italics).
70 MCL, M10/809, letter. The draft reply to Hudswell's letter is attached to the original.
71 For an excellent collection of these short notes, see NORO, PD 111/112, doctoring correspondence.
72 SRC, P3/5/39/9, George Bottomley to unknown parish official, 20 April 1829 (underlining in original; my italics).
73 NRO, 325p/193, letter.
74 NRO, 325p/193, letter 17.
75 NRO, 325p/193, letter 7.
76 NRO, 325p/193, letter 3.
77 LRO, PR 1349, miscellaneous letters.
78 Paid overseers long in office adhered more closely and consistently to the law, sought more advice and were more sceptical of appeals. How letters were received thus depended in part on the proportion of salaried officials. E. Hampson, *The Treatment of Poverty in Cambridgeshire, 1597–1834* (Cambridge: Cambridge University Press, 1934), p. 245, suggests that by 1833 some 50 per cent of Cambridgeshire parishes had a salaried overseer. By contrast, Northamptonshire boasted only a handful of paid officials at the same date. Across the letter sample, turnover of officials stood at around 43 per cent per year.
79 J. Taylor, *Poverty, Migration and Settlement*, p. 105.
80 Daunton, *Progress and Poverty*, p. 452.
81 A. Wilson, 'The Birmingham General Hospital and its public, 1765–69', in S. Sturdy (ed.), *Medicine, Health and the Public Sphere in Britain 1600–2000* (London: Routledge, 2002), p. 87; M. Ogborn, *Spaces of Modernity: London Geographies 1680–1780* (London: Guilford Press, 1998), pp. 98 and 232.
82 A. Ashby, *One Hundred Years of Poor Law Administration in a Warwickshire Village* (Oxford: Oxford University Press, 1926), p. 114, argues that overseers gained an intimate knowledge of the poor in places such as Tysoe.
83 R. Hunnisett, *Wiltshire Coroners' Bills 1752–1796* (Devizes: Wiltshire Record Society, 1981), pp. 24, 63, 86, and 97.
84 The data encompasses many instances of parishes responding to pauper complaints, adding weight to Thomas's view that the views of the poor had traction. See Thomas, 'The treatment of poverty', pp. 72.

85 Lees, *Solidarities of Strangers*, pp. 20 and 40; Marshall, *The English Poor*, pp. 224 and 252.
86 NRO, 249p/164, vestry minutes, 8 July 1829; LRO, DDX 386/3, vestry minutes, 28 February 1822.
87 LRO, MBCo 7/1, vestry minutes, 5 June 1793.
88 S. King and A. Stringer, '"I have once more taken the Leberty to say as you well know": The development of rhetoric in the letters of the English, Welsh and Scottish sick and poor 1780s–1830s', in Gestrich, Hurren and King (eds), *Poverty and Sickness*, pp. 69–92. Once again, however, there is no evidence that the threat of public protest, riot or other action by popular radicals infused the rhetoric of letters in those areas where such activity was strong or current.
89 MCL, M10/810, letter, 18 July 1839.
90 Thane, *Old Age in English History*, p. 113.
91 Eastwood, 'The republic in the village', p. 25.

Part II

The scale and character of medical welfare

4

Treating the sick poor: a quantitative overview

Introduction

On 27 July 1806, Samuel Tibbs, overseer of Aldbury (Hertfordshire), wrote to his counterpart in St Albans (Hertfordshire) authorising payment of 2s 6d to Mrs Narroway 'in her distress'. He added, however, that 'we [the vestry] do not think she ought to be in the distress she says she is in' and asked his fellow overseer to 'have the goodness to attend her, and if what she relates is true, I will thank you to inform me of that or anything else relating to her, wishing to do all that is absolutely right – proper and fair to be done'.[1] This sort of sentiment can be found often and repeatedly in vestry minutes and correspondence. Yet our understanding of the contours and complexion of medical welfare spending – of what in practice was right, proper and fair – is imperfect. That coming to an accommodation with the sick poor could be expensive is clear. A consolidated bill sent from Eton (Hertfordshire) to Wallingford (Berkshire) comprised:[2]

Relief to Cottrell's child for 22 weeks	£2 4s 0d
For attendance on Cottrell during his Insanity	£2 16s 0d
His funeral expenses	£1 6s 0d
Mrs Cottrell in her lying in	£2 0s 0d
2 letters from Wallingford	1s 0d
Sum	£7 7s 0d

Here the overseer wrapped up consequential relief, medical administrative costs, nursing, midwifery expenses and the costs of a funeral into a single medical welfare episode, and a bill which was of such magnitude that it must have significantly affected total poor law expenditure for Wallingford. The suggestion of Chapter 2 that we

need a wide definition of medical welfare spending is clearly played out here. But operationalising that definition and interpreting the results are complicated.

We have seen in earlier chapters that the sources used here exhibit problems of recording, accuracy and observation, such that we detect only a subset of sickness experience and thus a subset of medical welfare spending. Not all of the poor who were sick applied for poor relief, or at least not immediately, and relief claims often appear to have been fractured even where illness was not. Some people became ill when on poor relief for other reasons, making it potentially difficult to distinguish medical from other forms of welfare. Workhouse accounts in particular sometimes provide little detail on the reasons for spending, even though we saw in Chapter 2 that a significant proportion of institutional populations were likely to have been sick.[3] Anticipating these and other source problems, our dual task is to deliver the largest and most consistent possible representation of the experiences of the sick poor on the one hand and to differentiate as clearly as possible between medical welfare and 'normal' spending at the individual and aggregate levels on the other, matters to which we return below.

In the meantime, there are also potential problems of how to interpret the medical welfare spending we can identify in the sources. Three in particular loom large. Firstly, there is the problem of accounting for inflation. The general upsurge in poor relief expenditure from the late 1770s[4] represented a complex amalgam of the changing life-cycle focus of poor law resources,[5] increases in the scale of poverty and the periodicity of crises and inflation in the core components of welfare spending. The latter was particularly important during the 1790s and early 1800s. Indeed, Hastings argues for North Yorkshire that if we deflate headline welfare spending by trends in wheat prices then 'real' welfare costs remained roughly stable between 1790 and 1813.[6] He is not alone in this view.[7] Interpreting headline spending on medical welfare is, however, even more complicated than a simple deflation factor for wheat prices would allow. Across all available data it is clear that inflation hardly affected key elements of the medical packages offered to paupers. Doctoring contracts certainly rose in value over time, but, as Chapter 5 explores at greater length, this often reflected the increasing scale of the task judged in terms of the number of the poor or the frequency of their illnesses.[8] The costs of drugs, nursing,

attendance by midwives, false legs, trusses, alcohol, rents and a whole range of medical extras remained in the 1810s exactly as they had been in the 1780s. Only where relief was given in the form of clothing, food or fuel do we see significant inflation in headline figures. Even cash allowances for the sick seem to have been less prone to inflation than those given for instance to families, and to have been variably related to food prices or numbers of children. The problem then is not simply that there was inflation but that its differential impact serves to artificially mute perceived spending on medical welfare. For this reason, in some of the material which follows medical spending is subtracted from overall spending on the poor and a deflator applied to the residual, with the resultant figure used in calculating the share of medical welfare in overall relief.[9]

A second artefact of the data is that the seven counties which form the bedrock of this analysis exhibit radically different proportions of their populations claiming relief. In 1831, for instance, 17 and 15 per cent respectively of Berkshire and Wiltshire people were engaged in some way with the Old Poor Law.[10] This figure falls to 10 per cent in Northamptonshire and 4.5 per cent in Lancashire. To some extent the implications of this observation are wrapped up in discussion of regional and intra-regional differences below, but it is important to notice two subtle interpretational issues. Thus it is likely that the life-cycle, age and gender composition of those on relief varied between different counties, such that the envelope of people at risk of detection when they became ill would also vary;[11] equally, the impact of (demo-economic) crisis years on poor relief spending in general and medical welfare in particular is likely to have been much more dramatic in counties where the background level of dependence was nominally small. These are important cautionary notes.

Finally, for the purposes of this chapter our wide definition of medical welfare is applied to the records of the 117 communities whose operational data make up one major strand of the data outlined in Chapter 1. Like any conceivable subset of Old Poor Law records, however, the accounts of these 117 places are chronologically fractured. This reflects factors such as a transition to indoor relief policies and back again, 'farming' (contracting out the management of) the poor, inadequate contemporary record-keeping, patchy subsequent record preservation and deposit, and the closure of certain records as being

'too fragile'. For this study Berkshire parishes exhibit the most chronological truncation, notably at the lower end from 1750 and the top
end from 1828. By contrast Norfolk and Northamptonshire parishes
exhibit the most intra-period fracturing, with that for Norfolk in particular explained by the scale of workhouse provision and farming of the
poor. Figure 4.1 indicates that the most complete coverage is between
1770 and the mid-1820s.[12] Across the sample as a whole, thirty-four
communities have complete runs of operational data for the period
1750–1834. In the analysis of aggregate spending below, this group
is labelled the 'Core'. A further twenty-one communities have gaps of
less than ten years, and forty-three between ten and twenty years over
the same period. These sixty-four places – labelled 'Tier 1' and 'Tier 2'
respectively below – join with the 'core' communities to constitute the
base data for this chapter. A group of nineteen further places ('Tier 3')
have more than twenty years of missing data, and material from these
places is used intermittently in subsequent analysis.[13]

The accretion and depletion of the sample over time clearly have
potential consequences for how we interpret perceived spending patterns and trends. Not least, reading Figures 4.1 and 4.2 together shows
that the steep rise in perceived medical welfare spending from the mid-
1810s coincides with a falling-off in the number of communities with
complete records. An increased concentration of parochial resources

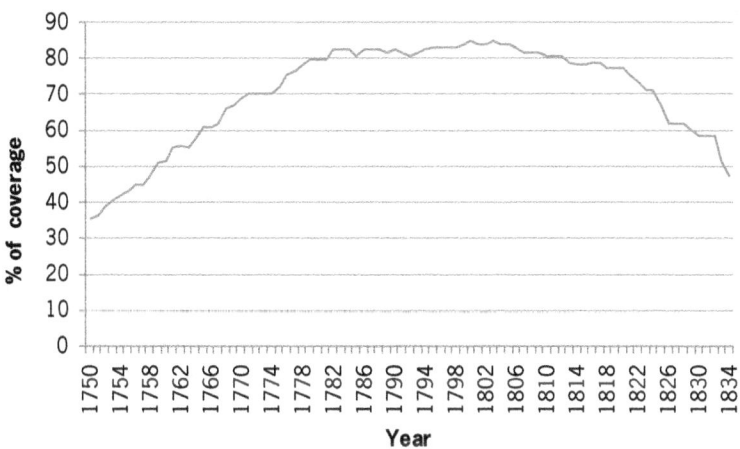

4.1 Chronological coverage of parochial data

on medical welfare spending may thus be either an illusory function of focusing on the best-documented parishes or a reflection of the fact that communities with the weakest spending record for medical care drop out of observation. Such interpretations would be misleading in three respects. First, where the coverage or quality of accounts drops off from the 1810s we often find balancing sources – vouchers, letters, vestry minutes – not available in earlier periods. These cannot make up for 20 or 30 years of missing overseers' accounts (and thus expand the Core and Tier 1 group of places) but they can and do offer independent testimony of an increasing concentration of parochial spending in the last decades of the Old Poor Law. Secondly, two of the communities with weaker spending records up to the 1810s (Calverley in West Yorkshire and Crick in Northamptonshire) have been the subject of prior family reconstitution, giving an enhanced level of surety about the reliability of interpretation. In both places we see a significant rise in medical welfare spending by the 1820s suggesting that compositional change in the sample is unlikely on its own to undermine the observations of this chapter. Finally, thirty-four of my communities have records that run consistently through the period, and more have records where the gaps are negligible. There is thus a consistent comparable spine across this period.

Against these backdrops, and in the absence of extensive family reconstitution, we need a multi-level methodology to apply the wide definition of medical welfare. A first step involves the at-face-value quantification for all 117 communities of spending on the categories noted in Table 2.2. Focusing particularly on overseers' accounts and vestry minutes, we count only spending which is specifically labelled as medically related. This yields a baseline level of community spending on medical welfare (for doctoring contracts, drugs, cash, etc.) and identifies a cohort of individual sick paupers for each place as recognised in these end-of-process sources. Because we are interested only in specifically identified spending, this first stage of data analysis is a basic counting, rather than record linkage, exercise. It yields, at community level, the minimum level of spending on medical welfare. A second stage involves working through the same data to discern whether illness for the individuals identified was repetitive, extending (to more serious illness/to other members of the family) or chronic (lasting more than one year). In effect, we create basic relief life-cycles for individuals. This

raises problems of name-orientated record linkage of the sort familiar to those who undertake family reconstitution in the English context. However, many officials took pains to distinguish those with the same forename and surname combinations, while other indicators within the sources themselves (payment levels, relationships) provide avenues for testing and confirming linkages. The survival of supplementary sources such as bills or correspondence can often help clarify which spending item relates to which individual. From this basis it is possible to discern whether payments made to an individual were likely to have been sickness-related even if they were not labelled as such. It also becomes possible to identify instances in which parishes bolstered the position of families with a sick member by making payments to other members of that family rather than to the sick individual herself or himself.[14]

This is not to argue that the process is either easy or always certain, as shown by cases where we find medical relief occurring late in a relief life-cycle and have to judge when the medical element really started. Yet the data is rich with cases such as Samuel White (resident in Halstead, Essex) and James Smith (resident in Woolwich, London). During the period 1825–1829, Samuel White's wife was confined three times, the family was beset with childhood diseases such as measles, and Samuel himself caught typhus. One of the children in the family was a cripple, other children died, and White's wife spent a period with mental illness.[15] James Smith between the years 1831 and 1833 had a wife confined, had three child deaths after lingering illnesses and looked after a further crippled child, and he and his wife were episodically sick.[16] In both cases, the sheer intensity of sickness means that we should regard all relief as medical welfare however it was actually recorded. Nonetheless problems of record linkage and the use of judgement about how allowances should be labelled[17] should lead us to read quantitative trends drawn from this analysis cautiously, a point to which I return below.

The effect of this stage of the data analysis is twofold: to identify 16,887 discrete individuals who received medical welfare across a spectrum from one-off to constant; and to increase significantly the level of perceived medical welfare spending at the level of communities. A third stage involves a change of focus to the supplementary sources (doctors' bills, correspondence, friendly society claim books, etc.) for each of the 117 parishes. Scouring these sources generates a separate list of poor

people who were ill or received forms of medical welfare, in particular capturing cases which may have had the most fleeting or fractured reference in accounts or not have been identified at all. These names are then linked to the existing cohort data from the second stage. While this process is neither easy nor certain, it has three broad effects on the data used for this chapter. The first is to increase the number of discrete individuals in observation (to 20,445) both by adding previously untraced people and breaking some of the prior assumed linkages in the second stage. Secondly, it increases perceived spending on medical welfare, a dual function of detecting more, often transitory, medical welfare payments and of changing the intensity of relief observed for existing personal profiles, which results in a larger part of their relief histories being classified as 'medical'. Finally, it increases perceived communal spending on medical welfare as a result of improved detection of doctoring contracts, workhouse spending, and greater clarity over the purpose of some unlabelled payments in overseers' accounts.

A final stage of data analysis requires a focus on 'pre-recording' sources such as pauper letters, overseers' correspondence and vestry minutes so as to detect medical welfare claims that were resourced but not recorded, or were dropped or rejected but later revived, or which resulted in relief different from that requested, especially where it bore no relation to the original claim. It is at this stage that we pick up families who requested medical relief but never had it recorded or instances such as that in Garstang (Lancashire) where doctors were continually reprimanded for treating individual paupers without authority from the vestry and then submitting accounts. Such bills named sick paupers but their cases were never recorded as medically-related.[18] This process further increases the number of discrete sick individuals detected and simultaneously inflates the level of perceived spending on medical welfare, locating individuals not previously identified as sick but also extending and intensifying the levels of spending in observation. In this way, we generate a set of individual relief histories (a final total of 26,324) of varying quality and coverage and a set of community spending profiles patterned onto Table 2.2. The latter represents the largest detectable subset of sickness and medical welfare expenditure, and one that can be re-constellated to explore spatial, typological or chronological nuance,[19] deliver dense community studies and produce anatomisations of individual strands of medical welfare.

At the root of the approach is a sense that we must understand medical welfare as a dynamic process, simultaneously contingent, constructed, contested and malleable. This is not, however, to underplay the uncertainties of the final data. Some communities have a richer source base than others even where chronological coverage is comparable, and may therefore exhibit higher medical welfare spending simply because of this richer observational data. There will definitely be some erroneous record linkage, though the use of letters, bills and other dynamic sources may help to minimise this, while the tendency of officials to pay small cash sums to sick vagrants probably means that we pick up this group rather well. There will also be some truncation bias: individual profiles at the start of the period will start in the middle of a sickness and relief history while those at the other end of the period will end artificially early. Moreover, in addition to all of the potential source and recording problems noted in prior chapters, we will have failed to identify some lump sum medical welfare payments in overseers' accounts because they were simply recorded under the name of a non-recurrent provider. False limbs, for instance, may be under-accounted in this analysis. For these reasons, it is important not to ascribe to the graphs and tables which follow more precision than they can bear. Broad trends rather than specific experiences are the order of the day.

On this basis, the next section provides a broad quantitative overview of the scale and nature of spending on medical welfare for the Core, Tier 1 and Tier 2 parishes, employing the wide definition outlined in Chapter 2. I then move on to consider spending profiles in the county-level and typological sub-samples, and to the wider question of how the composition of medical welfare changed over time or varied between community types. The chapter ends with an extended conclusion which in part focuses on the question, first raised by Chapter 3, of how much of the spending that we can trace was truly 'discretionary'. At its broadest extent, the chapter argues that medical welfare became an insistent and significant call on the resources of parishes. What was right, proper and fair by the 1800s was unrecognisable in scale and intent from the 1750s, and certainly after 1815 the crisis of the Old Poor Law was actually coterminous with a sharply rising trend of medical welfare. While there were regional and intra-regional variations in this experience, its relative uniformity has important implications for

the way we must understand the final decades of the Old Poor Law. The composition of medical welfare saw rather more variation over space, typology and time, but by the end of the period both county and typological parochial subsets coalesced around two different models, one wide and diverse, the other increasingly narrow and focused.

Medical welfare spending profiles

Employing data from communities encompassed by the Core and Tiers 1 and 2 categories, Figure 4.2 traces the proportion of total spending devoted to medical welfare across the period 1750–1834, weighted according to parochial population size. For the reasons explored above and in earlier chapters, the absolute level of medically related spending feeding into these calculations is likely to be undercounted. Moreover, the corresponding figures for total poor law spending as drawn from overseers' accounts have not been corrected for items (such as maintenance of bridges, contributions to country levies, militia payments) which have at best a tangential relationship to 'poor relief'. These expenditure categories were clearly delineated in some record sets but not in others, and no consistent correction process could be adopted. The 'true' importance of medical spending within the overall total is thus likely to be understated, particularly in the middle years of the eighteenth century when record-keeping was at its least proficient.

Nonetheless, the lessons of Figure 4.2 are important. Medical welfare absorbed at least 10–15 per cent of all parochial resources from the 1750s to the late 1780s, with a modest dip in the 1770s. Spending peaks during the 1790s and early 1800s are familiar from discussions of total poor law spending, where such increases have been related to unemployment and inflation occasioned by war and bad weather. The fact that medical welfare clearly increased faster than overall spending, reaching a peak of 18 per cent of all poor law resources in 1806, is significant and suggests either that sickness was increasing or that it was being used as an excuse to extend the welfare base. It is, however, the mid-1810s that mark the start of a transformation in the character and scale of medical welfare, such that at the advent of the New Poor Law from the mid-1830s at least 29 per cent of all poor law spending was applied in this way, and on a sharply rising trend. Figure 4.3, tracing the importance of medical welfare separately in the Core, Tier 1 and

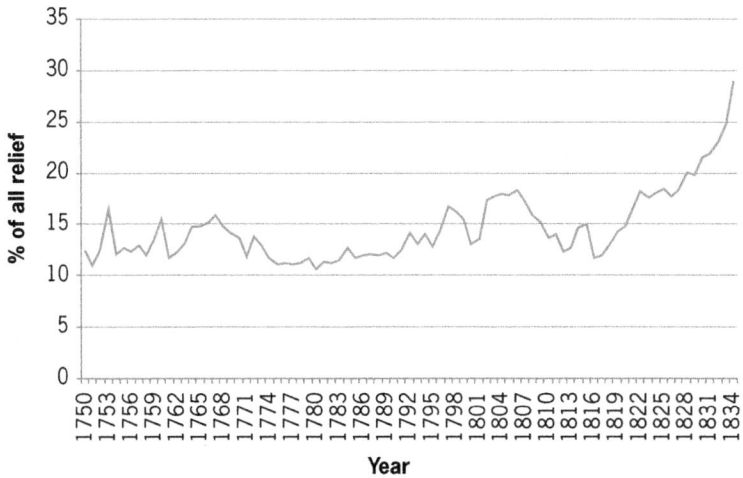

4.2 Relative importance of spending on medical welfare

Tier 2 parishes, suggests that these trends are not the product of chronological variations in the composition of the sample. While peaks and troughs are accentuated in the smaller sub-samples, the broad shape of the spending curve is relatively uniform, and more so when we account for the fact that data censoring for the Tier 1 parishes was heavily at the lower end of the chronological range. In particular the fundamental upsurge in medical welfare spending from the 1810s is common across all of the potential constellations of parochial data. This also extends to communities in Tier 3, where record-keeping was most interrupted.[20] Chapter 2 suggested an increase in both the frequency and duration of sickness which may have driven some, but by no means all, of this upsurge. The broad message from these figures, then, is that many more paupers were likely to have had more of their poverty 'medicalised' by the 1830s than was the case in the 1750s, something that is not obviously an artefact of the richness or coverage of the data or the methods used to generate it.

These broad trends become more complex where we apply a differential deflator for inflation across medical welfare and other forms of spending as outlined earlier. Figure 4.4 shows that all-sample peaks in the scale of medical welfare in the 1790s and early 1800s are

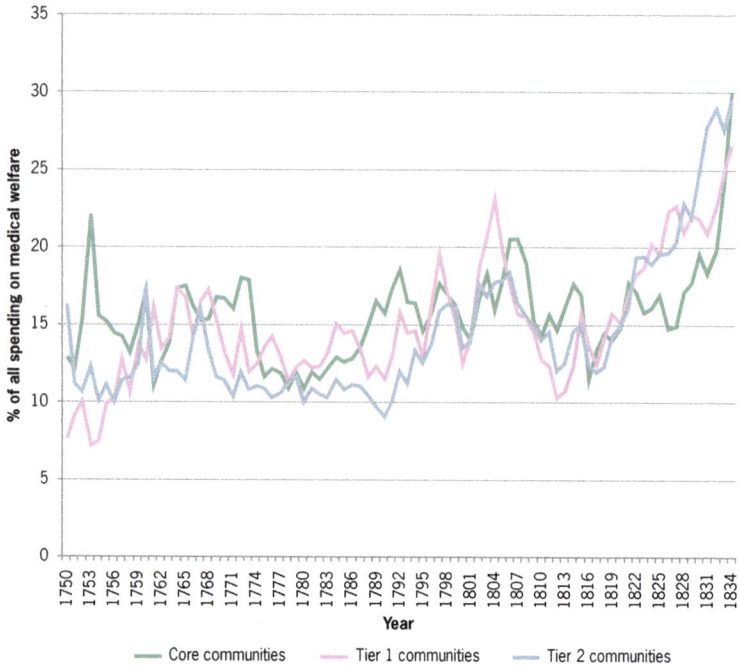

4.3 Relative importance of spending on medical welfare in Core, Tier 1 and Tier 2 parishes

considerably enhanced by this exercise. Intervening troughs remain, but the effect of deflating is to raise the base level importance of medical welfare systematically. The surge in such spending from the mid-1810s remains, even if masked by the scaling in Figure 4.4, but controlling for inflation suggests that this was part and parcel of a wider medicalisation of poverty starting in the 1790s. If we accept that even by the 1820s ambiguities in the underlying data mean that we are still detecting the minimum level of medical welfare, then it is possible that by the 1830s the majority of all welfare spending was medically related.

The composition of, as well as trends in, medical welfare spending for the Core and Tier 1 and 2 parishes provides an important framework for this chapter and the rest of the study. Figure 4.5 traces the distribution of spending between the categories outlined in Table 2.2.

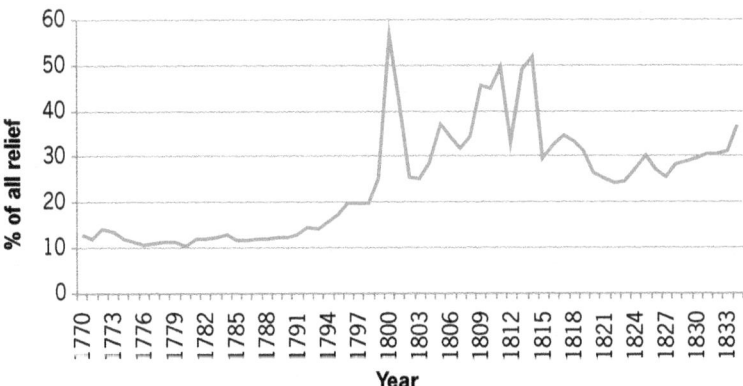

4.4 Relative importance of spending on medical welfare after deflation factors

A change in the importance of medical welfare from the 1810s was not ostensibly driven by expenditure on doctors, nurses and medical irregulars. While absolute spending on medical people rose throughout the period, the effect of parishes increasingly employing doctors in particular under contract rather than through *ad hoc* engagement was to contain costs relative to other aspects of medical welfare.[21] These matters, and the associated question of the wider role of doctoring and nursing in the medical lives of the poor, are taken up in Chapter 5. In the meantime, other features of Figure 4.5 are striking. Across the sample, parishes spent surprisingly little on drugs or devices, even before the advent of doctoring contracts from the 1780s, which often included these 'ordinaries' within the contract price.[22] In part, of course, this reflects a wider tendency for eighteenth-century and early nineteenth-century doctoring to be more art and attendance than science and drugs.[23] By contrast, welfare in the form of cash to the sick witnessed a sustained increase from the late 1780s. The fact that the aggregate cost of such medical allowances tended not to be particularly volatile over time may be read in several ways. The one preferred here is that there was both an increase in the number of paupers receiving them and an increase in the length of payment to reflect the increased duration of sickness traced in Chapter 2. Figure 4.5 also suggests that medical treatment and allowances afforded via the workhouse

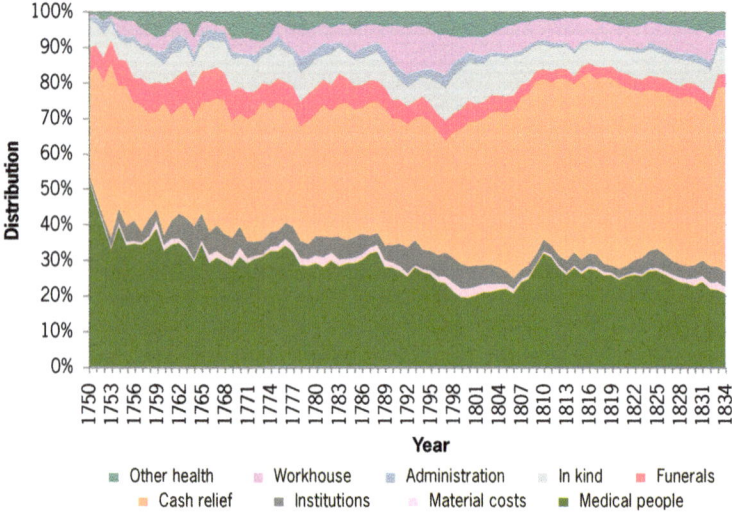

4.5 The composition of medical spending

were episodic as parishes experimented with various constellations of workhouse, poorhouse, nursing homes and parish houses. The particularly notable increase in resources accruing to workhouse care soon after Gilbert's Act in 1782 perhaps reflects the exogenous power of changes to legal possibilities in shaping local welfare practice.[24] Finally, funerals, institutional subscriptions and bills, and payments in kind all form a constant backdrop to the story of parochial medical welfare.

These are important observations. In some ways, however, this high level of aggregation masks as much as it reveals. A secondary litera-ture laden with debate over the existence of intra- and inter-regional variation in poor law spending and practice would lead us to expect significant spatial variation in the nature and scale of medical welfare.[25] Other aspects of the way that historians have traditionally made sense of the socio-economic dynamism of the period from the 1750s to 1850s – urban versus rural dichotomies; or the identification of indus-trial, arable and pastoral districts – might also lead us to expect the all-sample picture to be a rich amalgam of attitudes to and experiences of medical welfare. It is to such issues that we now turn.

Spatial, typological and topographical patterns

Figure 4.6 reconstructs the place of medical welfare in overall relief spending for the seven counties that underpin this study. At the start of our period, Northamptonshire, Norfolk and Leicestershire all spent lower proportions of their resources on medical welfare than was the case in the all-parish sample.[26] By contrast, Wiltshire, West Yorkshire, Berkshire and Lancashire were all above the average. While the differences between Leicestershire at the bottom of the distribution and West Yorkshire at the top are significant there is little across the sample to suggest systematic variation in attitudes towards medical welfare. Moreover, the consistency in the broad shape of the spending curves is notable. Two counties – Northamptonshire and Norfolk – experienced an enhanced spending peak in the 1760s, one that was consistently felt across almost all parishes in those samples. For Northamptonshire, the peak is explained by smallpox and responses to it (including enhanced cash allowances, employment of specialist nurses and the building of pest-houses or isolation wards) across the county.[27] Inoculation added significantly to parochial medical bills in the aftermath of the widely experienced outbreak of the mid-1760s, while the sharp decline in the spending curve thereafter reflects the more episodic and less spatially concerted impact of smallpox.[28] Similar peaks in Norfolk appear to reflect a toxic combination of widely experienced smallpox outbreaks, the particularly acute onset of summer fevers and a concerted move to workhouse building and use by Norfolk parishes during this decade.[29]

In the post-1760s period, spending profiles for Northamptonshire, West Yorkshire and (albeit with more pronounced peaks and troughs and a sharp but brief downturn rather than a plateau in the early 1820s) Lancashire can be patterned comfortably onto the wider sample. While Wiltshire does not seem to have experienced the 1790s peak in medical welfare spending common to other counties (instead seeing a more pronounced peak in the early 1800s), its profile too is consistent with the mean. Berkshire's spending profile was more volatile but there is a broad consistency with the Core, Tier 1 and Tier 2 sample until the mid-1810s. After this date the surge in importance of medical welfare spending familiar from all of the other country profiles is interrupted and put into reverse by the mid-1820s. This observation is partly

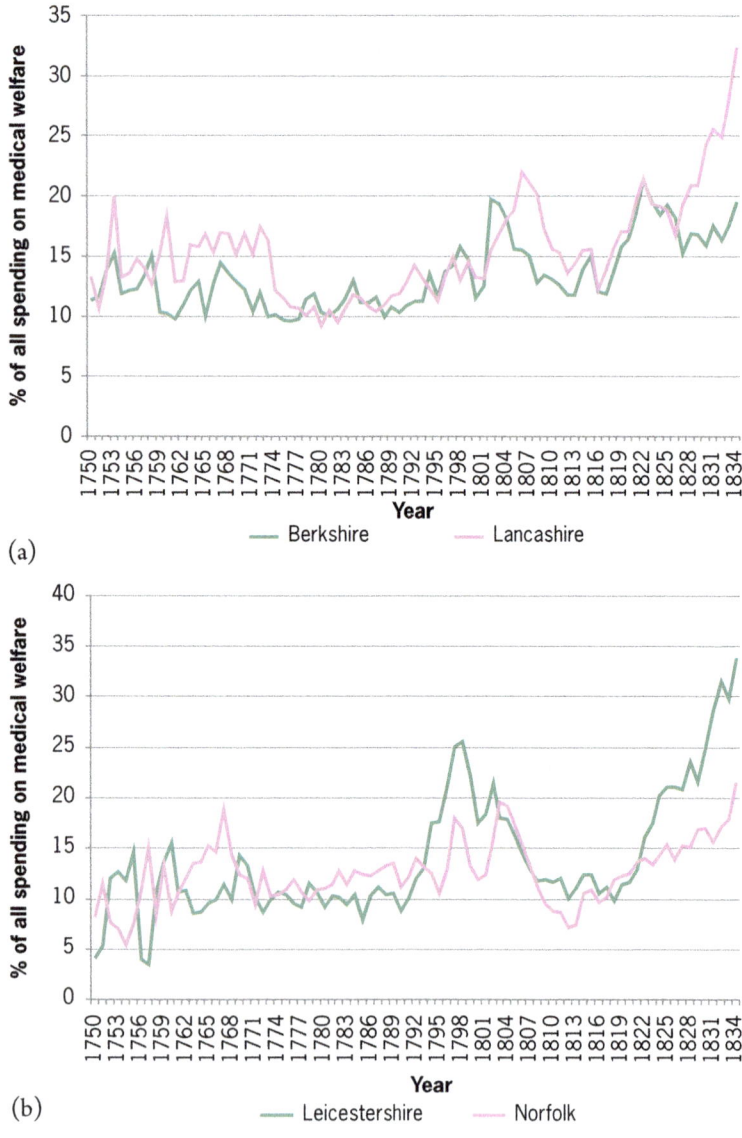

4.6 County spending profiles:
(a) Berkshire and Lancashire; (b) Leicestershire and Norfolk

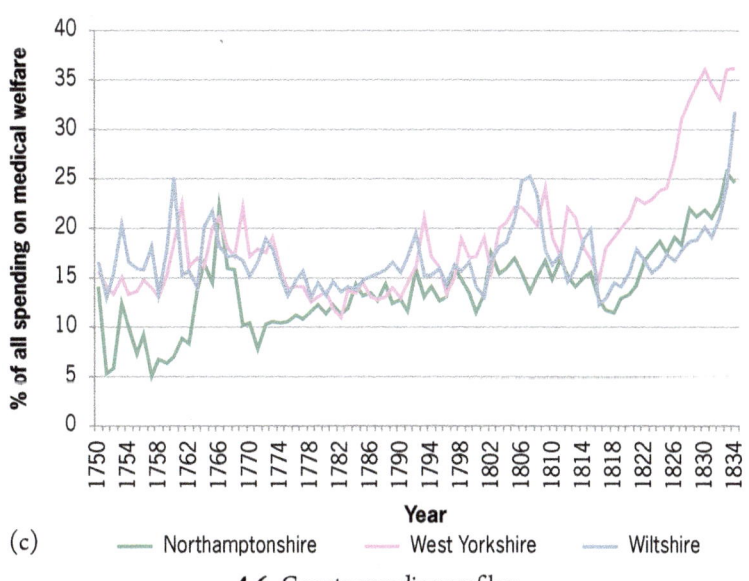

(c)   —— Northamptonshire   —— West Yorkshire   —— Wiltshire

4.6 County spending profiles:
(c) Northamptonshire, West Yorkshire and Wiltshire

explained by truncation bias at the later end of our period in Tier 1 and
2 parishes, but even allowing for this phenomenon Berkshire parishes
seem to have had a different experience of medical welfare in the very
last years of the Old Poor Law. Two other counties also demonstrate
some distinctive elements to their profiles. For Norfolk, the long
U-shaped pattern of late eighteenth-century medical welfare spending
observable in the wider sample is replaced by a gently rising profile followed by a dual peak in the 1790s and early 1800s, the latter succeeded
by a deep trough which, while developing into the sustained surge
from the 1810s also seen in other counties, leaves Norfolk parishes
permanently behind in the scale of its medical welfare spending. In
Leicestershire, parishes consistently spent only around 10 per cent of
their resources on medical welfare during the later eighteenth century.
The peak and trough of spending between the 1790s and early 1800s
familiar from other profiles were also more pronounced and smoother
than elsewhere, suggesting the consistency of the experience across the
county. As with other places, however, relative spending rose considerably from the 1810s, reaching the highest level of any county sample

by the 1830s. In short, while overall poor relief spending certainly did exhibit considerable inter-regional variations, the same cannot be said of the spending envelopes for medical welfare.

Of course, recent debates over the spatial dimensions of poor relief, visited in Chapter 1, have drawn attention to the scope for considerable intra-regional variation in welfare practice. Indeed, differences in the scale and nature of spending between proximate parishes in the same county could be more marked than those between counties and regions. Medical welfare is no exception, and every county encompasses outlier experiences. In Northamptonshire Thorpe Achurch spent 94 per cent of its resources on medical welfare in 1781 and never less than 23 per cent across the whole period. By contrast Crick and Ashby St Leger rarely spent more than 10 per cent. Leicestershire similarly had some very high rates of peak spending and correspondingly large parochial ranges. In Enderby, for instance, the lowest level of spending was 1 per cent of total parochial resources while the highest (in 1769) was 93 per cent. Ravenstone similarly varied between 1.5 and 77 per cent and Normanton between 4.5 and 71 per cent. At the other extreme, Thurcaston spent at most 32 per cent of its resources on medical welfare, with values usually well below this. The majority of parishes operated in a rather narrower range. For Berkshire, Stanford-in-the-Vale spent 51 per cent of its poor law resources on medical welfare in 1803 and at least 7 per cent in every year of the sample. By contrast, the range in Ardington was between 4 and 10 per cent, while that in Buckland was 2–14 per cent. In general, however, most Berkshire parishes varied in their (non-deflated) spending patterns in a fairly narrow spectrum of 9–33 per cent. Similar conclusions might be drawn for Lancashire (where most parishes varied between 10 and 40 per cent), Norfolk (where Holme Next the Sea and Warham both had peak spending at 62 per cent of overall poor law resources but the vast majority of parishes fluctuated in a much narrower range and at lower values than other counties) and West Yorkshire (where the spending profiles of almost all parishes sat within the range of 13–44 per cent). Wiltshire was in turn the most distinctive of all counties with the majority of its parishes demonstrating high peak medical welfare values – Sopworth at 79 per cent and Charlton at 69 per cent, for instance – and generally higher average values across the sample than those exhibited in other counties.

Detailed consideration of the datasets underpinning Figure 4.6 also reveals two further chronological aspects of intra-regional variation. Thus, only sixteen parishes across the sample had no significant surge in spending from the 1810s. Of these, seven were to be found in Norfolk, which does much to explain why average spending on medical welfare in this county lagged behind that elsewhere. However, the consistency of the surge in almost all parishes suggests a generalised and generalisable experience.[30] A second chronological feature relates to the decade from the late 1780s to the late 1790s. For most parishes in Leicestershire, Northamptonshire, West Yorkshire and Wiltshire this decade marked a permanent step-change in spending on one or more aspects of medical welfare, most commonly medical people and cash relief but also sometimes payments in kind, funerals, institutions and even administrative spending. As just one example, the Leicestershire parish of Enderby saw spending on medical people as a proportion of all spending double from 1794 and never return to its eighteenth-century levels. Episodic institutional engagement before 1796 became continuous institutional provision for the sick poor after this date. And the parish saw a permanent doubling of cash allowances from 1797. Berkshire and Lancashire parishes demonstrated no consistent tendency for this decade to mark a long-term transformation of medical welfare practice, while in Norfolk only five out of eighteen parishes experienced such tipping points. Norfolk, in other words, seems to occupy an increasingly distinctive place in the county-level complexion of medical welfare.

We can further explore the meaning of trends in the Core, Tier 1 and Tier 2 sample by re-constellating the parishes along typological lines (Figure 4.7), further detail of which can be found in the Appendix. The urban and industrial or proto-industrial profiles have clear resonance with the all-parish sample, and both seem less affected by the crisis of the 1790s than is the case with our small rural parishes, where the dual peaks of this decade and the early 1800s are experienced even for rural parishes in Lancashire and West Yorkshire. In turn and perhaps not unexpectedly given the disproportionate focus of this subset on the county, the small rural spending profile has strong patterning to Norfolk. All three samples, however, see sustained upsurge in spending during the 1810s, confirming once again the generalised increase in the importance of medical welfare from this date. Reshaping the

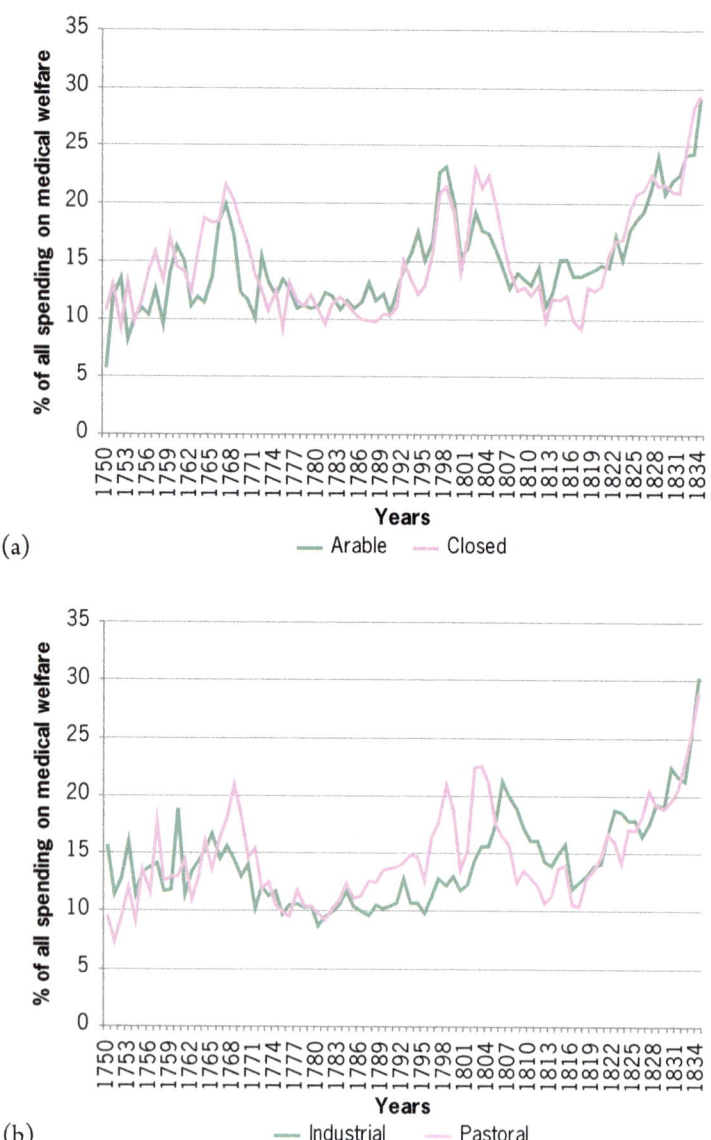

4.7 Medical welfare spending profiles of typological subsets: (a) arable and closed communities; (b) industrial and pastoral communities

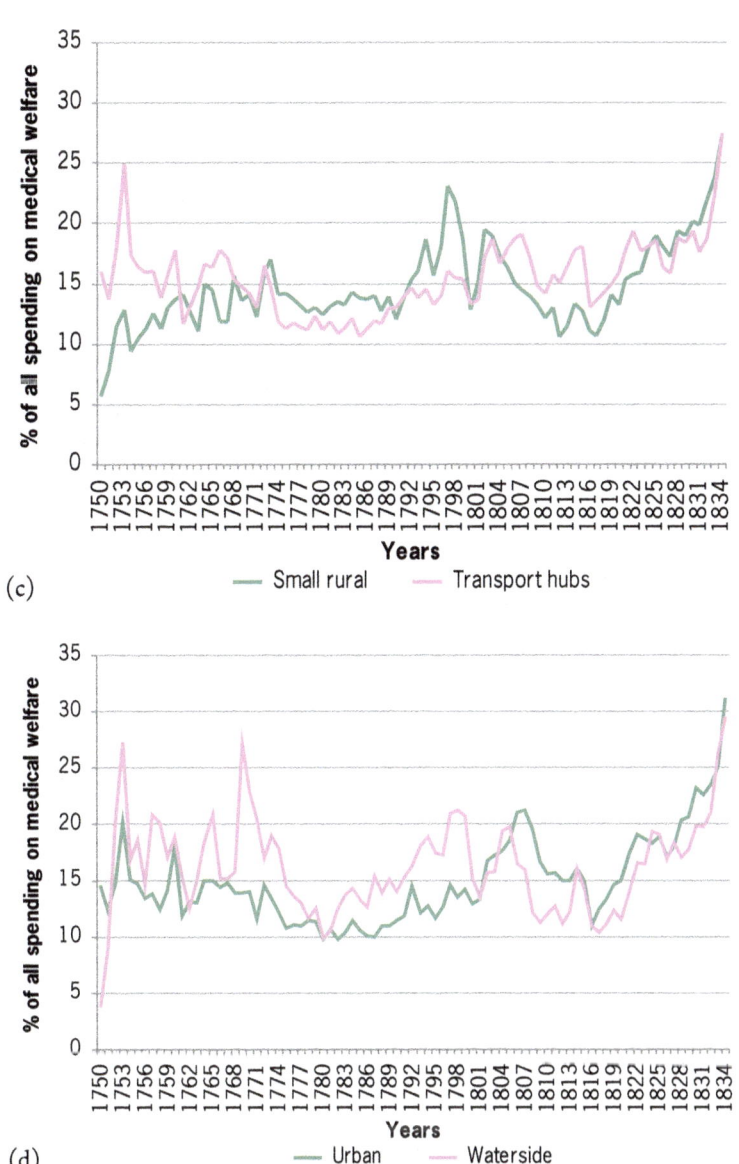

4.7 Medical welfare spending profiles of typological subsets: (c) small rural communities and transport hubs; (d) urban and waterside communities

'small rural' sample to discern pastoral and arable subsets amplifies the peaks and troughs but does little to question the broad shape of the spending profile in the all-parish corpus. A distinct 1760s spending peak in the pastoral sample (mirrored in the country profile for Northamptonshire as we have seen, and consistent across the entire run of parishes) suggests that smallpox was particularly keenly felt in these sorts of community at this time. Further refining the rural sample to identify communities which might be defined to varying degrees as 'closed' during all or part of the period (see Appendix) generates a distinctive spending profile up to the mid-1770s, with ostensibly steep rises in the importance of medical welfare. Such observations provide support for John Broad's view that a key distinction in terms of welfare scale and sentiment must be made between gentry and non-gentry parishes; the former appear to have reacted to sickness with vigour and generosity.[31] In any case, by the 1790s these communities seem to have returned to the broad patterning of the all-parish sample.[32] The really distinctive profile in these typological subsets is generated by those communities which sat on or became part of good transport networks, whether road or water. While spending curves look similar to those of the all-parish sample up to the later eighteenth century, at least when we allow for the volatility associated with a smaller parochial corpus, by the early 1800s a triple peak and trough motion means that the importance of medical welfare in overall spending remains roughly flat until a rapid and steep rise in the 1830s. How far this profile is an artefact of rapid population turnover in well-connected communities, turnover which makes it more difficult to consistently trace medical welfare and medical welfare recipients through poor law data, is unclear. Without variation, however, parishes in this subset spent disproportionately on 'exceptionals' – small but frequent allowances given to travellers, migrants and the significant numbers of people caught in the out-parish system – and such 'exceptionals' were rarely either renewed or explained.[33]

These observations of chronological and spatial nuance are important and will inform the analytical agenda for Chapters 5 to 9. At the macro-level, however, the striking thing about the differently constellated parochial samples is the consistency of pattern and trend. Norfolk sat at the lower end of the spending profiles, notwithstanding a period of catch-up late in our period. Berkshire parishes witnessed a

distinctive plateau in medical welfare spending during the later 1820s. On the other hand, alternative sub-samples – urban–rural, pastoral– arable and industrial–rural – do little to complicate the spending profiles for the Core and Tier 1 and 2 corpus. The systematic spatial variation that might have been expected, given debates about the regional and intra-regional character of poor relief, are largely absent. If there were notable differences between individual parishes within county samples in the scale and volatility of medical welfare spending, it is still the case that most communities followed the broad spending trends visible in the all-parish sample. Most importantly of all, the vast majority of parishes saw a strong upsurge in medical spending, both absolutely and in comparison to other forms of poor law spending, from the mid-1810s. Parishes across the typological range responded to increasing need and increasing medical possibility for the poor in more expensive and more sustained ways. When Samuel Tibbs wrote to his counterpart in St Albans noting that he wanted what was right, proper and fair in the case of the sick Mrs Narroway, he was giving voice to a genuine and increasingly expensive sentiment, clearly felt across our parochial sample: that medical welfare was a, or perhaps (bearing in mind that we have been able to quantify only a minimum level of such welfare) the, core issue in the closing decades of the Old Poor Law.

Yet if there were similarities in the trend and level of spending across the spatial and typological subsets, the existence of outliers to the county samples suggests the need for further work on the particularities of local medical welfare. Some of this is developed in later chapters, but it is also important to explore here the varying composition of spending between different parochial subsets. There are good historiographical reasons to expect significant variations in the importance of spending on doctors and nurses between southern urban areas replete with medical people and the smallest rural areas that were rather less well served.[34] Similarly, we might expect more payment in kind by parochial officials in urban-industrial areas or more frequent contributions to funeral costs in proto-industrial areas (which tended to have higher age-specific mortality rates) or in Norfolk with its much higher incidence of malaria and other fever-inducing diseases. And it might be reasonable to expect communities that were part of transport hubs to make more use of drugs and

devices (because they were easier to obtain) than those which were more remote. Figure 4.8 thus illustrates the complexion of spending in each of the seven counties.

The material requires sensitive interpretation; more volatility than in the all-sample equivalent of these graphs is to be expected given the potential for epidemics or other situational events to influence spending patterns in any single year. Differences in the strength and composition of the local medical economy of makeshifts (explored further in Chapter 9) might also influence the local and county-level complexion of medical welfare. The consequences of ambiguities in the sources are likewise magnified in smaller county samples. Hence in Methwold (Norfolk) a January 1819 entry in the overseers' accounts reads: 'Allowed Ed. Fuller for Ann Bitson being confined in the work-house and for his expenses for the midwife, and for the nurse and for his journey to Hockhold with her to sware the child, £1.' In the 1750s the spending items contained in this entry would have been separately accounted for; their elision by the early nineteenth century requires some inventive ascription to different spending categories which in turn are less precise than the figures attached to them suggest. The increasing practice of sharing bills between parishes has a similar effect: In the bills discharged column of Methwold's 1819 account we find the entry 'Paid Mr Roberts per bill attending S. Bones Child and Mr Cork of Cranwich paid the remaining part as being a *party* concern'.[35]

These caveats notwithstanding, Figure 4.8 provides some power-ful signposts. While absolute spending levels on doctors, nurses and others increased consistently in all counties, this was not reflected in the share of medical people in overall spending, as we have already seen. Two broad experiences coalesce at county level to generate the pattern of a slow decline followed by a plateau evident in earlier graphs. For Northamptonshire, Norfolk and Leicestershire medical people absorbed a relatively stable long-term average of 27, 26 and 22 per cent of medical welfare respectively. In Lancashire, West Yorkshire or Wiltshire,[36] the declining relative importance of spending in this area is clear, falling from more than 40 per cent in all three counties in 1750 to 19, 26 and 24 per cent respectively by 1834. The starkest movement is in Berkshire, which demonstrates the very highest concentration of medical welfare on medical people for any county in the early 1750s

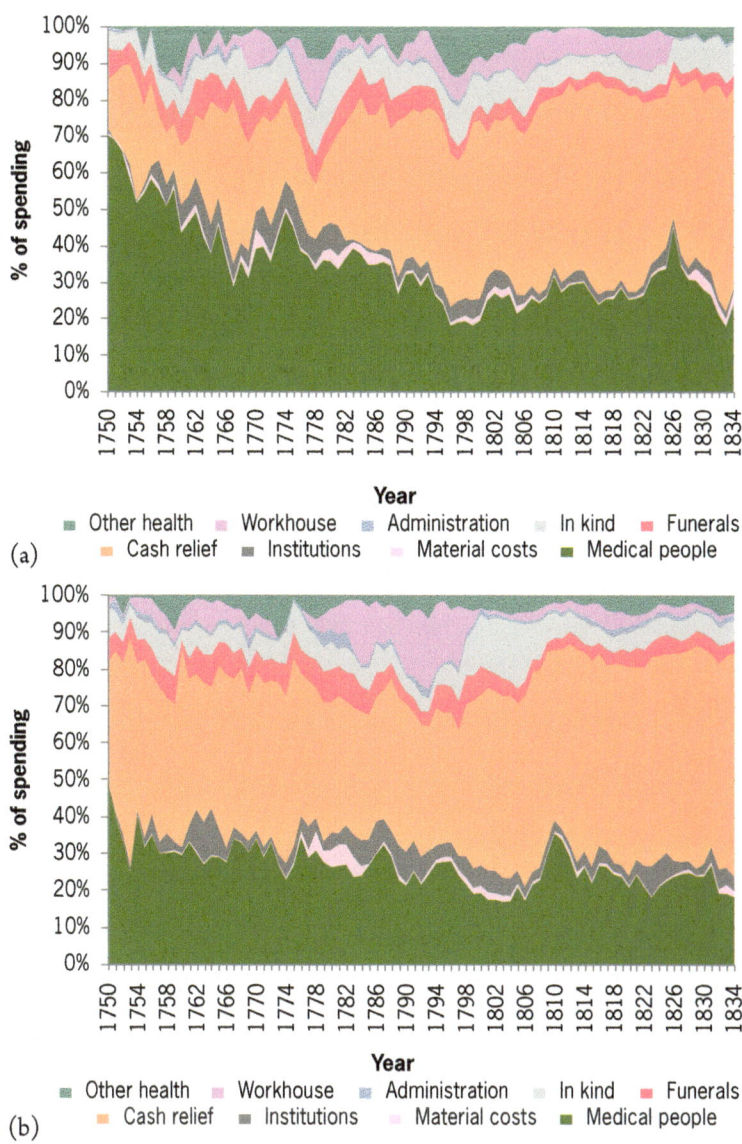

(a)

(b)

4.8 The complexion of spending in the county samples:
(a) Berkshire; (b) Lancashire

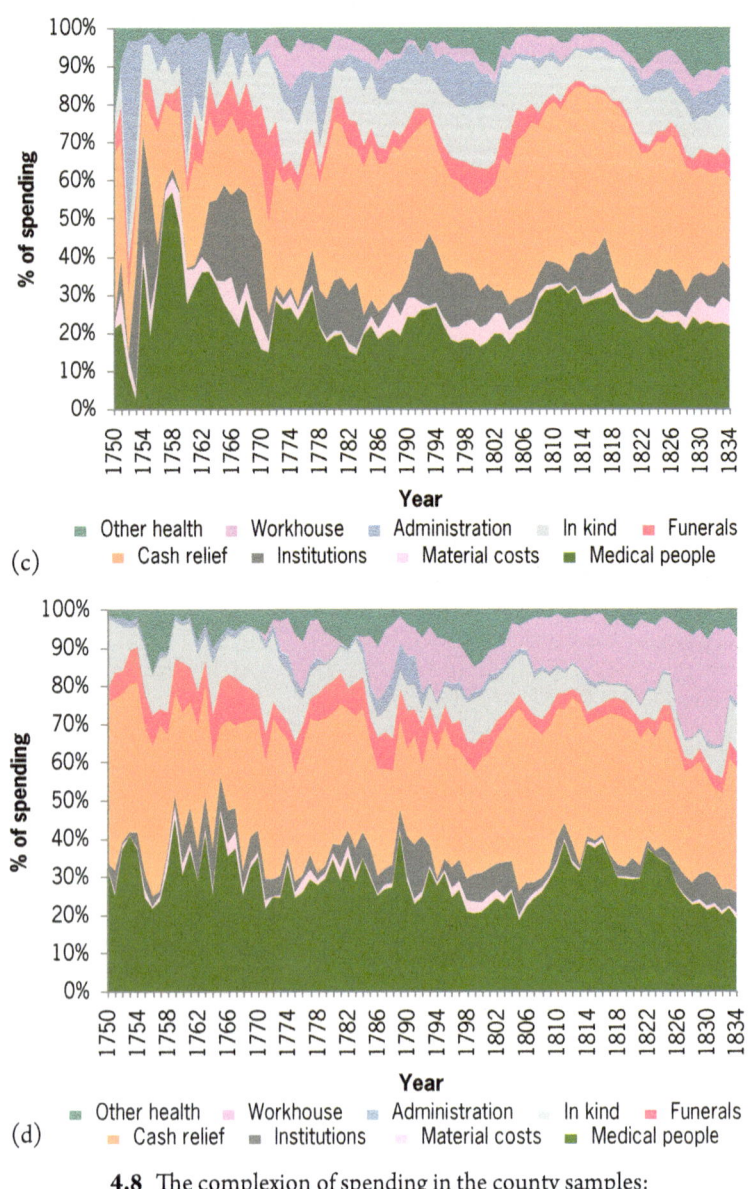

4.8 The complexion of spending in the county samples:
(c) Leicestershire; (d) Norfolk

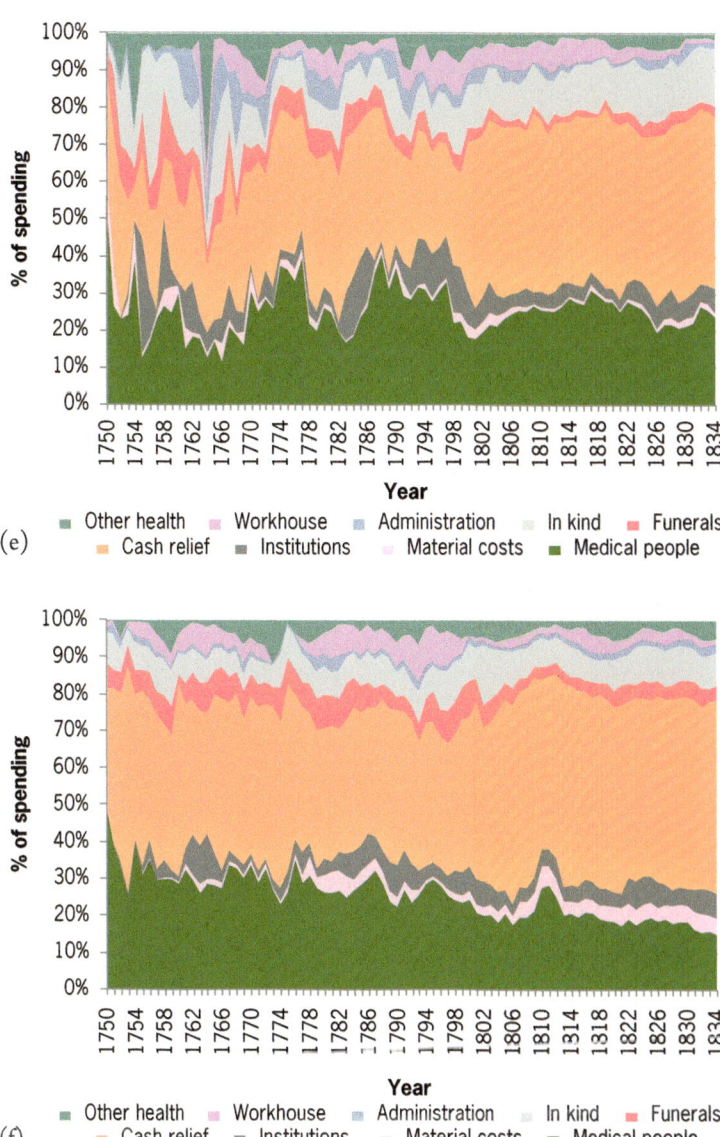

(e)

(f)

4.8 The complexion of spending in the county samples:
(e) Northamptonshire; (f) West Yorkshire

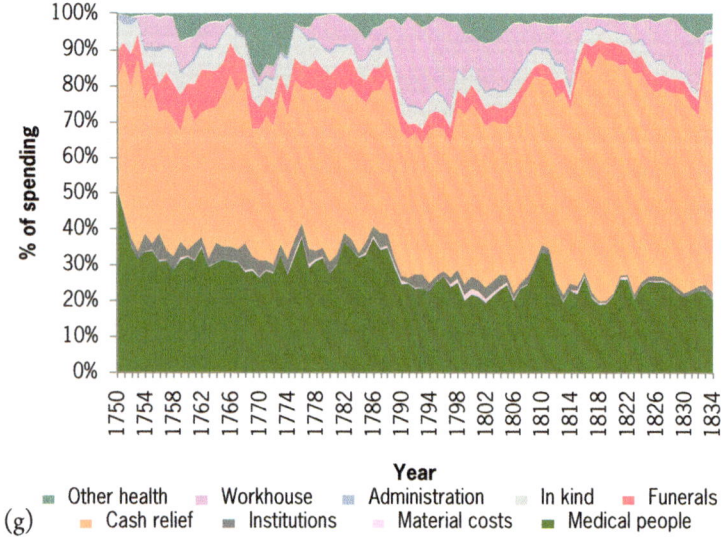

(g)

4.8 The complexion of spending in the county samples: (g) Wiltshire

but then shows a substantial relative decline and ultimately plateau. The complex nature of doctoring is explored at greater length in Chapter 5.

The county samples also fit neatly into two broad experiential categories in terms of engagement with institutions. In Northamptonshire this small but stable spending category represents the accumulation of consistent institutional engagement for difficult cases across almost all of the underlying parishes. Wiltshire and West Yorkshire parishes turned to institutions with even more consistency, seeing multiple sequential institutional solutions for both chronic and 'ordinary' sickness. By contrast, while most Lancashire, Norfolk and Berkshire parishes spent considerable sums on institutional care or advice (particularly after 1800), the regularity of such engagements at the level of individual parishes was at best episodic and at worst sporadic. Thus no Lancashire parish came close to the levels of institutional engagements paid for by West Yorkshire communities despite the common socio-economic roots of the two samples. We revisit these different cultures of institutional care in Chapters 6 and 8, where questions of

parochial knowledge, pauper demands, the availability of institutions and parochial sentiment are considered at length.

As we might expect from the wider historiographical literature, the place of workhouses as a locus and mechanism for medical care was complex. For the majority of parishes across the sample, engagement with workhouses was inconsistent. In Berkshire, Northamptonshire, West Yorkshire and Leicestershire we thus see a continuous (as parishes successively started and ended workhouse provision) but relatively small place for workhouses in overall medical welfare spending. For Wiltshire and Lancashire recourse to the workhouse by parochial authorities seems to have been considerable in the 1790s and early 1800s but rather less sustained before and after. This leaves Norfolk as the most distinctive of the counties; the trend for medical welfare to be increasingly provided via the workhouse can be seen in Figure 4.8.

It is, however, for the spending categories 'kind' and 'cash relief' that the starkest county-level variations emerge. Across all Core, Tier 1 and Tier 2 parishes there was an association between the growing importance of medical welfare and the rising share of cash payments. This pattern was duplicated in Northamptonshire, Lancashire,[37] Wiltshire, Berkshire and West Yorkshire. Yet neither Norfolk nor Leicestershire parishes witnessed any sustained change in the role of cash in medical welfare. This experience was widely distributed across the county samples, and officials in Norfolk in particular seem to have tried to cap cash allowances at the same time as they expanded the use of workhouses. In neither county was the growing importance of medical welfare spending after 1815 associated with a new wave of cash allowances. Meanwhile, payments in kind (food, rent, clothing) maintained a consistent if modest profile in the all-parish sample, and there was a (perhaps not unexpected) positive association in the underlying data between crisis periods such as the 1790s and early 1800s and this form of spending. At county level, however, distinct experiences manifest themselves: the stability of the whole sample is reflected in Lancashire, Leicestershire and Berkshire, while the dwindling importance of payment in kind in Wiltshire or Norfolk is more than balanced by sustained increase in Northamptonshire and West Yorkshire. Such spatial divisions have little foundation in conventional understandings of

the regionality of welfare under the Old Poor Law, and we return to them in Chapter 6.

Other differences between the county samples are less striking. With the exception of the decade from 1774, spending on drugs and medical devices in Lancashire was tiny, something replicated in Wiltshire and Norfolk. By contrast, Berkshire experienced several small peaks of spending on material costs, while Leicestershire and (particularly) West Yorkshire parishes seem to have had a sustained commitment to this area of spending. In turn, Leicestershire and West Yorkshire officials also seem to have spent more of their local resources on administration related to medical welfare than all of the other county samples put together. It would be convenient to draw an association between these dual experiences and the shared county roots in hosiery and woollen manufacture, but it is notable that parishes in Wiltshire, Northamptonshire or Berkshire with residual woollen or hosiery industries do not generate similar profiles in either material costs or administration.

Recasting the parochial samples along typological lines, both as a means of finding alternatively constructed medical welfares and by way of explanation of some of the trends noted above, is relatively unproductive. Figure 4.9 shows that the main features of the urban, industrial, proto-industrial, and transport hub subsets map easily onto most of the broad trends (the consistent presence of the workhouse, rising in crisis periods; the increasing role for cash allowances; a relative decline in spending on medical people; consistent engagement with institutions) flowing from the county samples. The contrast with the small rural subset is important. In these communities cash relief was important but remained roughly stable as a proportion of overall medical welfare after the mid-1780s. Indeed, the complexion of medical welfare spending in these areas was markedly diverse, particularly at the end of our period, compared to that in urban-industrial communities. The slightly rising profile of medical people in the spending profile for small rural communities was shared by the pastoral parishes with which they slightly overlap. Here and in the arable subset the advance of cash allowances was more pronounced over the period as a whole until the later 1820s, but both community typologies retained a diverse range of strategies for coping with pauper illness.

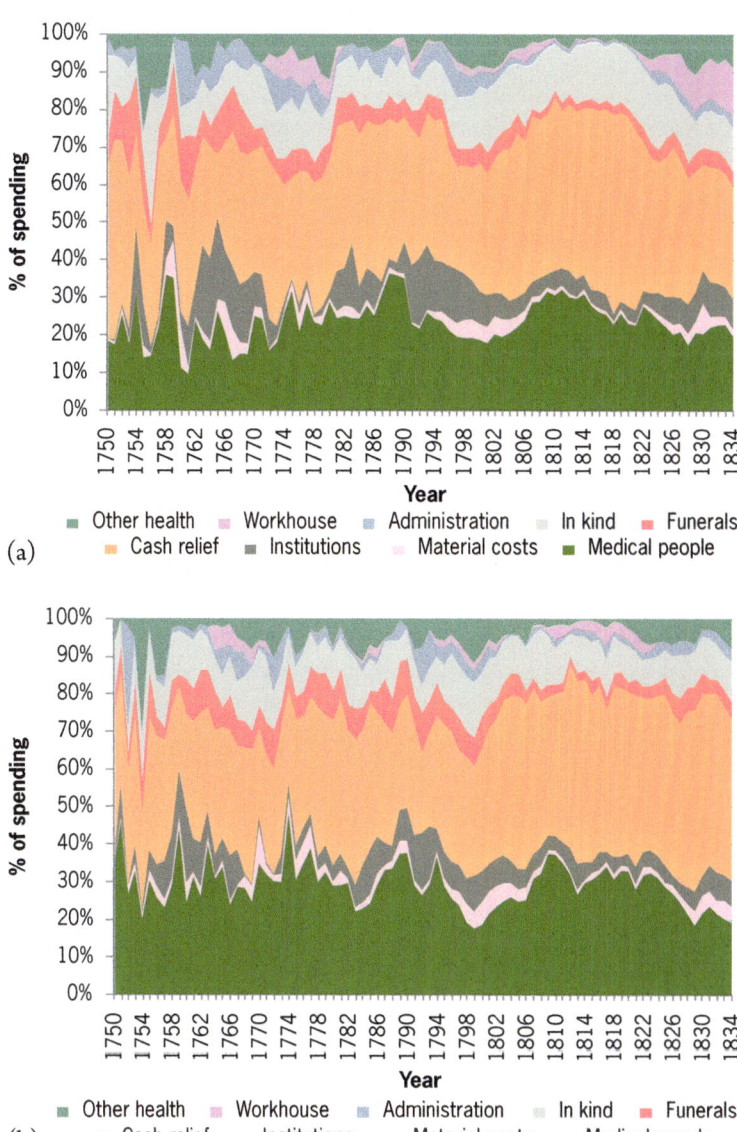

4.9 The complexion of spending in typological subsets:
(a) arable communities; (b) closed communities

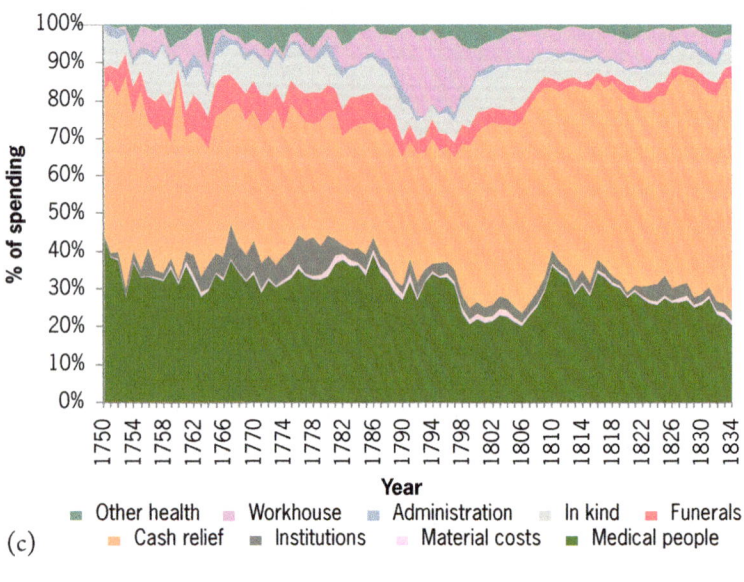

(c)

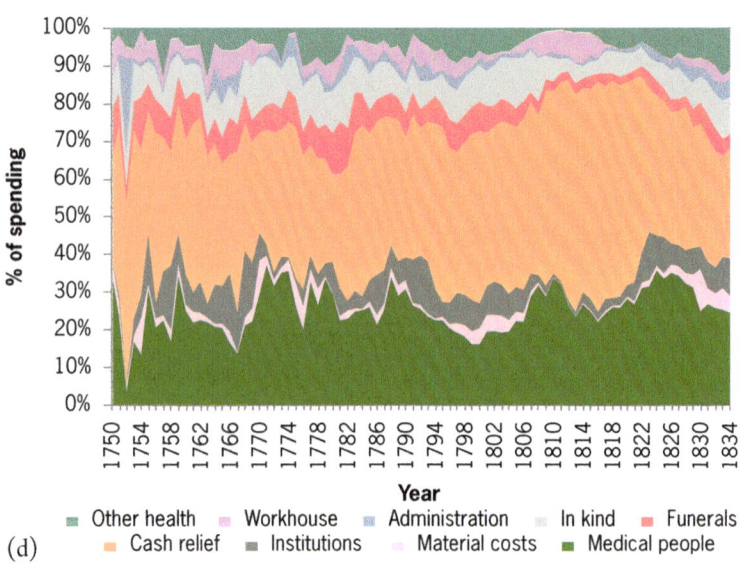

(d)

4.9 The complexion of spending in typological subsets:
(c) industrial or proto-industrial communities; (d) pastoral communities

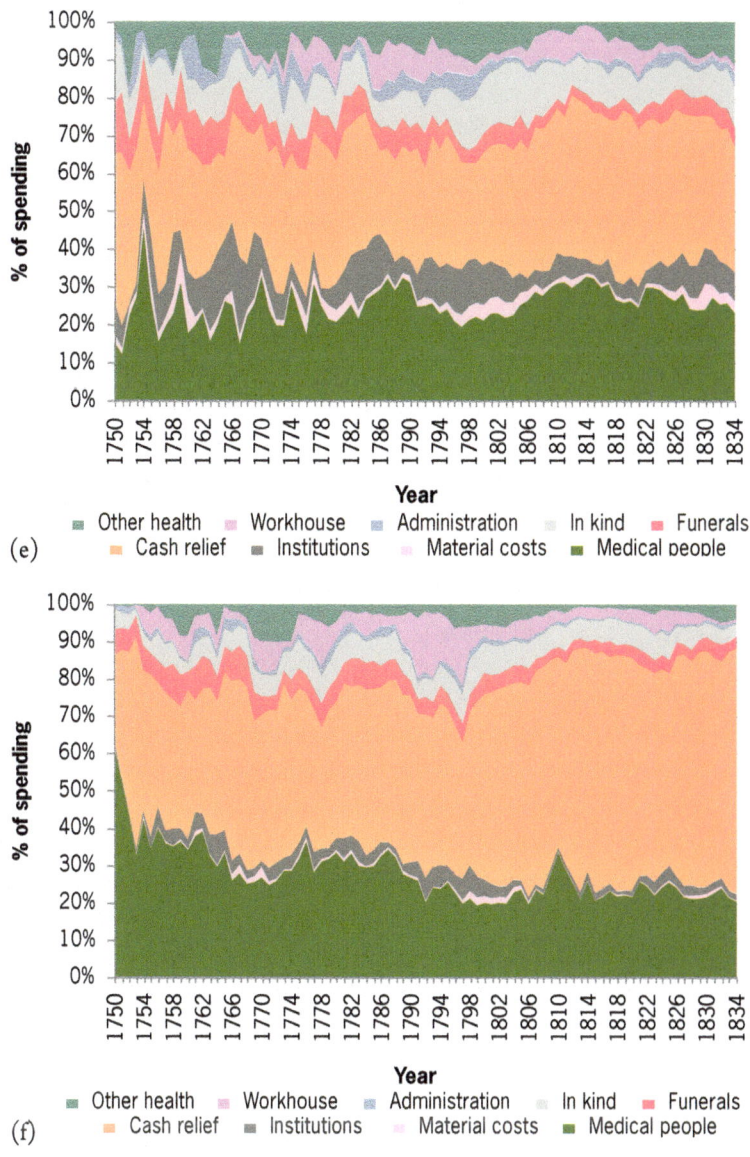

4.9 The complexion of spending in typological subsets:
(e) small rural communities; (f) transport hubs

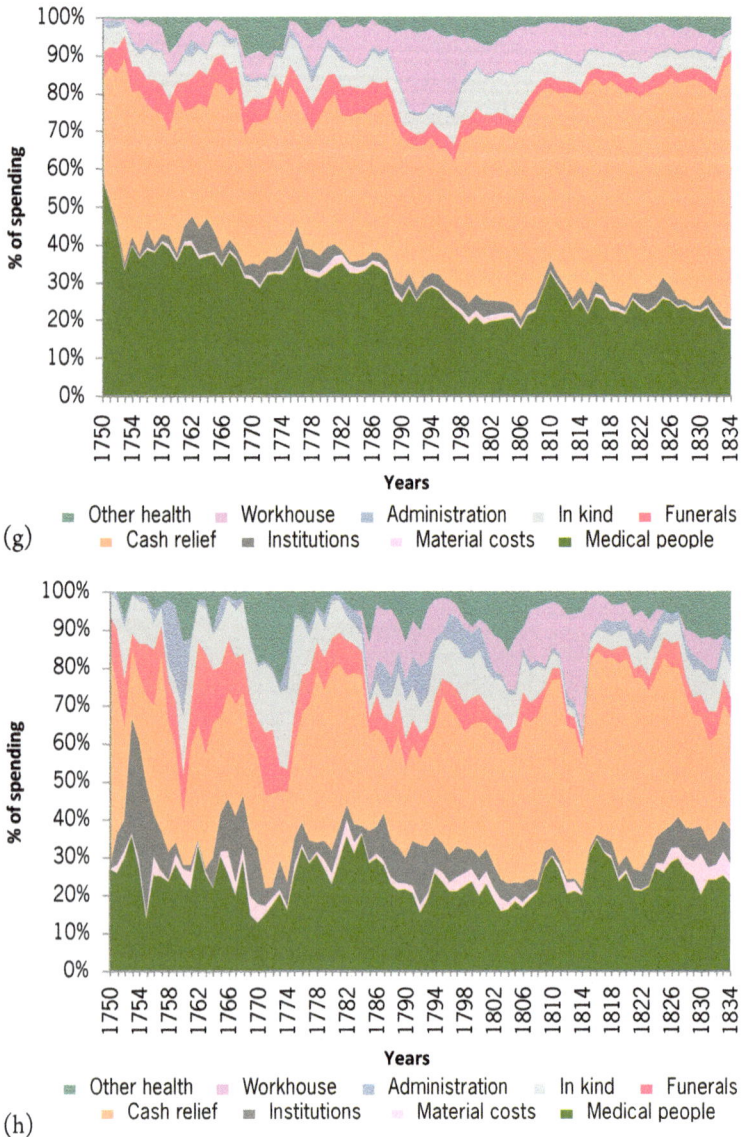

4.9 The complexion of spending in typological subsets:
(g) urban communities; (h) waterside communities

Conclusion

The lessons of this quantitative overview are simultaneously clear and complex. Medical welfare absorbed at least 10–20 per cent of total poor law spending from the mid-eighteenth century through to the 1810s, and probably rather more when we allow for the differential impact of inflation and the muting effect of source limitations that cause us to pick up only a subset of medical spending to balance easier-to-calculate total spending at parochial level. There were significant peaks (at over 20 per cent of total spending) and troughs (at less than 10 per cent), and these were accentuated in the smaller county and typological parochial sub-sets. Some of these experiences mirrored well-established wider trends in poor law spending. Even here it is notable that during the 1790s medical welfare spending rose as against total poor law spending even without applying a differential inflation correction. Other peaks – the county-wide smallpox crisis in Northamptonshire during the 1760s, for instance – and troughs were more situational. After 1815, there was across most of the sample a sustained upward surge in the importance of medical welfare spending. This is not, as I have argued above, the artefact of a parochial dataset that changes in composition. With the exception of some Berkshire parishes, the upsurge is consistently observed however we constellate the data. Whether other compositional effects – in particular the possibility that there was a shift in the type of person applying for or getting relief towards those (the aged, mothers, etc.) most likely to be sick – have explanatory power here must remain a moot point in the absence of extensive formal family reconstitution.[38] Chapter 2 suggested that there was a real upsurge in morbidity in the early nineteenth century, and this chapter suggests there was a balancing response from communities such that the 'crisis of the Old Poor Law' was clearly in part driven by an upsurge in medical welfare spending. There is little evidence to support Pat Thane's idea that by 1832 there was 'a strong framework of stringency' which had switched the calculation of what was right, proper and fair firmly from the interests of paupers to those of ratepayers.[39]

While there was every reason to expect either systematic regional variation or chaotic intra-regional and sub-sample variation in medical welfare, in practice it is the relative uniformity in aggregate spending profiles that is marked. There was more diversity in how parishes spent

their resources. In the majority of places, the importance of cash allowances rose notably over the period, and the upsurge in aggregate spending after 1815 was clearly linked to the provision of such allowances and the narrowing (but never the elimination) of other expenditure categories. For small rural communities and to a lesser extent the arable and pastoral parochial subsets, the diversity of spending – particularly payment in kind, engagement with institutions, 'other' medical welfare and workhouses – apparent in most places at the start of our period was maintained throughout.[40] By contrast while the absolute cost of doctors, nurses and alternative practitioners increased over the period, this was overtaken by other forms of support for the sick poor, and spending on medical people did not feed through as a dynamic force shaping the growing importance of medical welfare in most parishes. The county-level samples are, of course, a variable composite of rural, urban and industrial communities and thus tend towards the all-parish yardstick. Nonetheless distinctive features – the increasing importance of workhouses as a vehicle for medical welfare and consequently muted cash allowances for Norfolk; the fact that Wiltshire moved from the most diverse spectrum of medical welfare in the 1750s to the least by the 1830s; a plateau in overall spending for Berkshire in the later 1820s; or the fact that Leicestershire and West Yorkshire retain a highly diverse complexion of medical welfare at the end of our period – require more detailed exploration. So do the labels used here. Our expenditure categories are constructed as monolithic categories for the purposes of quantitative overview, but in practice they were anything but that. Some cash allowances, for instance, were applied to cases which would prove fatal on a spectrum between 'decline' associated with old age through to sudden illness as a result of epidemic disease. In contrast, other cash allowances were deployed to combat illness and accident across a non-fatal range running from broken bones through to midwifery. Where officers focused their allowances on this spectrum tells us much about the essential sentiment of parishes towards sick paupers, the central function of this important form of medical welfare and the way in which paupers experienced sickness. Such elaboration is a function of the later chapters of this study, each of which explores core elements of medical welfare.

Meanwhile, it is also important to acknowledge the lesson of Chapter 3 that not all of the spending represented in this quantitative overview

was likely to have been entirely discretionary. Both officials and paupers assumed that nursing and payments in kind would be given if
individuals and families suffered from smallpox. Requests of this nature
hardly ever appear in pauper letters and yet they are a heavy expenditure items in associated overseers' accounts. Paupers similarly assumed
that they or their wives, daughters and sisters would be granted a midwife or doctor at the birth of children. Joseph Ellerington's request to
Garstang (Lancashire) on 3 December 1816 is typical of the sentiment
across all of the counties considered here: his wife 'just going to lie in
and [he] wanting to know what doctor she is to have – that she must
fix on someone to wait on her during her confinement'. The fact that
this vestry and most others like it agreed – 'Resolved. That Joseph Seed
to speak to a Doctor to attend her'[41] – points to the essential lack of
discretion on this matter. Even in 'ordinary' illnesses many paupers
and their advocates elaborated an expectation of medical attention and
medically related relief as a parochial obligation. Thus on 30 January
1818 Mr Whitehead, John Daster and Stephen Packer, respectively
vicar, churchwarden and overseer of Twerton, collectively asserted
that Longbridge Deverill should respond to the out-of-the ordinary
expenses occasioned by the illness of Isaac Curtis. The parish seemingly agreed, directing on 4 February 1818 that it would recompense
the attendance of the Twerton parish doctor 'and they [the vestry]
will not have any objection to make such allowance for the attendance
of any other as may be deemed just and reasonable'.[42] Such language,
reflecting the words of Hertfordshire overseers at the start of this chapter, is the language of constraint.

Similar observations apply to funerals, where paupers and their
advocates left little room for manoeuvre in correspondence. When
Mr White wrote from Leicester to the parish authorities of Market
Harborough (Leicestershire) on 8 December 1823 to inform them
of the death of Mrs Bullington he noted that she had been dependent on her neighbours for nursing during a long illness and that those
neighbours were arranging a funeral but 'they were not willing to do
anything until we would give our word – my Father [h]as given orders
for a coffin as they wish to bring her tomorrow – I should be glad of a
line from you tomorrow morning as we don't wish to do anything till
we have recd. orders from you.'[43] In the face of such advocacy a generous contribution to the funeral was forthcoming, as we might have

expected given the analysis of Chapter 3. Indeed, the letter sample is replete with powerful expressions and assumptions of obligations. On 4 April 1816, Thomas Heywood, overseer of Lichfield (Staffordshire), wrote to his counterpart in Lilleshall (Shropshire) on the subject of Thomas Dorling. Pointing out that Dorling's allowance of 5s was insufficient, he enjoined, 'you must consider an Old man 73 years of Age with a wife past Business a lusty daughter continually in fits, requiring a person constantly with her, must be supported'. His successor, William Cartmale, took up this theme in January 1818. The daughter, he noted, 'has fits night and Day continually, & knocks & bruises herself to pieces, and not able by being Isaniated with the fits able to earn one farthing or even to be trusted out of doors'. In this circumstance, he argued, parishes should do 'more than common, certainly Parishes are much Burthened by Poor, but in downright necessaited Cases such as Old Lame, Blind and persons afflicted with Illness who can stand off I being a Parish Officer ought not to [have to] press you'.[44] There is much here to support Geoffrey Taylor's view that 'the poor were the responsibility of all sections of the community … they could not … be herded out of sight'.[45] While poverty and the enmeshing of the poor into a discretionary welfare system such as the Old Poor Law could be inferiorising and marginalising, it is not at once clear that the sick poor navigated their welfare with these sentiments in mind.

Of course, officials were sometimes sceptical of the 'necessary' claims occasioned by sickness. In August 1819, for instance, the overseer of Methwold (Norfolk) noted a claim from Thomas Tibbett 'being unwell *he says*'. Despite his scepticism, the overseer paid an allowance because, to return to the story with which we opened this chapter, he needed to be, and to be seen to be, 'fair'. While David Eastwood regards the mid-1790s as 'a staging post in the long and miserable decline in the fortunes of the labouring poor',[46] this review of the quantitative evidence suggests that parishes (albeit with gloriously rich local variation) responded forcefully, positively and in sustained manner to the claims of the sick poor even as they had the most incentive to mete out harsh treatment. What was 'fair' became more expensive, more expansive and of longer duration over the period considered here. The quality of entitlement rose[47] because in so far as the parish state can be conceptualised as 'a network of people, knowledge, power and material objects' it was an open network, susceptible to both rational argument

and irrational humanitarian sentiment in equal measure, at once rigid and fluid.[48] The robustness of entitlement also rose as long-standing expectations of action in severe cases of medically related need ceased to be a discussion point within and between parishes. Thus for many thousands of people with physical impairments in this sample, medical welfare never became a legal right, but it became a *de facto* right nonetheless. These complex individual, experiential and parochial pictures are both encapsulated and masked by quantitative analysis. The remaining chapters explore these complexities, seeking to create a 'meaning of medical welfare'.

Notes

1   HALS, D/P/90/18/1, letter.
2   BRO, D/P 139/18/49, undated letter and bill.
3   I apply an assumed sickness component of one-third to undifferentiated workhouse spending. This is the very minimum level of likely sickness spending in such institutions judged from the perspective of those places which do have detailed workhouse accounts.
4   S. King, *Poverty and Welfare.*
5   Broadly fewer women and older people and more men, families and younger people; see T. Sokoll, 'Families, wheat prices and the allowance cycle: Poverty and poor relief in the agricultural community of Ardleigh, 1794–1801', in Jones and King (eds), *Obligation, Entitlement and Dispute*, pp. 78–106, and French, 'An irrevocable shift', pp. 769–805.
6   Hastings, *Poverty and the Poor Law*, p. 9.
7   For wider context see G. Boyer, *An Economic History of the English Poor Law 1750–1850* (Cambridge: Cambridge University Press, 2008), and D. Baugh, 'The cost of poor relief in south east England 1790–1834', *Economic History Review*, 28 (1975), 50–68.
8   S. Williams, 'Practitioners' income', pp. 159–86.
9   I use Charles Feinstein's cost of living index as the deflator in this instance. The index has a base year of 1770, which explains the truncated analysis of Figure 4.4. See C. Feinstein, 'Pessimism perpetuated: Real wages and the standard of living in Britain during and after the Industrial Revolution', *Journal of Economic History*, 58 (1998), 625–58, at pp. 633–42 and 652–3.
10 King, *Poverty and Welfare*, p. 86.
11 The fact that allowance systems were both ubiquitous and short-lived means that we can put to one side traditional dichotomies such as the able-bodied versus sick. See Sokoll, 'Families, wheat prices'.

12 This coverage relates only to overseers' accounts. Many places with sizeable gaps nonetheless have long runs of other sources.

13 For a mapping of communities see the Appendix.

14 On reconstitution, see S. Ruggles, 'The limitations of English family reconstitution: *English Population History from Family Reconstitution 1580–1837*', *Continuity and Change*, 14 (1999), 105–30; S. Ruggles, 'Marriage, migration and mortality: Correcting sources of bias in English family reconstitutions', *Population Studies*, 46 (1992), 507–22; and E. Wrigley, 'The effect of migration on the estimation of marriage age in family reconstruction studies', *Population Studies*, 48 (1994), 81–97. The linkage exercise is of course substantial, involving in each instance the identification of the same individual within and between sources, both at the same point in time and over time. However, this is definitively not family reconstitution, and we cannot easily employ the conceptual and linguistic framework of that process. The key methodological architecture of family reconstitution is the creation of a family record and the probabilistic linkage of observable demographic events to it. This creates a base population into which one can link nominal data from other sources, and allows practitioners (because there is a definitive base population) to trace rates of 'success' or 'failure' in linkage practice. Creating relief profiles involves similar probabilistic decisions but using a wider suite of linkage variables, for instance the nature and scale of prior allowances to a person. But the process does not create a stable base population bounded by definitive events such as marriage or death; rather, linkage across time and source type creates a dynamic and fluid number of profiles and can change fundamentally the chronological and life-cycle range of the relief which attaches to any individual or family group. We cannot ultimately know how many individuals were receiving poor relief or medical welfare and for how long because the sources, even when linked, are incapable of delivering this certainty.

15 Sokoll, *Essex Pauper Letters*, No. 164, letter from Samuel White in Halstead to Mr Joselyne in Chelmsford, 20 June 1825. See also Nos 180, 182, 184, 193, 197, 207, 241, 242, 252 and 264, letters from Samuel White in Halstead to James Read, overseer of Chelmsford, June 1825 to February 1829.

16 *Ibid.*, Nos 2, 3, 4, 5 and 8, letters from James Smith in Woolwich to the overseer of Aveley, September 1831 to March 1833.

17 I rejected the idea of a threshold of medically orientated welfare over the pauper life-cycle or period of observation (say 50 per cent) that had to be met to consider all spending medically related, in favour of judgements on intensity based upon periodicity, duration and whether more than one family member was involved.

18 LRO, DDX 386/3, vestry minutes.
19 The utility of these variables is discussed by Langton, 'The geography of poor relief'. The sample has not been dissected according to the size of the rate base because the point where the rate was set was not always, or indeed often, linked to the scale of poverty. In many places rating records were not updated for many years. See Baugh, 'The cost of poor relief', pp. 53–4.
20 On the context of wider spending, and particularly spending after 1815, see Baugh, 'The cost of poor relief'; Lees, *Solidarities of Strangers*; P. Lindert, *Growing Public: Social Spending and Economic Growth since the Eighteenth Century* (Cambridge: Cambridge University Press, 2004), pp. 40–8 and 60–7; B. Harris, *The Origins of the British Welfare State: Social Welfare in England and Wales, 1800–1945* (Basingstoke: Palgrave, 2004), pp. 1–39; and French, 'An irrevocable shift', pp. 797–805.
21 For context see Marland, *Medicine and Society*.
22 See contributions to L. Curth (ed.), *From Physick to Pharmacology: Five Hundred Years of British Drug Retailing* (Aldershot: Ashgate, 2006) and Lane, *A Social History of Medicine*, pp. 46–7.
23 R. Porter, *Bodies Politic: Disease, Death and Doctors in Britain, 1650–1900* (London: Reaktion, 2003).
24 S. Shave, 'The welfare of the vulnerable in the late 18th and early 19th centuries: Gilbert's Act of 1782', *History in Focus*, 14 (2008), 14.
25 S. King, 'Welfare regimes'.
26 This observation applies even if we confine analysis to places with complete chronological coverage.
27 The importance of smallpox for spending profiles in individual parishes can be seen in the very fabric of Kibworth parish church in Leicestershire. A slate tablet on the wall celebrates the life of Lewis Powell Williams, a surgeon who died aged thirty-nine in 1771 and 'was the first that introduced into practice inoculation without preparation in this Kingdom'. See also J. Firth, *Highways and Byways in Leicestershire* (London: Macmillan, 1926), p. 211.
28 For wider context see Rusnock, 'Catching cowpox'; Thomas, 'The Old Poor Law', pp. 8–13; and Razzell, *The Conquest of Smallpox*.
29 On malarial-type fevers in Norfolk, see M. Dobson, *Contours of Death and Disease in Early Modern England*, 2nd edn (Cambridge: Cambridge University Press, 2010).
30 The surge is also observable in the parishes outside our core counties.
31 Broad, 'Parish economies of welfare', pp. 989 and 991.
32 The brief plateau in spending for the late 1820s amplifies into the Berkshire county sample, which is disproportionately represented in this collection of closed parishes.

33 S. Shave, 'The impact of Sturges Bourne's poor law reforms in rural England', *Historical Journal*, 56 (2013), 399–429.

34 Digby, *Making a Medical Living*; Loudon, *Medical Care*.

35 P. Warren, *Extracts from the Accounts of the Overseers of the Poor, 1807 to 1820: For the Parish of Methwold in the County of Norfolk* (Norwich: privately published, 1958).

36 Notwithstanding the fact that Wiltshire was very early in commissioning doctors: regular bills for apothecaries and doctors were recorded in Chippenham from the 1690s, and the parish entered into a contract with Dr Bushell as early as 1708. See F. Hinton, 'Notes on the records and accounts of the overseers of the poor of Chippenham, 1691–1805', *Wiltshire Archaeological and Natural History Magazine*, 149 (1933), 312–35.

37 Redford's assertion that even the worst cases of sickness attracted meagre relief in Lancashire is not supported here. A. Redford, *The History of Local Government in Manchester*, vol. 1: *Manor and Township* (London: Longman, 1939), p. 179.

38 I am grateful to one of the anonymous referees for this point. A consideration of the pauper letter sample outlined in Chapter 1 suggests very little change in the sorts of person applying for and getting relief, but this is only one sub-group of the parochial poor.

39 Thane, *Old Age in English History*, p. 155.

40 To some extent these typological variations may be an artificial reflection of the populations 'at risk' in the various subsets. Communities, many of them rural, with a significant proportion of their population 'normally' on or at the edges of poor relief were perhaps likely to adhere to a very different complexion of spending from those (often urban or industrial) communities where the 'normal' poverty problem was less severe.

41 LRO, DDX 386/3, vestry minutes.

42 B. Hurley, *Longbridge Deverill Poor 1816–1821 and 1825–1835* (Devizes: Wiltshire Family History Society, 2005), pp. 4–5.

43 LCRO, DE 1587/154/3, letter, 8 December 1823.

44 S. King, Nutt and Tomkins, *Narratives of the Poor*, pp. 292–6.

45 G. Taylor, *The Problem of Poverty 1660–1834* (London: Longman, 1969), pp. 3 and 18.

46 Eastwood, *Governing Rural England*, pp. 118 and 142.

47 Taylor likewise claims that the Old Poor Law was 'comprehensive in needs addressed'. J. Taylor, *Poverty, Migration and Settlement*, p. 9.

48 Ogborn, *Spaces of Modernity*, p. 232.

5

Medical people

Introduction

On 2 January 1833 H. J. Raines MRCSL wrote from Newport (Gwent, where he was parish doctor) to Beverley (Yorkshire) on the subject of John Scott's wife.[1] Having received a letter 'requesting me to discontinue my Attendance', Raines noted a serious relapse in her condition. Not content with this factual narrative,[2] however, he pointed out:

> You are probably aware that I have had, an extraordinary harassing, and fatiguing attendance upon this woman, for a long period, and as she has been, I may say, <u>entirely</u>, kept alive by medicines, she has taken a large quantity; indeed, I felt that I should not be doing my duty, either as a medical man, or a Christian, if I did not do everything in my power to alleviate her very Severe, and (excepting when under the influence of medicine) and incessant suffering, and I trust the Gentlemen of St Marys [parish, Beverley] will not think the account larger than the necessity of the Case warranted, when they consider my anxiety to preserve a life, for which I am morally, and legally responsible.[3]

The indignation of this letter is palpable, and the fact that Raines felt justified in launching a scathing attack on the overseer is important for this chapter. There are also other lessons. John Scott and his wife had been simultaneously and sequentially ill since September 1832, when she was noted to be 'hanging as it were between life & death'. Notwithstanding that, John Scott 'was troublesome before'[4] Beverley sanctioned considerable expenditure on medical care. This echoes the sense in Chapter 4 of doctors playing a more continuous role in parochial medical welfare over time. In addition to sustained attendance, the patient apparently required considerable quantities of drugs, while

the parish had also paid variously for nursing care in prior months. The costs of treating Mrs Scott (claimed in a single bill) were prodigious at nearly £11. Yet at the heart of this correspondence lay the question not of money, but of power. Raines felt it his professional, moral and Christian duty to treat the Scotts and clearly expected that such considerations would and should override parochial objections. For their part, officials in Beverley wanted to maintain ultimate power over how and when sickness was defined and what medical welfare should be attached to it. The fact that Raines's bill was paid in full perhaps suggests that the overseers themselves ultimately shared his views.

Such imperative is deeply ingrained into the vestry minutes, official correspondence and letters of epistolary advocates employed in this study. Thus, Charles Moore overseer of Clewer Mill near Windsor (Berkshire), was called by a local gentleman to see sixteen-year-old Mary Gibson, who was in 1832 'then dying in an out house belonging to him'. The gentleman suggested that 'she was so very bad unless immediate relief was afforded her she would not live the night, I found it exactly as was stated'. Moore:

> had her taken to our Workhouse, and sent for the Surgeon who attends our Poor, he said he thought she could not live, but by his great attention and I may add the assistance we had from everyone who could afford her relief, she is now perfectly recovered, from as bad a state of venereal disease as Mr O'Reilly [the parish doctor] ever witnessed.

He was certain that Tilehurst parish 'will without doubt pay the Surgeon and a moderate sum for the time she has been in our Poor House', which was substantial because 'it is not till wither this week that Mr O'Reilly would suffer her to leave the House as not being quite well'.[5] Clearly then here, within close sight of the New Poor Law, doctoring was firmly ingrained in the material, emotional and organisational culture of the Old Poor Law. Doctors were not, however, the only group that parishes and paupers turned to during 'normal' and epidemic sickness, and our spending category 'medical people' also includes nurses (professional, familial and neighbourhood), midwives, wise men and women, specialists in particular conditions outside the locality concerned, people in charge of healing spas and bonesetters.

In Chapter 4 we saw that Northamptonshire, Norfolk and Leicestershire spent a long-term average of 20 to 25 per cent of their

medical welfare on these medical people whereas in Lancashire, West Yorkshire, Berkshire and Wiltshire there was a decline in the spending category over the period. The broad aim of this chapter is thus to understand how the frequency, duration and cost of engagement between parishes and medical people of different stripes coalesced to generate these spatial patterns and, more widely, to look at the range and depth of provision at parochial level. The next section thus turns to the role of doctors in treating the sick poor. In particular I analyse the spread of doctoring contracts and the way they shaped the nature of treatment available to the poor. In turn, the chapter moves on to consider the complex question of nursing. It traces the character and cost of nursing in county contexts and highlights the differential regional evolution of nursing cultures, with all that this implies for the place of nursing within the overall medical welfare envelope. So-called irregular practitioners are the subject of the third main section of the chapter,[6] where it is argued that notwithstanding the rise of medical contracts, communities continued to turn to a rich array of irregulars. Finally, the chapter extends a discussion begun in Chapter 4 and suggests that paupers came to expect the deployment of doctors, nurses and other groups as a matter of course – even a matter of right – as they struggled with the consequences of sickness.

The doctor

Table 5.1 records the proportion of medical welfare resources and the proportion of the spending category 'medical people' absorbed by doctors in two periods (1750–55 and 1830–34) for the Core and Tier 1 and 2 communities and the county subsets.[7] In the former set of communities the rise in absolute spending on doctors does not translate to a rise in the proportion of all medical welfare resources accruing to them, though we do see a sustained rise in their share of spending on medical people.[8] This does not of course mean that doctors advanced in every parish or that the chronological path to their greater use was linear. In fact, it is possible to construct five broad categories of parochial engagement: communities in which the use or retention of doctors was limited and episodic;[9] those places which moved fluidly between contracting doctors,[10] more *ad hoc* usage and back again; parishes with doctoring contracts which either stuck to them rigidly or only

Table 5.1 The importance of doctors as a spending category

Level	1750–55		1800–34	
	% of medical welfare	% of medical people	% of medical welfare	% of medical people
All parishes	14.2	36.0	15.9	72.1
West Yorkshire	13.9	33.2	11.0	39.2
Leicestershire	12.6	36.0	14.9	73.0
Northamptonshire	18.8	41.6	19.2	74.2
Lancashire	13.7	36.4	16.7	77.9
Berkshire	14.0	35.5	7.8	38.6
Norfolk	19.9	41.2	23.1	83.8
Wiltshire	16.0	39.0	22.0	78.4

Sources: 98 Core, Tier 1 and Tier 2 communities. See Chapter 4 and Appendix.

used a small cohort of additional practitioners; communities which issued doctoring contracts but also engaged with lots of other medical practitioners, including specialists; and parishes where the doctoring contract was a small part of parochial engagement with local, regional and national medical men, irregulars and institutions. The changing composition of parochial arrangements within this broad categorical structure does much to explain the county-level spending profiles outlined in Table 5.1 and goes some way to constructing an explanatory framework for wider county trends in spending on medical people.

Contemporaries would have noted profound changes in the nature and scale of doctoring over our period. In 1750 only eight parishes employed any form of traceable doctoring contract. Chippenham (Wiltshire) contracted Jane Mortimer for the year 1753 at a salary of £15. She was one of four surgeonesses employed in the 1750s and 1760s.[11] Contracting also had deep roots in closed parishes like Geddington (Northamptonshire) and Holkham (Norfolk).[12] Most other places employed doctors on an *ad hoc* basis in relation to individual paupers, outbreaks of epidemic disease or as a precautionary measure to provide inoculation.[13] Indeed, few communities in the 1750s and 1760s escaped years or sequences of years in which the bills of doctors had a substantial material impact on overall poor law spending. Thus Dr Barry inoculated 426 poor people in Chippenham

in 1779 at an extra cost to his contract of £53. Further inoculation campaigns in 1785 and 1793 cost £48 and £73 respectively. At the opposite end of the country, dealing with the sickness of Thomas Layfield and his family absorbed fully 10 per cent of the total poor relief resources for Easington (Lancashire) in 1762.[14] If anything these *ad hoc* bills understate parochial spending on doctors, given that such men and women charged additional fees for administrative duties[15] and that they may have been contracted to the early workhouses and by those who episodically farmed the poor under terms which are very difficult to trace directly in the written record.[16] Nonetheless, it is clear that most places at this early date were orientated to our first category of parochial relations with doctors.

By 1834, and as might be expected from contemporary accounts of doctors accumulating local institutional and parochial positions,[17] the situation with doctoring contracts was reversed.[18] On the eve of the New Poor Law just fourteen parishes fell into our first category and had no recent or current contracts with local doctors.[19] Most rapidly in Berkshire, Wiltshire and West Yorkshire, and with Lancashire and Norfolk lagging by the later eighteenth century, communities in the county subsets advertised, negotiated, agreed and re-negotiated doctoring contracts with vigour and purpose. In turn, there was surprisingly little variation in the timing and completeness of the spread of doctoring contracts between the different typological subsets: While urban areas such as Trowbridge had already contracted with local doctors by the early 1750s, other urban communities, Wellingborough or Bradfield for example, lagged significantly behind their rural or industrial counterparts. The propensity to turn to doctors was not related in any simple way to their probable number in the local medical marketplace,[20] and nor was there any clear association between exploding poor relief bills and the decision to contract.[21]

As Samantha Williams has observed, the bare bones of the doctoring contract in terms of structure and duties were shared within and across counties.[22] For the eighteenth century, most excluded from the fixed price some combination of smallpox cases, midwifery, amputation and (less commonly) broken bones.[23] There was rather wider variation in the spatial limits of such contracts. Some required attendance upon or correspondence with all parochial paupers wherever they might reside, while others focused entirely on the parochial boundary. Hybrid

agreements required doctors to attend or otherwise see to patients in a small number of proximate parishes or within a certain radius. By the nineteenth century, and very clearly by 1834, doctoring contracts across the sample fell into four distinct categories. First were those where doctors (individually or in concert) had managed to maintain a broad sweep of exclusions and thus keep up the real value of their contracts. Secondly, there were contracts where scope and exclusion moved fluidly between years, a reflection of competition on the one hand and local particularities on the other. Thus in May 1805 the vestry of Swanage (Dorset) engaged Robert Davis for a year at £25 to provide medical services both to that town and to the poor of Swanage in neighbouring Langton and Studland, with only midwifery excluded. By 1811 the same doctor had a contract valued at £35 and excluding smallpox, midwifery, venereal disease and all attendance outside the town boundary.[24] The remarkable Northamptonshire parish of Crick saw the spatial extent of contracts rise or fall with almost every renewal, normally by just the odd mile.[25] Thirdly, we can find sixteen all-inclusive arrangements. Thus the vestry at Diss (Norfolk) agreed in September 1818 to consider 'the application from the surgeons for an increase of Salary'. After some debate the ratepayers approved an increase to £60 but removed all exclusions and, particularly, 'difficult cases of midwifery'.[26] Finally, some twenty-one parishes exhibit broad hybrid contracts like that agreed in 1813 between the Northamptonshire parish of Guilsborough and Dr Henry Bullivant to provide medical services for paupers or those 'who do not in consequence of such sickness require other parochial relief'. The contract excluded 'all accidents, all cases of contagious fever, smallpox and all cases of midwifery' and all attendance on the out-parish poor. This standard list was, however, augmented by a further set of clarifications: 'we do not consider the said Henry Bullivant as bound to confinement at home by this agreement any more than under general professional engagement', a statement which suggests prior tensions with parish doctors over their availability when called.[27] Other doctors settled on a contract price but agreed to accept less if there were fewer sick paupers in the year ahead than they had contracted for. Of course, both parishes and their doctors could potentially move frequently and rapidly between these very different types of contract, but what is striking about the sample as a whole is the relative stability of the contractual form at the level of individual parishes.

This is not to say that the process of contracting was always harmonious, particularly when it came to fixing remuneration. Nonetheless, and
perhaps surprisingly when set against a literature which has emphasised
the competitive nature of the medical market at local level, the average
value of doctoring contracts rose over time in every county except West
Yorkshire. Interpreting this trend is more complex than it looks, not
least because rising contract values often reflected the increasing scale
of the task judged in terms of the number of the poor, the frequency
of their illness and (certainly by the 1820s) a tendency for parishes to
demand fewer exclusions. These caveats notwithstanding, the stipend
associated with doctoring the poor rose by about 120 per cent between
the early 1800s and 1834, with no obvious relationship between con
tract values and particular typological subsets of the parochial data.[28]
In Bickerstaffe (Lancashire), the remuneration attached to doctoring
contracts remained stable at £2 2s throughout the period 1769–1800,
rising by a third in 1800 and further doubling by the 1820s.[29] For
Wellingborough (Northamptonshire) a remarkably complete set of
contracts shows a rise in fixed price from £15 in 1802 to £59 in 1833.[30]
These observations do not of course mean that contract values were
stable year on year. Where the job attracted significant competition or
new entrants, parochial authorities were often quite successful in driving down costs.[31] In Swanage, for instance, the arrival of Dr Pink put
pressure on the incumbent Dr Davies and drove the value of the contract in 1815 down to £21, a sum which was maintained until 1818.[32]
Yet making reduced contract values stick over the medium term was
not always easy. In Long Buckby (Northamptonshire), for instance,
Charles Allen and William Dix agreed in 1827 to take the contract for
medical attendance on the poor 'exclusive of all journeys out of the
parish' at a sum of £36. By 1830, the arrival of two further doctors in
this small town had driven the contract value down to £30, and in 1832
Drs Bull and Dix declined a renewal of their contract at £35. For 1833
medical attendance at Long Buckby was thus provided at distance by
Edward Swan from Weedon, who agreed to deal with smallpox and
midwifery cases within his contract price.[33] The opposite side of the
experiential spectrum is represented by Oundle in Northamptonshire,
Calverley in West Yorkshire and Garstang in Lancashire, where communities maintained long-term relationships with individual doctors
or small groups of them on a rotational basis. In these places we witness

a significant inflation of contract values and a clear sense in which 'outside' practitioners found it very difficult to obtain a foothold. On balance, while the cost of doctoring contracts remained relatively modest given the scale of treatment involved, and certainly a modest part of overall poor relief spending,[34] there can be no doubt of their growing importance in parochial medical welfare.[35]

If the vast majority of our parochial sample from the 1810s onwards maintained fairly regular doctoring contracts, few relied entirely on such services.[36] At their most extensive, additional doctoring relationships were rich, colourful, prolonged and often expensive. Officers in Methwold (Norfolk), for instance, sent paupers to doctors in Wilton, Northwold, Swaffham, Mundford, Hingham, Brandon, Hockhold, Southery and Tofts and on numerous occasions to Dr Waters at Downham Market. This was in addition to a retained doctor on a contract escalating from £11 in 1804 to £22 in 1820, and additional payments for the attendance of specialist bonesetters and 'tappers' for the dropsy.[37] Every county sample can boast similarly extensive local relationships. The Leicestershire parish of Oxendon, for instance, used sixteen named doctors, three unnamed doctors and assorted irregulars in addition to contracted medical men between 1758 and 1834.[38] In places, these relationships could be very long-term. John Beech, overseer of Essington (Staffordshire), wrote to his counterpart at Thrapston (Northamptonshire) regarding the perennial pauper Joseph Richards on 25 August 1829. Richards had 'strained his side' and Beech had allowed cash relief, but when the complaint did not get better after two weeks he 'sent him to the surgeon that attended him [in Walsall] when his side was first bad several years ago as I considered it would be the least expense' to have him treated by someone familiar with the case.[39] Nor were parishes by the early nineteenth century reticent about sending paupers with persistent problems further afield. When Mr Blackshaw wrote from Northwich (Cheshire) to his overseer counterpart in Preston (Lancashire) noting that 'James Boyyer is gone to Manchester to the Doctor that he has a Cancer on his neck and nun of the Doctors in Northwitch cant cure him', he was elaborating a common experience.[40]

Overall, then, the central message of the data is that doctors (contracted and in various *ad hoc* relationships with parishes) played a more frequent role in the sickness lives of the poor by the last decades of the

Old Poor Law. How far this equated to 'better' or more comprehensive treatment is a moot point. There are good reasons to be sceptical. Contemporary publications buzzed with the need for reform.[41] Some historians have argued that parish contracts were awarded to the lowest bidder on the harshest terms, which in turn fed through to lowering standards of care for the poor. We can garner intriguing perspectives on this issue from overseers' correspondence: Robert Fifield wrote from Chiddingford (Surrey) to Tilehurst (Berkshire) on 18 February 1825 to apologise for delayed payment of a sum meant to support a bastard child he had fathered while visiting the parish. He explained that 'as I am only an Assistant, you may easily conceive that cash is not very plentiful, owing to the very small salary given by Surgeons. Indeed, many Assistants may be procured for their bread and lodging only'![42] Even if criticism of the system has been overdone (there is, as we have seen, very little evidence of a drive to the bottom in terms of contract values[43]), inherent flaws in the contracting system may have compromised the quality or regularity of care. Most importantly, it is clear that doctors accumulated multiple contracts which may have stymied their engagement with individual paupers and parishes. Thomas Grant of Litchborough doctored eleven Northamptonshire parishes between 1774 and 1793.[44] Similarly Dr Leete held contracts with eight Northamptonshire parishes. The record in our sample was held by Robert Alexander of Halifax, who serviced no fewer than fourteen West Yorkshire townships and communities. The meaning of the 'parish doctor' was thus likely to have been very different in these county samples from that in Wiltshire, where such overlap was rather rarer.

In one sense of course it is very difficult to test the actual quality of treatment afforded to paupers. Doctors under contract did not have to itemise their engagements or the nature of the treatment provided. Activities excluded from contracts did generate additional bills but in areas such as midwifery these often equate to no more than a claim for attending X during labour. By the 1820s and 1830s even *ad hoc* doctoring engagements frequently resulted in bills which simply detailed the name of the patient, the number of journeys made and the cost of unspecified medicines or other treatments. To some extent this trend was balanced by more detail in bills on surgical cases and aftercare as invasive treatments gained credence and effectiveness over the

Table 5.2 Dr Edgar's bill to Chippenham (Wiltshire), 1783

Date	Item	Cost (s/d)
6 August 1783	A journey	2/6
	Fever powders	3/0
7 August	A journey	2/6
	Fever powders	3/0
10 August	A journey	2/6
	Powders	3/0
14 August	A journey	2/6
	Powders	3/0
16 August	A journey	2/6
	Powders	3/0

Source: WRO CL/CHI/22, doctoring bill, 1783.

period.[45] Even in the eighteenth century, however, bills give us only the most superficial flavour of the nature and effectiveness of treatment as opposed simply to its frequency. A typically dull bill was sent by Dr Edgar to Chippenham in September 1783 for treatment of Thomas Framling and is reproduced in Table 5.2.[46]

Yet where more detail is forthcoming it does much to confirm that paupers had access to palliative and placebo 'medicines' across much the same range as independent patients and of a sort familiar from the commonplace books maintained and updated by lay families who practised extensive self-dosing.[47] Thus, Dr Swinsen charged Brington parish (Northamptonshire) 2s 6d for attendance; the rest of his bill for May 1784 to February 1785 included vomits (at 6d apiece), chamomile flowers (2d), Peruvian julep (2s per draught), antimonial drops (6d per bottle), saline powders (3s per set of six), sudorific draughts (8d each), anodyne mixtures (variously 1s 6d to 3s), pearl barley (6d per paper) and basalmic solution (at 2s per bottle), as well as the costs of dressing and compresses.[48] The same doctor billed the parish of Crick for a prodigious '39 leeches set on' Mary Slynn in 1774.

Switching attention from doctoring bills to our letter corpus, we get a clear sense that both doctors and parishes went to considerable lengths to provide an expansive medical service for the poor, as the stories opening this chapter may have suggested. Thus Dr Simpson wrote from Hutton Cranswick (North Yorkshire) to Beverley on

3 November 1832 to detail the dreadful case of 'a little Boy of the
name of Gray', whose brains had been dashed out by the kick of a
horse fracturing

> the Cranium of skull nearly the middle of the Forehead to nearly the
> right ear the Brain itself being Exposed to view throughout all that extent
> and in one part was actually lacerated and protruded in small raged
> pieces.

Dr Simpson despaired of his life, but his paying 'Every attention to the
Case' had brought the boy to a state where 'if He get over the acute
inflamation [sic] consequent on like accidents He will recover but the
danger is and must be great for a few days'. He would, Simpson promised the overseers, 'do my utmost and under charges of moderation'.[49]
The unwitting testimony of paupers in their own letters also provides
considerable evidence of intense attention by doctors working within
the limits of contemporary medical knowledge. Philip James wrote
from Leicester to Uttoxeter (Staffordshire) on 12 June 1834 asking for
further cash relief. He felt that 'if I could have better Support I should
soon get Round, Being Bled so Often & Blisterd & leeched it has left
me so very weak that I might Never get the Better of it without help'.[50]
    This is not to argue that care was universally good, nor as timely as
required. Paupers sometimes complained about the ineffectiveness of
institutional sojourns. We can also find first- and second-hand evidence
of complaints against individual doctors. William Hargreaves complained to the vestry of Calverley (West Yorkshire) that the attentions
of the contracted doctor had made his situation 'so much the worse',
while John Mason of Rothersthorpe (Northamptonshire) complained
that Dr Swinsen had treated him 'no better than a dog'.[51] Parishes too
might fall out with their own doctors and those of other parishes about
attendance and treatment. It is for this reason that we see sentiments
such as that from Dr B. Bell FRCSE in a letter to the Hulme overseer
Joseph Ballard in 1837 which requested that 'in order to avoid mistakes,
messages, if possible [should] be sent early in the day and in writing'.[52]
On the other hand, doctors also gained plaudits from both parishes
and their paupers. Dr Davis was given 'a present of two guineas' in May
1811 'for his extraordinary services' to the poor of Swanage in the last
year.[53] In Somerset, the overseer of Twerton noted the positive commentary of paupers on the treatment afforded by Dr Williams in 1832,

while his counterpart in Mells (Somerset) commended the 'unstinting duty' of Dr Willis when renewing his contract.[54] Similarly, on 15 April 1801 the vestry of Wellingborough presented Mr Richard Lettice with £5 5s for 'his assiduous attendance upon the poor in a very sickly year', while in Norfolk, three parishes voluntarily supplemented the annual stipend of the doctor because the prior year had seen so much sickness.

Judged in the round, it seems clear that paupers could access increasingly frequent and probably more intensive doctoring as our period progressed. More pauper lives and more of those lives were medicalised and doctored as part of the general upsurge in medical welfare in the last decades of the Old Poor Law. To echo Chapter 4, what was 'right, proper and fair' by the 1820s was intimately tied up with access to doctors. In turn, the fees of doctors absorbed more of the resources devoted to medical people over time, even as the relative importance of this spending category in the overall parochial fell from 30–40 per cent of medical welfare spending in the 1750s to only 20 per cent by 1834. Yet there were spatial nuances in this experience. Norfolk parishes demonstrated the most *ad hoc* arrangements, falling significantly and permanently behind other counties in terms of doctoring contracts. Paradoxically, such arrangements drove higher costs, especially when allied with the tendency for Norfolk parishes with contracts also to consult a wide variety of other local and regional medical men. Doctoring here thus became (as we shall see below) more and more central to the spending category of medical people. At the opposite extreme, Berkshire, Northamptonshire, Wiltshire and West Yorkshire were early adopters of doctoring contracts. Even in these places, however, the meaning and consequence of contracting could vary significantly. The propensity of some Northamptonshire communities to supplement contracts with resort to local, regional and national medical men meant that doctors still absorbed more of the spending on medical people over time. In Berkshire, by contrast, a tendency for parishes to stick closely to doctoring contracts and to supplement them in limited ways meant that doctoring as a component of medical people fell progressively over the period. Here, as we shall see, nursing was the dynamic spending category, and this was also true of West Yorkshire. One further observation complicates this assessment and suggests that we pick up only a subset of the doctoring afforded to the poor. As Roy Porter has argued, 'few who needed

medical attention would have gone without. And that includes even the very poor. Physicians and quacks alike often made a point of treating poor patients gratis, out of charity.'[55] We return to this matter at length in Chapter 9. For now, and however it was fashioned, there is substantial empirical support for Porter's assertion that 'being treated by the doctor became a way of life'.[56]

Nursing

As with doctors, the absolute amounts spent on nurses and nursing rose over time, though with distinct county profiles.[57] Thus for much of the period Norfolk parishes were spending less than one quarter of their Berkshire counterparts on nursing, while in the 1820s West Yorkshire communities were spending at least triple that of their Norfolk or Lancashire counterparts.[58] Within this broad framework, in most places and at most times the scale of nursing expenditure was not linked systematically to that on doctors, drugs, cash allowances or other elements of medical welfare. Nursing was, in other words, a discrete service. This is exemplified in a letter from William Boon, overseer of Kettering (Northamptonshire), to his counterpart in nearby Thrapston. Reflecting on the case of George May, Boon noted that his wife 'has been confined to her bed for this last six weeks and has scarcely had one days health for this year past so the poor man is obliged to have a woman constantly with her and he being so disturbed at night almost disables him from work'.[59] The parish was asked to consider an allowance to support May because of his wife's sickness, but the nursing response to such sickness had been happening for perhaps one year prior to the application.

The Old Poor Law was by far the biggest non-familial provider and funder of nursing care in England.[60] It is thus surprising that while our understanding of (particularly later) nineteenth-century nursing has become increasingly sophisticated, the same cannot be said of nursing practice in the thousands of communities that were the locus of welfare before 1834.[61] Jeremy Boulton's study of the parish of St Martin-in-the-Fields from the late seventeenth century to the 1720s suggests that between 11 and 18 per cent of total parish spending, as well as almost one third of all 'extraordinary' allowances, was absorbed by a small cohort of nurses, most of whom provided care in *de facto* nursing

homes.[62] Yet historians have had both little and little positive to say about poor law nursing. Samantha Williams's study of two Bedfordshire parishes (Campton and Shefford) identifies 102 'carers' who were retained for broad nursing duties. Almost all were employed on an irregular basis and poorly paid, with the majority themselves becoming dependent upon poor relief at some point in their life-cycle.[63] Anne Borsay suggests that eighteenth-century and early nineteenth-century community nursing (including but not confined to poor law nursing) 'was less abject than conventional wisdom alleges' but can draw on little empirical material.[64] Perhaps inevitably, the image of the poorly paid, untrained, ineffectual and amateur (often pauper) nurse has become a leitmotif in relation to the care offered to the poor.[65]

Table 5.3 begins a process of reassessment. As might have been expected given the growing importance of doctors traced above, the proportion of medical welfare and medical people spending devoted to nursing fell over the period when all parishes are considered together. While this picture seems to have varied little across the typological spectrum, there were striking county-level differences. In Berkshire (7.3 per cent) and West Yorkshire (7.2 per cent), nurses still absorbed a significant proportion of medical welfare resources by the 1830s. By contrast, relative spending on nursing had fallen heavily in Norfolk (2.1 per cent) and Lancashire (2.4 per cent). Explanations for this

Table 5.3 The importance of nurses as a spending category

Level	1750–55		1800–34	
	% of medical welfare	% of medical people	% of medical welfare	% of medical people
All parishes	17.4	41.4	4.8	21.0
West Yorkshire	24.2	44.1	7.2	33.4
Leicestershire	18.9	40.4	4.8	20.0
Northamptonshire	12.6	32.4	5.2	21.1
Lancashire	17.9	42.2	2.4	11.1
Berkshire	22.0	47.3	7.3	37.4
Norfolk	14.1	31.2	2.1	8.1
Wiltshire	21.6	46.5	4.1	16.4

Sources: 98 Core, Tier 1 and Tier 2 communities. See Chapter 4 and Appendix.

picture are by no means simple but three models of parochial commitment to nursing can be observed. In Norfolk, for instance, we encounter parishes like Scottow or Bressingham, the former with its sometimes substantial but always at least low-level spending on nursing and the latter with nursing the most common form of welfare next to cash. For such communities nursing was clearly written into the very fabric of poor relief. Other counties had their equivalent communities. In Wiltshire, for instance, both Sopworth and Hardenhuish spent more than 8 per cent of their medical welfare on nursing across the period. While most parishes falling into this first model were rural or rural-industrial in character, towns too could see nursing written into the fabric of poor law expectations. The urban parish of Trowbridge, for instance, spent less (just over 2 per cent of medical welfare resources per year) but it did so consistently across the period. A second model is exemplified by the Norfolk parish of Thetford St Cuthbert or the West Yorkshire parish of Guiseley, where spending on nursing was more substantial than elsewhere when it did occur but also more intermittent. Salhouse in Norfolk and the town of Wellingborough represent a third model. In the former, nursing as a category of relief disappeared altogether from 1809, while in the latter such spending was at best patchy. Parochial commitment to nursing as a form of medical welfare thus ranged on a spectrum between fragile and invulnerable in the last decades of the Old Poor Law. Higher spending levels in Berkshire or West Yorkshire and lower levels in Norfolk or Lancashire in part reflected the distribution of the parochial sample across this spectrum. Crudely, Berkshire had more parishes with a consistent and consistently high level of spending than did Norfolk. This is at best, however, a mechanistic explanation for the patterning we observe. In practice, counties differed significantly in the number of nurses they employed, the range and duration of their duties and the wages paid to them. This seems to have had little to do with differences in levels of sickness between parishes and counties and much more to do with ingrained nursing cultures.

Figure 5.1 provides a minimum quantitative overview of the scale of the nursing labour force in the seven counties. With 6.6 and 4.9 discrete nurses employed per parish per year, the Berkshire and West Yorkshire figures are somewhat higher than Williams found for Campton (1.04) or Shefford (0.94).[66] Norfolk and Lancashire parishes, by contrast,

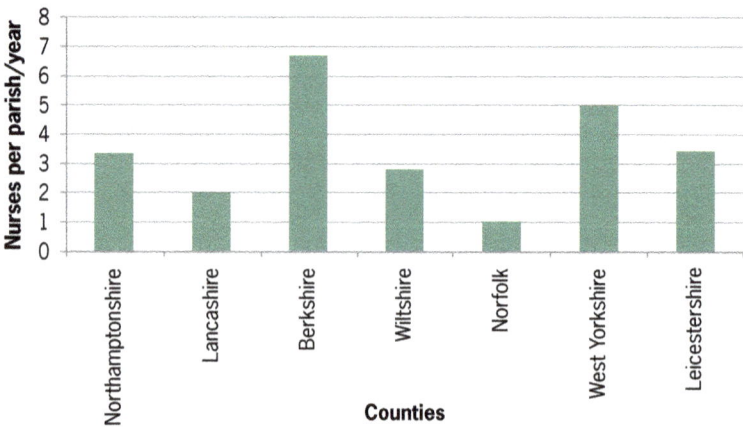

5.1 The scale of the nursing labour force in seven counties

employed many fewer people, an observation which is even more striking when set against the observation above that some places in these
parochial samples were consistent employers of nurses. The close fit of
Norfolk to the Bedfordshire figures begins to suggest a wider 'eastern
England' model of poor law nursing. These sorts of variations are in
turn more fully exemplified if we switch our attention to the range of
nursing duties that communities would support. Figure 5.2 thus traces
the proportion of nursing events that can be ascribed to certain kinds of
nurse for the period 1750–1834.[67] As Williams observes, few parishes
were without a person taking up multiple nursing roles within any given
year or time period. However, 'professional' parish nurses were particularly common in Berkshire, Northamptonshire and West Yorkshire.[68]
Such, for instance, was Mary White of Ardington (Berkshire), who
nursed three or four patients a year through the 1790s and early 1800s.
Moreover, just as Berkshire had a larger cohort of professional nurses
than other counties, so the range of their activities was also wider. Lucy
Goodwin of Ardington provided regular midwifery services, medicines, boarding for sick parishioners and strangers and general nursing
services to a substantial core of the sick poor in the parish. While she
was never called a surgeoness, her activities suggest that she fulfilled the
role.[69] Women such as this were occupied as nurses rather than simply

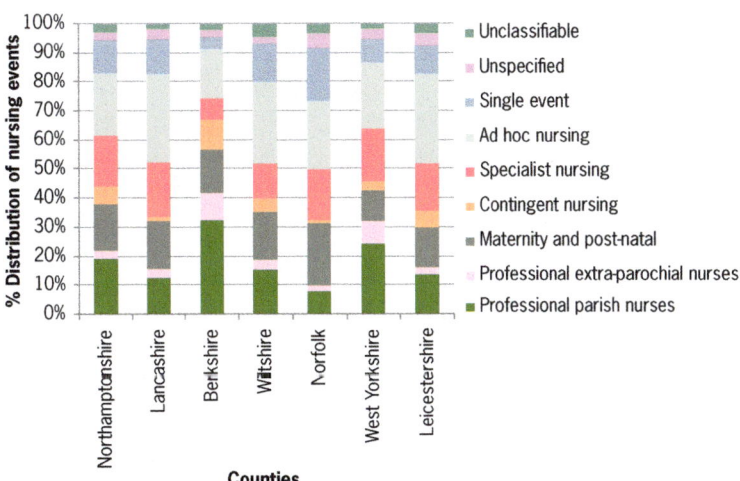

5.2 The proportions of nursing events accruing to different kinds of nurse

providing nursing labour. If the relationship was not always consistent at parish level, judged in the round counties and communities that witnessed greater reliance on professional nurses were also those devoting larger proportions of the spending category 'medical people' to nursing.

We must, however, distinguish the 'professional' group from a smaller but nonetheless very important subset of nurses who travelled between parishes. While this activity was often closely associated with epidemic disease cases, officials were also willing to use such nurses for other aspects of sickness. In Berkshire, for instance, Mary Hatt was engaged by at least four different parishes in the late 1820s, while other Hatt women were to be found as midwives and nurses in other Berkshire parishes, a *de facto* nursing dynasty. Overseers generally made a clear distinction between the role of these extra-parochial nurses and the more proximate nursing labour force. In 1805 at Burghfield (Berkshire) Elizabeth Money, a woman who had provided *ad hoc* nursing services in the past, was paid 5s 'for attending on Sarah Turner *after* the [professional] nurse was gone'.[70] For all of the counties analysed here there is evidence of the existence of a professional extra-parochial nursing network. Even in Norfolk, rural parishes such as Forncett

St Peter routinely brought in nursing labour from outside.[71] There was in turn a positive relationship at parish level between a tendency to employ extra-parochial nursing and the absolute and proportionate spending on nursing, helping to explain some of the intra-regional differences highlighted thus far and suggesting that ingrained commitment to nursing could develop in some parishes and not others.

Professional nursing also overlaps with the 'contingent nursing' categorisation of Figure 5.2. In Northamptonshire, Wiltshire and Berkshire, bills issued by doctors provide an indication that they could engage their own nurses and charge the parish for out-of-pocket expenses in this regard. We can be more precise about another aspect of contingent nursing: that in formal or informal institutional settings. On 29 September 1812, for instance, the vestry of Peterborough St John took out a fire insurance policy (£150) for a 'newly erected building used as a nursery and on a new building adjoining used as a place of confinement' at Westgate in the town; given the insurance amount it was clearly substantial.[72] Other parishes converted existing buildings or carved nursing areas out of workhouse accommodation. The workhouse book of Bray (Berkshire), for instance, recorded on 24 April 1792 that 'the upper right hand front Garret be reserved as a sick room, into which all persons deemed ill by the Apothecary shall be removed, and a proper steady person appointed as a nurse'.[73] The fact that parishes in Northamptonshire and Berkshire, irrespective of wealth or socio-economic typology, were more likely than parishes elsewhere to provide nursing in institutional settings explains at least part of the variation between the county datasets in the proportion of resources devoted to nursing services. Moreover, contingent nursing was also provided by way of parishes buying service and space in the houses of parishioners. At its lowest level this involved the boarding-out of individual sick paupers, but multiple boarding was surprisingly common. In Caversham (Berkshire), Mary Clisby was paid in the 1790s and 1800s for providing board and lodging for the sick in her own home, for attending and taking in sick travellers and for hiring out nurses who were clearly in her employ. We can find similar examples in all of the counties analysed here, though being nursed in the homes of others was much more common in Berkshire and West Yorkshire than in other places, especially Norfolk where such provision was rare. The nursing homes were not on the same scale as those traced by Jeremy

Boulton in London, but communities that used or hosted such nursing homes tended to devote more of their resources to nursing than parishes that did not.[74]

Other forms of nursing highlighted in Figure 5.2 exhibit less spatial diversity. *Ad hoc* nursing care in response to sudden need was commonplace. In all counties such care was recorded in the overseers' accounts alongside that provided by more regular nurses for the same person. Hence, in Bray in January 1818 Mrs Hearn was paid 24s for nursing Widow Haines, but Widow Brown was given an additional 3s for 'assisting the nurse'.[75] Specialist nurses employed to deal with epidemic disease, especially smallpox, typhus and the diseases of childhood, sit at the opposite extreme. Smallpox nurses were paid at a considerably higher rate (10–12s per week plus board and lodging even for nurses living within the parish appears normal) than those employed for regular or inter-parish nursing.[76] It thus follows that parochial susceptibility to smallpox and other infectious disease of the sort we see in eighteenth-century Northamptonshire was a driver of the regularity and scale of expenditure on nursing and the importance of nursing in medical welfare.[77] Much, however, also depended upon the constellation of nursing rather than simply its volume. In those parishes and counties (such as Berkshire or Yorkshire) where multiple simultaneous and sequential nursing in a combination of specialist-*ad hoc*-professional-single-event was deployed for bouts of sickness, nursing expenditure tended to be higher absolutely and proportionately.

Table 5.4, dealing with average pay for nurses, explores another aspect of this explanatory frame. Of course, reconstructing pay rates for nursing services is difficult. Within and between parishes, nurses were paid both by the week or month and by episode, and their pay was variously supplemented with perquisites. Rates of pay also varied according to whether nurses were expected to look after individuals or families, and whether they were providing other aid than just nursing. In Caversham, for instance, one nurse was paid extra for giving up her bed. Moreover, in all of the parishes analysed here except those in Lancashire, overseers made a distinction between ordinary nursing and that conducted during the harvest, for which extra pay was given. In August 1825 at Warham (Norfolk), Hannah Basham was given 'extra in harvest time doing for the old people as usual 5s', while Widow Green was paid 7s 6d for providing nursing for her family and 'Loss of

time made no Gleaning'.[78] Another subtle influence on the level of pay
for nursing was the question of whether an illness was expected to lead
to a death, for which nurses were paid more than when a patient was
expected to recover. Thus in Ardington in 1798 Nurse Ballard was given
1s 6d per week over two weeks for 'looking after' John Clark, but Mary
Brown was given 13s per week for providing nursing 'Eleven weeks at
several [times]' to the same person prior to his death. Nor, perhaps,
should we forget that some professional and semi-professional nurses
were actually paid even when they were not working. In Bray Mrs Lock
was retained at 3s per week.[79]

Against this backdrop, Table 5.4 suggests notable county-level differences in the range of nursing pay. Berkshire, West Yorkshire and
Northamptonshire parishes (on average and across all types of activity)
paid their nurses more than parishes in the other counties, particularly
their counterparts in Norfolk.[80] Thus, postnatal nursing across a range
of Berkshire parishes was paid at double the rate that can be traced for
Norfolk or Wiltshire communities, something that also applies to general nursing and attendance on the insane poor.[81] Moreover, Table 5.5
suggests that there were also substantial differences in the duration
of nursing between the county samples, with parishes in Berkshire
and West Yorkshire in particular engaging nurses for longer than their
counterparts in Wiltshire or Norfolk. Longer terms of general and
chronic nursing allied with simultaneously longer periods of attendance, waiting and other more casual forms of nursing reflects the fact
the Berkshire (and Northamptonshire and West Yorkshire) parishes
were particularly likely to engage more than one nurse to provide care
for an individual. The Berkshire and Northamptonshire parishes also
demonstrated the longest periods of chronic nursing, while in Norfolk
and Lancashire the juxtaposition of long-duration nursing care by relatives with the lowest figures for 'looking after' and chronic nursing
probably points to a rather heavier reliance on cheaper family labour
for long-term care than in the other counties. Norfolk parishes were
the only ones to consistently use girls (often but not always relatives of
the sick) as nursing labour, with average pay somewhat below that for
adult nurses.

Understanding the complexion of nursing for the sick poor is thus
complicated. A remarkable lack of variation between communities
on a typological basis is overlaid upon considerable spatial variation

Table 5.4 Rates of pay for nurses in the county samples (shillings)

Nursing	West Yorkshire	Leicestershire	Northamptonshire	Lancashire	Berkshire	Norfolk	Wiltshire
Smallpox or specialist*	18–30	16–30	20–5	12–38	20–7	13–20	18–25
Postnatal*	4–12	2–8	2–7	1–7	3–9	1–5	1–3
Cleaning, waiting or seeing to	1–9	1–11	1–8	1–5	1–6	1–4	1–3
Attending	1–4	1–4	0.5–2	0.25–4	0.5–3	0.5–1.5	0.25–3
Nursing by relatives	1–4	1–4	1–7	1–22	1.5–10	1–6	1–11
General nursing	2–6	2–6	1–6	0.5–6	2–7	1–3	1–3
Mad nursing*	8–41	2–37	6–31	4–38	12–40	6–23	6–16
Harvest nursing supplement*	1–3	4–6	4–6	0	4–5	2–4	3–5
Chronic nursing	4–10	3–12	2–10	0.5–8	4–10	2–6	2–9
Other	1–16	0.5–16	1–5	0.5–10	3–6	1–3	1–4

Notes: Nursing categories marked * represent payment range per episode. In other cases the table tries to control for differences of duration by presenting payment ranges per week.
Sources: 117-parish sample.

Table 5.5 Durations of nursing (days)

Nursing	West Yorkshire	Leicestershire	Northamptonshire	Lancashire	Berkshire	Norfolk	Wiltshire
Smallpox or specialist	24	17	25	18	26	16	20
Postnatal	3	3	4	5	4	3	3
Cleaning, waiting or seeing to	36	22	22	8	38	9	34
Attending	16	10	11	9	14	7	12
Nursing by relatives	7	18	17	22	13	26	16
General nursing	17	11	13	8	18	6	14
Mad nursing	46	39	42	51	64	30	37
Chronic nursing	59	52	58	20	82	34	41
Other	9	6	4	3	14	5	6

Sources: 117-parish sample.

Notes: Where the duration of intermittent long-term nursing is not exactly specified the average weekly pay for that type of nursing is used to fix duration. Payments for 'nursing' without nominal data are excluded.

in the scope, scale, cost and duration of nursing. A sense that differences in spending within and (particularly) between counties might reflect ingrained cultural and policy attitudes towards the nursing of the sick poor – an idea in the minds of some officials that they had basic obligations to provide a comprehensive nursing service for the sick – clearly emerges. This was certainly the case in most Berkshire parishes, where nursing labour was not casual, residual or cheap.[82] By contrast in Norfolk nursing tended to be provided at the less intensive, less professional and less expensive end of the policy spectrum. Norfolk communities did not lack the money or the nursing networks to adopt a different approach; they lacked the history of action and the will to change. Parochial officials – and particularly those who remained in post for some time – were remarkably powerful guardians of normative standards.

Irregulars

Perhaps unsurprisingly given *ad hoc* parochial commitment to doctors between the 1750s and 1780s, medical irregulars made an appearance in every set of overseers' accounts at the start of our period.[83] Abington parish (Northamptonshire) was buying papers of 'Phisick' from the druggist William Johnson of London as early as 1778.[84] Widow Smith first appeared at Welton (Northamptonshire) in 1774 'for salving and dressing John Collins leg'. Thereafter, she was paid consistently in the accounts, applying ointments and other medicines purchased in bulk from apothecaries and, increasingly across the later eighteenth century, for 'doctoring' and bleeding.[85] No parish in the entire sample used irregulars more than Crick. By 1760, Mrs Underwood was the primary medical attendant upon the poor, notwithstanding the fact that the parish turned almost every year to male doctors. She administered bark, wormwood, eye drops, Daffey's elixir and physic, used leeches and undertook venesection. Where she failed in medical care, her husband made the parish coffins! Other Crick irregulars included Mrs Whitnell, who supplied fever powders, bark and Hooper's Pills and acted as a midwife as well as being the first point of call for curing the itch.[86] More widely, irregulars absorbed 38 per cent of spending on medical people in the parochial sample between 1750 and 1790. As with nursing there was no sustained typological variation in the

propensity for parishes to engage irregulars. Spatial variation was more marked. Parishes in Northamptonshire, Leicestershire and Lancashire spent proportionately more on this group than other counties. By contrast Berkshire spent little on this group, while in Norfolk there are less than 40 references to irregulars across the whole eighteenth-century sample. The Norfolk parish of Lyng was, however, the only one to employ a phrenologist, with Mr Vassaw retained to examine lumps and bumps in 1803.[87]

There are good reasons to expect significant change in this picture over time. On the face of it, doctoring contracts gave little financial incentive for parochial officers to stray beyond the local medical man. Where they did, as we have already seen, there is evidence of engagement with other doctors in the same locality or region. Attempts at national and local level to drive out the quack are also well known.[88] Yet there were countervailing influences. Better postal services and new ways of advertising allowed irregulars to consult by post as effectively as doctors.[89] In 1766, for instance, 'Messrs Negus and Church' were sending diagnoses and medicines by post from London to the Norfolk parish of Scottow.[90] In turn, some irregulars achieved regional or national notoriety. Thus when in October 1806 the Chorley vestry determined to send Thomas Partington's son to Dr Taylor of Heywood near Bolton (the 'Witworth doctor') 'to get his opinion upon whether his hand can be cured', they were following the path of vestries and overseers across Lancashire, Westmorland, Cheshire and Yorkshire who sent paupers to see this famous bonesetter.[91] In the Midlands, the parishes of Geddington, Braunston, Islip, Woodford Halse, Pilton, Brafield, Ashby St Leger, Stoke Albany, Welton, Abington and Crick all sent paupers to 'the Welford doctor', also known as 'the water doctor'. The Leicestershire parish of Oxendon had a substantial reliance on this irregular, Dr Orton of Welford, from 1781 to 1834, including seventeen individual cases in 1793 alone, while Woodford Halse sent six cases in 1808.[92]

Nor did other groups of irregulars succumb to the pressure of doctors expanding their remit as fast or completely as much of the established literature would suggest. In midwifery, for instance, it is certainly true that many more births were delivered by male doctors in the nineteenth century than had been the case fifty years earlier.[93] Indeed, some of our parishes fit the historiographical model rather

well. At Bickerstaffe (Lancashire), for instance, female midwives were at least an annual and usually a multiple annual expense in the 1760s and 1770s, with events paid in the range of 2–5s.[94] In the 1780s the rise of doctoring contracts all but eliminated the female midwife, who was replaced by lower-level female nursing and attendance during 'lying in'. Not until the very end of 1790s did midwives make a re-appearance, and then they were paid at a third or half of the rate accorded to their male doctoring counterparts undertaking the same work as an exception to contract.[95] Yet female midwives remained a core part of provision in almost half of parishes, especially in Norfolk and Berkshire.[96] Indeed, there is evidence that paupers demanded traditional female practitioners and that parishes were sometimes obliged to turn back to this group having made alternative arrangements. Thus, in July 1803, Mary Tootell was to 'be employed as midwife at the [Chorley] workhouse for the future', which suggests some dissatisfaction with the parish doctor.[97] Irregulars also held on in other areas of activity. Widow Palgrave was paid in October 1797 for 'Nockalating' two children,[98] while across the entire sample (but particularly in Northamptonshire) cures for 'the itch' and 'scald head' fell disproportionately to medical irregulars. Moreover, there were forty-two references across all county samples to leech providers, with this group – consisting of farmers, fishermen and other local tradespeople – increasing in number over time.

The nineteenth century was also to bring a considerable expansion in the number of quacks, druggists and others even in the smallest of places, widening the scope of the medical market. This issue is taken up at length in Chapters 6 and 9, but in the meantime it can be stated that it would be very strange indeed if parochial officers in some places at least did not respond with reference to a wider palette of medical people. Thus, while Norfolk parishes may have employed few irregulars, they sourced large amounts of drugs in order that the poor might dose themselves. Across the country in east Northamptonshire the Rothwell-based quack Abbey Heygate produced an extremely expensive 'medicine' which was sold to five other nearby parishes. In 1824, Rothwell parish itself paid £2 4s 6d for a course of the medicine intended for self-dosing by Mrs Payne.[99] Nowhere was resort to quacks and druggists stronger than in West Yorkshire, where townships were spending significant sums each year on medicines obtained from providers in Leeds.

These emblematic examples, set against the complex parochial relationship with doctors noted above, demonstrate that parishes did (and perhaps had to) continue to engage irregulars on some scale even in the 1820s and 1830s. This process was facilitated by stable or falling unit costs across almost all services and products, a fact that allowed officials to commission more treatment events even when the relative place of irregulars in the spending category medical people declined after the 1790s. As an analogue to the doctoring typologies outlined above, it is possible to trace three broad parochial attitudes. First, there were places which completely or largely dispensed with irregulars. We have seen that Norfolk could boast a particular concentration of such parishes, but individual parochial examples can be found in all of the county sub-samples. Bickerstaffe and Easington (Lancashire) dispensed almost entirely with irregulars from the 1780s, as did Syston and Normanton (Leicestershire) from the early 1800s and King's Sutton and Wellingborough (Northamptonshire) from 1810.[100] A second group of parishes turned to irregular providers and treatments episodically alongside doctors and nursing care. Such attitudes dominated the parochial landscape in Leicestershire and (at a lower level of total cost) Berkshire, Lancashire and Wiltshire. Finally, a suite of communities maintained the diversity of approach seen in the 1750s. Among Norfolk parishes, for instance, Forncett St Peter stands out. The parochial authorities consulted eight different doctors in the 1760s in addition to Dr Jones, who was under contract at £4 per year. Across the period 1750–1800 they also retained Samuel Farrow (for bonesetting), Joseph Snelling (a farmer who cured scald head), the irregular eye doctor Mr Townifoot of Norwich, Mr Graty (for the itch), Mrs Brown (for blistering) and the Rev. Dr Cookson for poultices. Between 1800 and 1834, parochial officers turned to eleven further irregulars, including Mrs Brice for amputations and Mr Penn for applying his 'special' poultices to cure the itch.[101] Forncett was, however, unusual among Norfolk communities, and parishes with the greatest diversity of approach were disproportionately concentrated in West Yorkshire and Northamptonshire. This situation speaks to a developing theme in the chapter, that of the existence of ingrained local cultures of medical care. It is to this matter that we finally turn.

Pauper attitudes and local cultures

Parochial policy on the requisite constellation of doctors, nurses and irregulars was influenced by the expectations of the poor and their advocates. When John Hall, writing from Chelmsford to Colchester (both Essex) on 6 May 1816, noted that 'you know Sir Every Poor has a Doctor Allowe^d them', he was expressing a sense of right and analogous parochial duties which spans the spatial and typological dimensions of the data.[102] Both those whose sickness drove them into the arms of the poor law and those who became sick while poor assumed, by the early nineteenth century, that a doctor could and would be paid for. The immediacy of the poor's perceived right to doctoring is best demonstrated in the 1829 census of Warmsworth (Yorkshire), where the entry for John Firth, his wife and his five resident children was accompanied by a note that he was ill and that his wife had 'gone for doctor on [the] river'.[103] In turn, the volume of doctor's testimony added as postscripts to letters or in the form of short notes on particular cases sent to parochial authorities suggests that by the 1800s the poor had come to invest the status of doctors with totemic power in their engagements with officials. The crisis of the Old Poor Law was associated with the growing provision of medical welfare, but within that also with the increasing medicalisation of the lives of poor people at the hands of doctors.

Of even longer duration was an assumption, shared by officials and paupers in most places, that family and neighbourhood nursing would be augmented or substituted with care from nurses paid by the parish. James Brown, the clerk of King's Lynn (Norfolk), wrote to the overseer of Oxford St Michael parish on 28 November 1769 on the subject of the eighty-six-year-old Sarah Doe. Noting her to be a 'Decent clean Woman', he asked Oxford to increase her weekly allowance of 2s because 'she is obliged to have a Woman to assist her and what is 2s a Week for two people to live on'.[104] Exactly similar sentiments were expressed at the opposite end of our period by John Sharpe, who wrote to Shipton-under-Wychwood (Oxfordshire) from Brighton (Sussex) on 27 March 1832. He claimed that his wife was unwell and that he must have a doctor and nurse. Unable to afford one himself, he demanded that Shipton provide the means, noting that 'I know this parish [Brighton] allow'd him [a neighbour] 15/- a week & paid is

doctor with but one child.'[105] Even officials in Norfolk recognised the utility of providing nursing, though they paid those nurses relatively poorly, retained girls rather than women and disproportionately used the labour of other paupers.

My letters give no sense that paupers and officials had a shared understanding of rights to attendance by irregulars. Nonetheless, vestry minutes, *ad hoc* comments in accounts and the correspondence of officials do show that parishes expected and were expected to respond creatively to medical emergencies such as broken bones and difficult births. Even where these things were covered by a doctoring contract, the immediacy of the need (officials in West Yorkshire, for instance, generally distinguished between broken bones and those where the fracture was 'bad') might drive recourse to an alternative provider. It was, however, after recourse had already been taken to contracted and local doctors that irregulars came into their own. Long histories of the receipt of medical welfare at the individual level were frequently punctuated or tailed by the attendance of irregular providers either *in situ* or at their places of residence. It is hard to escape the feeling of exasperation or desperation with which such accounting entries were written.

Yet, as the experiences of Norfolk (with regard to nursing) and Leicestershire (with regard to doctoring) parishes show, a generalised sense of right masks subtleties in the extent to which it could be realised. Across all parishes there was an assumption that paupers would have exhausted their own means in order to pay the bills of medical people. Indeed, paupers and advocates made sure that they pointed to this fact in their correspondence with officials. At the start of our period, on 24 March 1754, Thomas Bayer wrote 'At your desire (being old Neighbours' from Watford (Hertfordshire) to Oxford saying that he found 'no likelihood of Silvester Wife's recover[ing] for some time'. Bayer further noted that Silvester's husband 'has been obliged to sell most of his Goods, part, he says, payed the Docto'r Bill'.[106] At the other end of our period Elizabeth Stephenson wrote to Beverley on 3 June 1832 saying that her daughter had been 'very hill and not able to do any thing this last fortnight'. Asking for 'somthing more in Addison [sic] to what you have aloud', she noted, 'I have been obligd to break into my rent to get her suport.'[107] There were also, of course, local and regional particularities affecting the construction of pauper rights to doctors and nurses. Letter writers from the north seem to have assumed that

they needed to specify the depletion of their own resources in more detail than those in the south or Midlands.[108] They certainly also had to be alive to the pitfalls of having proximate family. When Thomas Green applied to the Halliwell vestry for relief on 3 October 1816 'having a lame son', the ratepayers concluded that because Thomas was in work he 'shall allow his son Jno a sufficient maintenance with him and that the overseer visit them occasionally to see same done'.[109] Indeed, across northern England, the exploration of legal obligations on kin to care for each by parish officers was more regular and more determined than elsewhere.[110] In part reflecting these attitudes, but also a negotiating strategy more widely, paupers in the north and Midlands were much more likely to seek partnership in paying for medical people than were those from Wiltshire or Berkshire. This theme is taken up at greater length in Chapter 9, but an emblematic example is John Gann, who applied to Oundle (Northamptonshire) for help for his wife's sickness. The vestry, in replying to the overseer of his host parish, noted that 'it is not usual for the Parish to do so [pay an allowance] where the man has 12/- per week in a constant place and only one child. But in their case they do it on account of the good character given by you of the man & the unfortunate situation of his wife', awarding 2s 6d per week '*towards* the expense required by his wife's illness'.[111] These important subtleties notwithstanding, the correspondence of overseers, advocates and paupers shows that there was a shared understanding by the early nineteenth-century, if not earlier in many places, that parishes would and ought to ensure that the sick poor had access to a basic landscape of medical people. As Jonathan Thorpe, writing from Leeds (West Yorkshire) to Rothersthorpe (Northamptonshire) in October 1809, noted, 'the Gentlemen here order the medicals [doctors] at the least of trifles and so you must make an order [for a doctor] to help this youre poor parishioner as the light fades on my life'.[112]

Conclusion

Geoffrey Oxley has suggested that 'There were good [economic and moral] reasons why medical treatment should have been extended to the poor as soon as it became available.'[113] There is much evidence to support the idea that parishes saw attendance by medical people as a core part of this implicit contract with parishioners. Spending on

other elements of medical welfare increased faster than that on doctors, nurses and irregulars across our period. Indeed, the landscape of medical people was less varied, and arguably less chaotic, by the 1830s than it had been in the 1750s. Doctoring contracts brought a tighter order to this landscape at the same time as they contained relative costs and established a more dominant role for doctors themselves in this broad spending category.[114] Yet it was still a rich patchwork and one surprisingly immune to typological variation. In particular there is no evidence at all of urban–rural dichotomies which underpinned the experience of the local and regional medical market by middling consumers. Moreover, a focus simply on amounts spent at the all-parish level masks some very complex constellations of doctors, nurses and irregulars in individual parishes and for particular counties. At one end of the spectrum, Norfolk parishes clearly came to have an early reliance on contracted and *ad hoc* doctoring at the expense of nursing and the engagement of irregulars. Berkshire officials, by contrast, came to rely rather more on nursing as a core response to sickness, with doctors less prominent as a spending category.

This sort of representation is, however, in itself problematic, both because of the deflationary influences on the costs of doctors and irregulars noted above and because significant doctoring and nursing bills were 'hidden' in cash allowances given to the poor. The key observation for this study is thus that overseers, paupers and advocates assumed a right to access medical people on a scale and spectrum that would not have looked out of place for the labouring poor or indeed the lower middling orders. This is not to assume that such provision was of high quality, but even here the lack of complaints about doctors and nurses in the considerable corpus of correspondence available is striking. The nature of pauper experiences of medical welfare, however, also depended on where the provision of medical people by the parochial authorities sat in relation to other spending categories and within the wider economy of makeshifts. It is to these issues that the rest of this study turns.

Notes

1 For the structure of the medical profession, qualifications and regulation, see R. O'Day, *The Professions in Early Modern England, 1450–1800: Servants of the Commonweal* (London: Longman, 2000).

2 On the propensity for doctors to deliver short factual narrative in their engagement with officers, see S. King and Jones, 'Testifying for the poor'.

3 EYRO, PE1-702-80, letter (underlining and crossing-out in the original).

4 EYRO, PE1-702-38, letter, 23 September 1832.

5 BRO, D/P 132/18/15/35, letter. Moore assumed the parish would wish to act even though the cause of need was venereal disease. On public attitudes towards venereal diseases, see Siena, *Venereal Disease*. In other cases the treatment of venereal disease took the form of loans. See for instance the agreement between Alice Haslam, Sarah Haslam and the overseer of Little Bolton (Lancashire) for the loan of £1 1s to pay Dr Barrow's bill 'for curing the said Sarah of the French Pox'. BALS, ZZ/238/1/130, agreement, 11 March 1763.

6 The term 'irregular practitioner' itself is fluid since the boundaries between those considering themselves surgeons and apothecaries and other providers were often blurred. See Loudon, 'The vile race of quacks', pp. 106–28; R. Porter, *Quacks: Fakers and Charlatans in English Medicine* (Stroud: Sutton Publishing, 2000); and D. Porter and R. Porter, *Patient's Progress*, pp. 96–116.

7 The label 'doctor' will be used in its widest possible sense, since there is much evidence that neither poor law officials nor paupers made much distinction between different types of practitioner.

8 Exactly comparable data is difficult to extract from the existing historiography, but see Marland, *Medicine and Society*.

9 Lane, *A Social History of Medicine*, pp. 49–50, claims that this experience was primarily associated with small rural areas. For a more nuanced reading relating to East Bedfordshire, see S. Williams, 'Practitioners' income', p. 168.

10 'Contract' means a recorded agreement between one or more practitioners to provide medical services to parishes or communities with an element of fixed price rather than any sliding scale or per capita agreement.

11 WRO, 811/126, overseers' accounts. On the label 'surgeoness', see A. Wyman, 'The surgeoness: The female practitioner of surgery 1400–1800', *Medical History*, 28 (1984), 22–41.

12 The concentration in these counties has nothing to do with enhanced availability of doctors in comparison to other counties. See J. Lane, 'The medical practitioners of provincial England in 1783', *Medical History*, 28 (1984), 353–71, at p. 355.

13 This experience can be seen more widely. Northallerton and Richmond had no contracts until 1776 and 1788 respectively. See Hastings, *Poverty and the Poor Law*, p. 14.

14 LRO, PR 2995/1/13, overseers' accounts.

15 The charge of 2s made by the 'midcall man' in Northampton to attest the overseer's conclusion that the illness suffered by the Tebbot family 'is of no common nature' and 'arises from the want of all the common necessities of life' was an administrative expense and one common across the sample. See NRO, 110p/138/15, letter, 24 October 1830. Other administrative expenses abound: Dr Sinclair of Hulme billed the parish for 'Examining pauper lunatics and writing certificates as to their state of mind'. MCL, M10/810, bill.

16 S. Williams, 'Practitioners' income', pp. 162–3, sees a 'prominent' association between increased recourse to doctoring contracts and the extension of workhouse provision. There is little evidence for this in the current sample. However, the Walthamstow vestry resolved on 24 April 1769 that welfare was to be paid only to those in the poorhouse and that 'no Relief be granted to Any of such poor Persons but from the Apothecary', whose contract does not survive. See J. Gibson, *The Walthamstow Charities: Caring for the Poor 1500–2000* (Chichester: Phillimore, 2000), p. 41.

17 By the 1820s and 1830s there was fierce contemporary debate over the practice of contracting doctors on the one hand and the accumulation of local positions by doctors on the other. See for instance T. Hodgkin, *On the Mode of Selecting Medical Men for Professional Attendance on the Poor of a Parish or District* (Lindfield: The Hunterian Society, 1836).

18 Digby, *Making a Medical Living*, p. 119, and S. Williams, 'Practitioners' income', pp. 170–4.

19 On the difficulty of discerning whether a contract actually existed see Ramsbottom, 'Christopher Waddington's peers', p. 135.

20 This is a surprising trend given that in 1783 only five other counties had more doctors than, say, Norfolk. See Lane, 'The medical practitioners', p. 355.

21 S. Williams, 'Practitioners' income', pp. 162–4, by contrast, finds that in east Bedfordshire the primary reason for moving to contracts was to contain or reduce spending as parochial finances came under 'exceptionally heavy pressure in the latter half of the eighteenth century'. See also Marland, *Medicine and Society*, pp. 58–9.

22 S. Williams, 'Practitioners' income'.

23 Lane, *A Social History of Medicine*, p. 50, sees all-inclusive contracts as common and exclusions 'occasional' in Warwickshire. Precisely the opposite is true in this sample.

24 DRO, PE/SW/VE1/1, vestry minutes.

25 NRO, 92p/117, Crick memorandum book.

26 NORO, PD 100/88, vestry minutes.

27 NRO, 143p/106, contract draft.

28 Unsurprisingly given the larger sample size, the definitive step-like nature of increased remuneration (after 1806) and relative stability (after 1815) found for east Bedfordshire by Samantha Williams is not duplicated here. S. Williams, 'Practitioners' income', pp. 177–8.

29 LRO, PR 418/1, overseers' accounts, and 422/1, overseers' accounts.

30 NRO, 350p/162, overseers' accounts.

31 It is largely for this reason that we see an inconsistent relationship between contract value and the size of the parochial population. See S. Williams, 'Practitioners' incomes', pp. 167.

32 DRO, PE/SW/VE1/1, vestry minutes.

33 R. Lilly, *An Account of Rural Medical Practice from the 18th Century Onwards in Long Bucky, Northamptonshire* (Dunton Bassett: Volcano, 1993), pp. 25–7.

34 A point also made by Lane for Warwickshire, which had a slower take-up of contracts. See Lane, *A Social History of Medicine*, p. 50.

35 For further context see *Administration & Operation of the Poor Laws 1833* (London: Fellowes, 1833), pp. 3, 39, 63, 65, 70, 72, 74, 75 and 132.

36 In contrast to east Bedfordshire, where contracted surgeon apothecaries met 'most of the medical needs of the poor' and had their contracts renewed annually. See S. Williams, 'Practitioners' income', pp. 160, 183.

37 Dropsy equates to water-retention. Warren, *Extracts from the Accounts*.

38 NRO, 251p/25–29 and 36/1–19, overseers' accounts.

39 NRO, 325p/194/142 and 143, letter and certificate.

40 CRO, P143/19/9/153, undated letter, probably 1821.

41 See for instance J. Hulbert, *Farming the Sick Poor and Other Observations on the Necessity of Establishing a Different System of Affording Medical Relief to the Sick Poor, than by the Practice of Contracting with Medical Men or the Farming of Parishes* (London: Longman, 1827).

42 BRO, D/P 132/18/12/25, letter.

43 Crowther, 'Health care and poor relief', p. 209, suggests that West Yorkshire doctors were remunerated generously and that the role of parish doctor was attractive. This perspective is shared by Lane, *A Social History of Medicine*, p. 50.

44 NRO, GI 375, volume of surgeons' accounts 1774–93.

45 See P. Stanley, *For Fear of Pain: British Surgery, 1790–1850* (Amsterdam: Rodopi, 2003).

46 WRO, CL/CHI/22, bill.

47 See contributions to R. Porter (ed.), *Patients and Practitioners: Lay Perceptions of Medicine in Pre-Industrial Society* (Cambridge: Polity Press, 1985), and D. Porter and R. Porter, *Patient's Progress*.

48 NRO, 49p/151, bill. See also J. Lane, 'Eighteenth century medical practice: A case study of Bradford Wilmer, surgeon of Coventry, 1737–1813',
Social History of Medicine, 3 (1990), 369–86.

49 EYRO, PE1-702-62, letter.

50 S. King, Nutt and Tomkins, *Narratives of the Poor*, p. 277.

51 WYRO, BDP 17/84, guard book; RPC, letter, 14 May 1815.

52 MCL, M10/814, letter, 3 June 1837.

53 DRO, PE/SW/VE/1/1, vestry minutes.

54 SRO, D/P/Twn/9/1/1, copy letter book 1832–33; D/P/Mls/13/2/9,
letter book 1826–35.

55 R. Porter, 'The patient in England', p. 94.

56 Ibid., p. 100.

57 There are considerable ambiguities over how to define what a nurse was,
to understand what he or she 'did' and to consistently trace nurses in the
sources. In particular there were subtle overlaps between doctoring and
nursing. When Dr Fred Bluntington wrote to the overseers of Hull on
the subject of Xerxes Bishoprick, who had been suffering from a cold and
bronchitis, he noted that he could not say anything about the state of the
family at home because 'I have not visited Xerxes at his own house; (for
he has Mended at my Surgery)'. EYRO, PE1-702-130, letter, 6 April
1836. However, overseers' accounts are replete with entries where the
detailed composition of a bill for 'nursing widow X' might comprise
carrying, washing, mending, childcare, nursing, attending, 'doing for'
someone and laying out the dead body all in one consolidated block.
This suggests that officials maintained a very expansive definition of
the duties associated with the label 'nurse', and that they could make a
distinction between regular 'nurses' and the providers of *ad hoc* 'nursing
services'. A broad definition of status and duties underpins the following
discussion.

58 S. Taylor, 'Aspects of the socio-demographic history of seven Berkshire
parishes in the eighteenth century' (unpublished PhD thesis, University
of London, 1987), p. 397, suggests that the proportion of all poor law
resources devoted to nursing in seven Berkshire parishes fell from a slim
1.7 per cent in the 1760s to a tiny 0.006 per cent by the early 1800s.
S. Williams, 'Caring for the sick poor: Poor law nurses in Bedfordshire
c.1770–1834', in P. Lane, N. Raven and K. Snell (eds), *Women, Work
and Wages in England 1600–1850* (Woodbridge: Boydell and Brewer,
2004), p. 165, sees a similar linear decline for Shefford (from a more healthy
4.8 per cent in the 1790s to 1 per cent by the 1820s) and a slightly more varied
trajectory for Campton (where the figure fell from 2 per cent in the 1770s to
0.6 per cent in the 1780s before rising and then falling to just 0.2 per cent in

the 1820s). For our sample, Berkshire devoted the highest percentage of its total welfare spending to nursing over the period (0.95 per cent), while the equally rural Norfolk devoted the lowest (0.22 per cent).

59 NRO, 325p/193/12, letter, 29 August 1824.

60 This dichotomy is important. When Elizabeth Dowling wrote from London to the overseer of Peterborough at an unspecified date in early 1834 to say that her mother had undergone a paralytic stroke, she confirmed the ubiquity of family labour: 'she cannot move herself only as I lift her about, she does everything as she lies, her money [an allowance from the parish] will hardly by [sic] soap and extra fireing without my labour'. NRO, 261p/244, letter 14.

61 See Hodgkinson, *The Origins*; C. Helmstadter and J. Godden, *Nursing before Nightingale, 1815–1899* (Farnham: Ashgate, 2011), pp. 1 24; P. Williams, 'Religion, respectability and the origins of the modern nurse', in R. French and A. Wear (eds), *British Medicine in an Age of Reform* (London: Routledge, 1991), pp. 234–47; and A. Borsay and B. Hunter, 'Nursing and midwifery: Historical approaches', in A. Borsay and B. Hunter (eds), *Nursing and Midwifery in Britain since 1700* (Basingstoke: Palgrave, 2012), pp. 8–9.

62 J. Boulton, 'Welfare systems and the parish nurse in early modern London, 1650–1725', *Family and Community History*, 10 (2007), 127–52.

63 S. Williams, 'Caring for the Sick Poor', pp. 141–69.

64 A. Borsay, 'Nursing, 1700–1830: Families, communities, institutions', in Borsay and Hunter (eds), *Nursing and Midwifery*, pp. 27–9 and 37–9, quote at p. 29; C. Hallett, 'Nursing, 1830–1920: Forging a profession', in Borsay and Hunter (eds), *Nursing and Midwifery*, does not mention the Old Poor Law at all.

65 There is evidence in the underlying data for this viewpoint. In August 1751 the Wimbledon vestry determined that if any pensioner was fit enough to work but refused to do so, they would have their allowances rescinded. F. Cowe, *Wimbledon Vestry Minutes 1736, 1743–1788* (Guildford: Surrey Record Society, 1964), p. 22. In our sample, only a small proportion (22 per cent) of nurses employed on any basis were, at the point when they started nursing, paupers.

66 S. Williams, 'Caring for the sick poor', p. 165.

67 S. Williams, 'Caring for the sick poor', p. 152, talks of three types of carer; the categories employed here are more numerous, reflecting the complex nursing structures and experiences that emerge when considering multiple parishes across county boundaries.

68 S. Williams, 'Caring for the sick poor', p. 158. Borsay and Hunter, 'Nursing and midwifery', p. 21 suggest that 'professionalisation' was a product of

the later nineteenth century. Since 'professional' is a perceived as well as an ascribed and claimed status, I use the term here to reflect parochial employment policies which might indicate trust, skills or other yardsticks of worth.

69 See O. Davies, 'Female healers in nineteenth-century England', in N. Goose (ed.), *Women's Work in Industrial England: Regional and Local Perspectives* (Hatfield: Local Population Studies, 2007), pp. 229–31.

70 BRO, D/P 29/12/4, overseers' accounts (my italics).

71 NORO, PD 421/132, overseers' accounts.

72 NRO, 261p/256, vestry minutes.

73 BRO, D/P 23/18/3, workhouse book.

74 For other examples, see M. Fissell, *Patients, Power, and the Poor in Eighteenth-Century Bristol* (Cambridge: Cambridge University Press, 2002), pp. 61 and 66.

75 BRO, D/P 23/18/3, workhouse book.

76 See also Fissell, *Patients, Power*, p. 106.

77 Ibid., p. 96.

78 NORO, PD 552/66, overseers' accounts.

79 BRO, D/P 7/12/1, overseers' accounts; D/P 23/18/3, workhouse book.

80 S. Williams, 'Caring for the sick poor', p. 157, suggests that in 1837 Norfolk parishes were on the higher end of the spectrum. These findings also contrast with S. Taylor, 'Aspects', who sees rather more parsimony in his sample of Berkshire parishes.

81 Berkshire and Northamptonshire also seem to have had a particular tendency to employ male nurses for insane patients. Such nurses invariably cost more than their female counterparts.

82 See also M. Pelling, 'Thoroughly resented? Older women and the medical role in early modern England', in L. Hunter and S. Hutton (eds), *Women, Science and Medicine 1500–1700* (Stroud: Sutton, 1997), pp. 63–87.

83 There is no single definition of irregulars but the group runs across spectrum from quacks to local wise men and women.

84 NRO, 1p/166, overseers' accounts.

85 NRO, 356p/28, vestry minutes.

86 NRO, 92p/122–4, overseers' accounts.

87 NORO, PD 374/56, overseers' accounts.

88 Loudon, 'Medical practitioners', p. 226; I. Loudon, 'The nature of provincial medical practice in eighteenth-century England', *Medical History*, 29 (1985), 1–32.

89 For an overview, see Wild, *Medicine-by-Post*.

90 NORO, PD 145/47, overseers' accounts.

91 CPL, Vestry Minutes, and J. West, *The Taylors of Lancashire: Bonesetters and Doctors 1750–1890* (Worsley: Privately Published, 1977). For context see R. Cooter, 'Bones of contention? Orthodox medicine and the mystery of the bone-setter's craft', in W. Bynum and R. Porter (eds), *Medical Fringe and Medical Orthodoxy, 1750–1850* (London: Wellcome Trust, 1987), pp. 158–73.

92 NRO, 251p/25–9 and 36/1–19, overseers' accounts; 251p/23, vestry minutes. There is nothing in the data to support Digby's assertion that traditional, folk and irregular healing survived largely in the north and rural areas by the early nineteenth century. Digby, *Making a Medical Living*, p. 64.

93 For background, see A. Wilson, *The Making of Man-Midwifery: Childbirth in England 1660–1770* (Cambridge, Massachusetts: Harvard University Press, 1995), and A. Tomkins, 'Demography and the midwives: Deliveries and their denouements in north Shropshire, 1781–1803', *Continuity and Change*, 25 (2010), 199–232.

94 This range of fees was a constant across northern England at the time.

95 LRO, PR 418 and 422, overseers' accounts.

96 Tomkin's sense that midwives could be part of packages of support which was extensive even if not expensive is borne out across this sample. Tomkins, 'Demography and the midwives', p. 126. See also Lane, *A Social History of Medicine*, p. 48, who finds local female midwives to have been delivering the majority of babies in Warwickshire.

97 CPL, vestry minutes.

98 NORO, PD 145/47, overseers' accounts.

99 NRO, 284p/189, vestry minutes, 28 February 1824.

100 For context see Lane, *A Social History of Medicine*, pp. 51–3.

101 NORO, PD 421/132–7, overseers' accounts.

102 Sokoll, *Essex Pauper Letters*, p. 301.

103 DHC, DD/BW/Local/58, Warmsworth census, 9 February 1829.

104 ORO, PAR Oxford St Martin 211/5/C1/1/36, letter.

105 ORO, PAR 236/5/A13/2/3, letter.

106 ORO, PAR Oxford St Martin 207/5/A7/5, letter.

107 EYRO, PE1-702-49, letter.

108 S. King, 'Regional patterns'.

109 BALS, PHA 1-3, Halliwell township books.

110 The contrast with Norfolk is particularly important. Parishes here explored the potential of familial support but they also tended to pay for such support with a regularity which we do not see in northern parishes.

111 NRO, 249p/216, letter, 30 April 1834 (my italics).

112 RPC, letter, 11 October 1809.

113 Oxley, *Poor Relief*, p. 65.

114 Most remarkably in the whole sample, the contract agreed by East
     Dereham with Dr Woods in 1805 was at a lower stipend than its first
     contract with a doctor agreed in 1753. NORO, PD 86, overseers'
     accounts.

6

Wider medical welfare

Introduction

On 19 March 1834 George Taylor, proprietor of the 'Norwich Truss Manufactory', sent a printed bill to Wighton (Norfolk). Enclosed with the bill was an 'Improved Double Truss (38 inches)' ordered for John Ladell at the cost of £1 5s. A handwritten addendum expressed hopes that the truss:

> may suit your workman and as I conclude his Hernia is bad, I have sent two [extra] springs in case the main springs are not strong enough, which can be applied by sliding off the casing and letting the extra springs embrace the main one. Also to keep the truss steady, have put to it under straps to pass under round the thigh and button on the stud in the front pad, these need not be used if the patient can do without. Any alteration shall have the best attention of Sir, Your obt servt G Taylor
>
> Should the patient after a time not be able to get on <u>well</u> with it if he could come up by a carrier for the greater part of the day, I am confident of giving him relief.[1]

A small rural parish was willing to respond to a debilitating case of hernia by buying an expensive truss from a specialist manufacturer. In this, it was keying into a wider socio-technological movement that had come by the 1830s to see deformity and bodily decay as by degrees remediable.[2] Wighton was not alone among Norfolk communities. Denton regularly purchased adult and child trusses, which ranged on a cost spectrum from 4s 6d to (for a double truss) 25s. When a hernia grew or shrank or the truss became worn, repairs and alterations were done in Norwich, and the parish was consistently ready to meet the partial cost of trusses where individuals and families had themselves

found resources before applying.[3] Other examples abound. As early as 22 November 1777 Forncett St Peter was paying Noah Nichols 'for carrying Wm Kerrison twice to Norwich after a truss', while at the other end of the period, in July 1831, overseers were paying 11s for 'Loveday's Truss, Kemp bringing them [from Norwich]'.[4] Nor did parishes just turn to Norwich; several bought steel trusses from makers in Reepham and Salhouse. There is no doubt that some purchases were driven by exogenous factors – in Lyng, for instance, discharged hospital patients seem to have carried with them demands from doctors that trusses be provided[5] – but most were discretionary and part of a wider package of support for individuals experiencing 'rupture'. Nowhere is this clearer than in Scottow, where between 1801 and 1834 Robert and John Kemp, John Thistle and Thomas Grimes were provided with multiple trusses, including some from local makers, others from Norwich and (in March 1830 for John Thistle) a 'patent Double Truss' from London at the cost of 22s plus carriage. These and other individuals also received cash allowances in their own right or to support families, the services of doctors, clothing, fuel, rent payments and 'sundries'.[6] There is clearly much here to support Anne Crowther's view that in some places at least the Old Poor Law provided a comprehensive medical service.[7]

The picture for other counties is more varied. In Wiltshire, Chippenham St Andrew purchased trusses between the 1740s and 1770s, but mainly for children and hardly at all after 1776.[8] Trowbridge likewise purchased trusses for those with 'broke belly' in the period between the 1740s and 1760s, including 'fustian belly trusses' and steel spring versions. Most were made up locally by Mrs Fryer from material purchased by the overseer. Children again figured strongly as recipients during this period, after which there is little evidence of further purchases for any pauper.[9] Marlbrough St Peter purchased 'elastic trusses from Messrs Pinkney and Maurice' in the 1790s as part of long-term relief packages for most of the individuals concerned, but never for children.[10] Outside these larger communities, however, evidence for the provision of devices like trusses is almost non-existent. Sopworth spent 10s on a truss for Mrs Peracilla Barton in 1816 but this is the only reference in an otherwise complete set of poor law accounts.[11] For most of rural Wiltshire there is no evidence at all. This polarity is repeated across the country: industrial parishes in counties such as Lancashire

spent money on trusses and other devices while their equivalents in West Yorkshire did not; rural communities in Berkshire purchased trusses while very similar parishes in Leicestershire did not. Some of these spending patterns reflect differences in the nature of labour (and thus susceptibility to 'broke belly'), the penetration of friendly societies (where benefits might include devices) and local knowledge of advances in surgical techniques.[12] Yet, and as the tendency for a handful of communities across the sample to spend significant sums on trusses for children suggests, we can also detect a difference of sentiment between parishes.[13] Against this backdrop, the current chapter explores the range and depth of spending on wider elements of medical welfare. Some of the big themes of Chapter 4 – the inexorable rise in the importance of cash allowances, the limited quantitative importance of spending on drugs apparent in some counties, the fluctuating and in some places modest provision of in-kind benefits, and the highly volatile 'other' category of medical welfare – are central to the chapter. It seeks both to explore broad trends but also to give an insight into significant spatial differences in the complexion if not level of spending.

Drugs and devices

Chapter 4 suggested that the provision of drugs and devices by parochial officials absorbed a modest part (just 1–2 per cent on average) of the medical welfare budget across the period, though rather higher rates for Leicestershire and West Yorkshire were also highlighted.[14] Interpreting this observation is by no means simple. Thus, all Norfolk parishes blurred the boundary between drink and drugs, systematically purchasing brandy, beer, porter, wine, rum, gin and unspecified 'liquor' for the sick, presumably as a form of pain relief. At the individual level the amounts could be significant. In Warham Mrs Smith received six pints of wine over eight days in 1773, while in 1821 'Standgroom's and Woodrow's children' shared three and a half bottles of wine at a cost of 15s 9d. The parish of Holme Next the Sea paid for three gallons of gin for William Bull in 1776, while Tower's wife was allowed a prodigious amount (23s 9d worth) of beer when ill at Scottow in April 1807.[15] Some of this alcohol was provided 'by order of the doctor', but most was supplied direct by overseers.[16] The contrast with other counties is profound: in so far as it was ever supplied as a drug, alcohol as a general

category of spending tended to fall off sharply after the 1750s. There are colourful examples of individual supply – the fifteen gallons of gin provided over two weeks in 1792 for John Ward of Syston (Leicestershire), for instance[17] – but by the late eighteenth century most parishes in most counties reserved purchases for those in their last illness or individuals and families afflicted with smallpox.[18] More widely, it is not always obvious whether the purchase of other foodstuffs for paupers and their nurses was for nourishment or as basic ingredients of remedies.[19] Thus Norfolk parishes uniformly provided oatmeal for poultices, while their Berkshire and West Yorkshire counterparts supplied bread.

Other contextual complexities abound. Most obviously, the unit cost of medicaments and many medical devices remained relatively stable over the long term. It was thus possible for paupers to be accessing more drugs even as the relative importance of the spending category in overall medical welfare remained small or fell.[20] The question of whether this was the representative experience is, however, entangled with problems over the visibility of drugs and devices in overseers' accounts. As chapter five suggested, even at their most expansive the bills of doctors and apothecaries provide evidence only of a patchwork of purges, blisters, drops and unspecified pills.[21] Sometimes there was no detail at all. In 1768, Warham (Norfolk) paid 8d for 'sundry goods from the apothecary', while at the other end of our period in 1825 the vestry at Rothwell (Northamptonshire) paid Mr Carpenter the apothecary £8 15s according to his contract but then £35 'additional for his extra trouble during the fever' in the town, without any breakdown of material provisions.[22] Even accounting entries for nursing might be misleading. In 1793, for instance, the Berkshire parish of Shellingford paid Mrs Horton for 'attending Mary Turvey'. A separate voucher indicates that attendance in this case meant provision of leeches, a draught and a purging mixture.[23]

Clearly, then, the parochial and county profiles outlined in Chapter 4 capture only a subset of spending. It is nonetheless possible to discern three broad sources of medicine and device supply for the poor.[24] The first was essentially local or homemade, something which is perhaps not surprising given deeply ingrained traditions of self-dosing on the one hand,[25] and the fact that 'A practitioner's materia medica ... tended to comprise those botanical specimens which could be grown or collected locally' on the other.[26] At their simplest and most ubiquitous these

remedies comprised poultices and salves, either pre-packaged or in the form of ingredients to be made up. In March 1763, Forncett St Peter purchased 'sulphur, tragle [treacle], bark, lard for to cure goody Clark and her children of the itch 1s 4d'.[27] Similar purchases later substituted vinegar for sulphur. Local supply also extended to pain relief (alcohol and opium) and various purgatives.[28] Officials in Caversham (Berkshire) had a particular take on local supply, copying cures for scald head and the itch from *Primitive Physic* into their accounts for 1785. This was part of a determined effort to provide local drugs on a considerable scale, even extending to filicic (a drug made from the roots of ferns) for extended treatment of worm infestations.[29] Unwitting testimony from the records provides further evidence of the local horizon in Caversham; an 1821 entry in the overseers' accounts noted that Hetty Reade had her ferry fees paid for going 'over the water after medicines for Sarah Lloyd'.[30] More widely, if payments for unspecified 'medicines' and 'drugs' equated to local supply then this source would dominate the spending category across all subsets of the data.[31]

Local supply also extended, as we have already seen in the case of trusses, to medical devices. Crutches and 'rolers' (walking frames for those with broken or crippled limbs) were ubiquitous across all counties, while both Berkshire and Wiltshire purchased episodically 'Girdles' or 'quicksilver Girdles' for the cure of the itch and King's Evil.[32] Some wooden legs were also locally made or repaired. In Chorley (Lancashire), a vestry of March 1817 resolved that 'James Rogerson's stump be surveyed' by the overseer prior to the purchase of a wooden leg.[33] At the other end of the country, parish officers for Englefield (Berkshire) purchased one wooden leg a year for Thomas Knight from a suite of local carpenters.[34] For those with deformed rather than absent limbs, parishes often sought local solutions. At Caversham in 1810, Mr Scott was paid £1 6s for reducing the dislocated ankle of John Newman's child and a local cordwainer was paid extra for a single new shoe. Constant dislocations and even more frequent single shoes thereafter suggest that the parish was responding to a case of club foot.[35] Nowhere, however, was such provision more ubiquitous nor more local than in West Yorkshire, where parishes regularly purchased special shoes, 'high shoes' and assorted support instruments such as splints and leg braces, presumably in an effort to get those with physical impairments into sustained work. It is important in this context to note

that local supply did not always (or in Leicestershire usually) equate to 'cheap' or low quality.

Local provision notwithstanding, most parishes also turned (episodically or more regularly) to a second source of supply: the wider regional market.[36] The overseers of Stratford-sub-Castle St Lawrence (Wiltshire) purchased Squary's Mixture from Bath and Dutch Drops (salted liquorice) from Salisbury in 1809 as well as ordering fifteen unspecified medicines from Bristol and Bath in the 1810s.[37] Norfolk parishes made multiple orders for twenty-three discrete medicinal products from Norwich, Ipswich, Downham Market and Bury St Edmunds between the late 1790s and 1820s, including St Anthony Pills and Gully Lotion. Some of these regional remedies were extraordinarily costly. In Salhouse, for instance, 'Dilly Drops for Girl Fuller' cost 33s in 1789.[38] Parishes in West Yorkshire seem to have been particularly likely to access medicines in the regional market, though often at the end of a sustained period of support for sick paupers and their families. Recourse was also had in extremis to the anti-rabies draughts brewed by the Parker family of Brownsholme (Lancashire),[39] but more regularly to saltwater draughts from Fleetwood and other areas of the Lancashire coast, Bushey Drops from Preston, Camphire Salve from Leeds, Hardy Steel Pills from Bolton, Jamaica Drops from Liverpool and Mackle Pills from Wakefield.

In turn, and as we saw with truss makers at the start of the chapter, parishes also turned with regularity to reputed regional device makers. While the provision of wooden legs was surprisingly rare in Norfolk, most other counties turned to regional suppliers. At Welton (Northamptonshire) the vestry paid a Northampton supplier 5s in December 1788 for a pair of wooden legs intended to fit the child Susannah Mann. They were replaced in 1793, 1794, 1798 and 1802, with each replacement more expensive than the last, presumably as the girl grew into young adulthood.[40] The overseers at Trowbridge purchased several wooden legs for 'Whitcomb's girl', paying 14s in 1791 for 'A wooden leg and carriage from Bristol'. In 1819 they spent the extraordinary sum of 42s plus sixpence carriage from Bath on a wooden leg for 'Eliz Franklin's boy', while in 1823 they purchased legs for both young people simultaneously at a cost of 51s.[41] And if parishes in West Yorkshire tended, as we have seen, to buy wooden splints and leg braces, those in the south and Midlands favoured iron or steel devices.

The overseers of Hinton Waldrist (Wiltshire), for instance, purchased leg irons for adult and child paupers, presumably for cases of rickets or club foot.[42]

Finally, parishes had occasional and sometimes concerted recourse to the national drug and device market as officials supplemented, circumvented or substituted the work of their contracted doctors. Forty-two parishes record the purchase of bottles of Daffy's Elixir.[43] Some, like Stanford-in-the-Vale (Berkshire), turned to this well-established palliative with regularity. In general Berkshire parishes were more likely than any other in the sample to turn in this direction. Other medicines appear less regularly but we can find sustained recourse to Star's Ointment, Ward's Paste (for piles), Morison's Pills, Stoughton's Cordial, Cordial Balm of Gilead, Solomon Drops and Stead Pills.[44] Frequent referrals by parishes to specialist doctors outside their immediate region, as traced in Chapter 5, must also have involved proprietary medicines. In turn, recourse to national device makers was also increasingly common, perhaps as a response to the advertising revolution of the early nineteenth century.[45] Stratford-sub-Castle St Lawrence paid the London truss maker William Beach 'for attending and applying a double truss to J White' in January 1831, while Trowbridge paid 'John Cox as part of the expense of a steel apparatus [supplied by the Reading corrective instrument maker John Gale] for his son he being a cripple' in 1824. Stanford-in-the-Vale turned as early as 1768 to Henry Tomey of London for leg irons in the case of William Joyes, and was purchasing 'Bango trusses' by mail order from London in 1804.[46] Leicestershire parishes were particularly likely to commission devices from national suppliers, including frequent purchases of straitjackets, calipers, trusses, steel stays, steel belts, head stays (frames for those with neck injuries) and corrective boots.

In short, the potential landscape of drugs and devices for the poor was extremely and perhaps increasingly rich.[47] Nowhere is the colour of this picture sharper than in Northamptonshire. To take one example, in addition to its doctoring contract the parish of Crick purchased bark, salts of wormwood, physic, Genova cream, 'stuff' for eyes, fever powders, Hooper's Pills, physic, oatmeal, Trooper's Ointment, iron pills, Salts of Steel, mercurial physic, worm mixture, Ormskirk medicine, Norton Drops, syrup of rhubarb, syrup of violets, mustard, Daffy's, Oil of Rum and Southam Mixture. This range of drugs, many of

them regionally purchased and part of a wider package of support for individuals, would not have looked out of place in the suite of remedies offered to middling families in most doctoring account books. Yet if Northamptonshire offers a sense of the rich complexion of parochial supply, we have seen that overseers generally spent only a tiny part of their medical welfare resources on drugs. The picture in Wiltshire is particularly striking. Here, spending on drugs and devices (as well as payment in kind outside smallpox epidemics or last illnesses, and other support payments such as rent) was effectively capped by the extraordinary reach and expense of hospitals in Salisbury, Bristol, Bath and other major towns. Cash payments as a component of overall medical welfare were correspondingly inflated by caution money, transport, clothing and subsistence for paupers going to, at or returning from institutions. We revisit this aspect of Wiltshire experience in Chapter 8. For now, the cash element of the Wiltshire spending was also inflated by a tendency, more keenly felt than in other counties, for overseers to make cash awards to paupers so that they could buy their own drugs and devices rather than providing them direct. Similar trends and levels of spending at county level thus mask very different attitudes towards the role of the parish in providing drugs and devices. We see this too at the other end of the spectrum. Significant spending in West Yorkshire was driven by recourse to local device and regional drug providers, often as part of a package of support which included nursing, cash and funerals. Similar spending levels in Leicestershire were driven by extensive parochial engagement across the local, regional and national piece, and often with discrete purchases rather than drugs and devices forming part of a package. Such differences point once more to the existence of multiple ingrained cultures of medical welfare at local and regional level.

Cash allowances

The idea that similar county or typological trends might be underpinned by very different parochial sentiment also extends to cash payments.[48] Chapter 4 suggested that the central change in spending patterns over time was an increase in the proportion of medical welfare given as cash allowances.[49] This experience was reproduced in all of the county subsets except Leicestershire and (to a lesser extent) Norfolk,

though even in these places cash generally constituted the single biggest element of medical welfare. At parochial level, places like Upavon St Mary (Wiltshire) or Pennington (Lancashire) focused almost all sickness relief on cash allowances after 1800. Moving beyond these broad observations is complicated by elongated detail in overseers' accounts on the one hand and their lack of transparency on the other. In contrast to the provision for the unemployed and those with large families, there was no obvious 'going rate' for different types of sickness.[50] Indeed, the notable thing about the endless list of payments that underpin the quantitative analysis of Chapter 4 is just how adaptable allowances could be. They varied from a matter of pence for vagrants falling sick on the road to cases like Michael Ellat, who was paid 14s 10d 'at severall times' and then a further £3 2d 'at severall times his family being much out of health' by the parish officer of Easington (Lancashire) in 1757. A single sickness episode had absorbed 4.4 per cent of the entire poor relief bill for the town in that year.[51] Just as there was no representative sickness allowance, so there was no typical profile of recipients. Parishes like Clitheroe (Lancashire), Calverley (West Yorkshire) and Belgrave (Leicestershire) paid relief direct to those aged fourteen to sixteen, who stood between childhood and independent youth, whereas the majority of parishes paid cash allowances for young people to parents or other guardians and carers. Some parishes seem to have been particularly proactive with cash and other support for those with mental and physical impairments, whereas others were not.[52] Moreover, and as we saw in Chapters 2 and 3, recorded cash allowances were the end of a process such that understanding their meaning and intent is complex. Thus the sick William Sumner applied to the Tarleton (Lancashire) vestry on 4 March 1834 asking for a cash allowance of 5s per week and 40s towards a rent payment. The vestry allowed him only '4s per week for a few weeks his family sick'.[53] Alice Wakefield applied for relief at Garstang (Lancashire) on 6 August 1816, her husband having run away and she under 'a series of ill health which has reduced her to her present distress'. Because she had a sixteen-year-old daughter in work, the application was declined and Wakefield was 'offered the workhouse if dissatisfied'.[54] Towards the end of 1816 a renewed application met with success. In both of these cases, then, a recorded cash allowance tells us little about either the sentiment of parishes or the experiences of paupers.

These issues mean that our figures for the importance of cash allowances boast more certainty than they should. Nonetheless, it is possible to discern five broad experiences of cash payments. Similar magnitudes of cash expenditure at parochial and county level are generated by very different combinations of such experiences, with important consequences for our understanding of the character and role of medical welfare.[55] Thus, and firstly, most cash allowances to the sick were, and were meant to be, transient. In some communities sickness payments were calculated on a daily basis from as early as the 1780s, clearly pointing to their transience in the minds of officials. This expectation was often inscribed into the words of accounting or vestry entries themselves. In October 1810 the Chorley vestry decided that 'Alice Crompton [was to] be allowed necessary relief during her and her child's sickness and that the overseer call on them frequently', a signal that officials expected relief to be curtailed as soon as possible. The same vestry in February 1811 determined that 'Jane Hodgson be allowed some temporary relief during her sickness'. For Easington, the transient and situational nature of much relief is indicated by the frequent accounting entry 'more at several times' next to consolidated entries, while in Garstang we find the notation 'to be casually relieved'.[56] The language of transience was less marked in the southern counties of Berkshire and Wiltshire,[57] but even here there is no escaping a sense of officials hoping that rapid casual relief would prevent something more serious, regular and costly. Thus, while Dorothy Marshall suggests that in the south and Midlands an allowance of only 1s to 1s 6d 'must have been very much in the nature of mockery', George Rudley's 1s payment at Shellingford (Berkshire) in 1801 was calibrated to the fact that he had spent '1 day ill'.[58] Moreover, it is clear from both pauper letters and advocate correspondence – which often asked for unspecified cash amounts or 'trifles' – that the sick poor themselves actively sought transient allowances. And such payments meld seamlessly with a related type of transaction – the cash gift – which seems to have remarkable traction in a handful of parishes spread across the spatial and typological sample.

Where transient sickness payments were renewed they merge subtly into a second major type of allowance: those (both for new applicants and for people who sought supplements to existing payments) that were time-limited or conditional. Vestries frequently added rhetorical riders to decisions: 'X be allowed relief during his sickness'; 'X

be allowed 2s a week until he is able to work'; allowances to be paid
only 'while in cure' or 'until her recovery'; 'some further assistance
to be made when she lays in'; relief paid conditionally on inspection;
and most frequently payments limited to a certain number of weeks
or days. This sort of rhetoric speaks keenly to the desire of officials to
control the scale and pace of medical relief. It was also a shared rhetoric
with advocates. Thomas Heath wrote from Overton (West Yorkshire)
to Billington (Lancashire) on the subject of John Shawe in September
1828. His concluding remark that 'I trust, Sir you will see the purpose
of augmenting his weekly allowance 1/0 during his illness' is typical
of many hundreds of letters which sought supplemental, time-limited,
relief. Similar sentiments can be found in pauper letters, but are often
supplemented there, as we saw in Chapter 3, with a genuine or rhetoricised sense that the people anticipated recovery and actively sought
time-limited payments in consequence.

Unsurprisingly, there is little system to the scale, distribution or
longevity of such cash payments. In northern England much appears
to have been left in these terms to the discretion of officials. By way
of example, Mrs Parkinson of Walton (near Preston, Lancashire)
attended the Garstang vestry in November 1815 wanting 'some further
relief she receives 3/6 per week out of the town, she is nearly blind and
very infirm'. It was resolved that the overseer 'allow her a trifle more if
he deems necessary'. The worry that discretionary trifles might begin
to add up is perhaps demonstrated by a resolution of the same vestry
in June 1816 that 'no increase in pay shall be granted or allowed to any
pauper without the sanction of the committee'.[59] Defined payments
might be graduated and could be given to those in work as well as to
people who were incapacitated. When Lambert Heaton applied for
relief because of ill-health on 17 May 1788, the Halliwell vestry calculated that the family had 9s a week in income and 'It appears suspicious
that the family gets more than the above otherwise they could not
have subsisted.' An allowance of 2s was granted but 'only until the man
recovers his health'.[60] Some years later, in December 1800, the Chorley
vestry considered the case of Peter Longworth, 'who has 6 children
under 14 years of age and earns 18s a week'. Notwithstanding such
earnings the vestry allowed '4s a week whilst said Peter Longworth
is unwell and also have 2 flannel waistcoats'.[61] Against the backdrop
of relatively small average cash allowances in Lancashire, the size of

these payments is significant and points to the fact, already discussed in Chapter 3, that overseers in even the most parsimonious counties saw utility in concerted action on sickness.[62] And while these examples are drawn from Lancashire, their core lessons apply across the parochial piece. This is well illustrated in the case of Robert Ball of Hinton Waldrist, who received eight weeks of sick pay in 1816 but broken into three distinct phases which traced the course of his illness and consequent poverty: '2 weeks 16s, 3 weeks 31s, 1 week 5s, 2 weeks 13s'.[63]

Yet Ball's experience points to a wider question: when did an allowance cease to be time-limited or conditional and instead merge into a third – open-ended – allowance category?[64] Parish officers themselves often had trouble in locating and policing this threshold. In June 1824 the Garstang vestry resolved to relieve Thomas Huntingdon 'during the time that his hand shall continue lame but not to exceed in such relief after the rate of 5s and the like sum for next week'. This resolution came on top of annual episodes of sickness-related need from 1822. By December 1824 a clearly exasperated vestry resolved that Huntingdon was to have 5s 'on account of the present state of lameness in his hand – but to inform him that no further allowance will be given'.[65] Hope and apparent resolution was in vain; within a year the man was a regular 'pensioner'. This experience maps onto persistent and universal attempts in pauper letters across the spatial, typological and chronological dimensions of our sample to rhetoricise their conditions from periodic sickness up to permanent inability and decline. In turn, and as I have argued elsewhere, this was a rhetorical landscape shared with officials, vestries and advocates, all of whom accepted that physical and mental impairment, the decline and withdrawal from labour associated with extreme old age, care of children with impairments, the loss of a mother or father and the episodic recurrence of diseases could and should result in regular cash support.[66] The human face of this shared landscape of understanding may be George White, who began his relief history at Caversham in 1782. He was awarded cash relief for his own illness, then that of his family, followed by repeat personal payments as his original sickness recurred. The same pattern, with most payments in the winter months, persisted for eleven years.[67] Or we might tell the story of Barnard Sewell, who wrote from Workington (Cumberland) to Greystoke (Westmorland) in 1822 to say that 'my time is over for laber'. At seventy-four he had 'fought the world fareley', and in his

decrepitude he asked the vestry to 'consider we cannot live on the air'.[68] None of this means that cash payments were adequate, but in all of the counties analysed here there is an inecapable broad sense that the sick poor were treated with more generosity in terms of regular allowances than other groups of the long-term poor.

This conclusion extends to a fourth type of cash allowance: that linked to demographic crises, final illnesses and serious accidents, and often part of a wider and expensive package of care. When Samuel Moore broke his leg at Geddington (Northamptonshire) on 25 May 1765 he was attended by the doctor (who also had a beer allowance of 2s 2d) at a cost of £2 4s. Thereafter Moore's bed was modified to accommodate the break (1s 6d) and he received almost daily payment of 1s until 17 June. Such payments were then consolidated to an allowance of 5s per week for a further fifteen weeks, 4s for the next four weeks and 3s per week for the final three weeks. The parish also paid for crutches and to have his bed changed back again. Over the same period, Moore's wife received a further £1 8s 10d for family clothing. A five-month recovery from a broken leg had thus cost the parish £10, a substantial proportion of total cash payments.[69] The letters of paupers and epistolary advocates also show, however, that sometimes the onset of ill-health was so sudden or serious that individuals just acted in commissioning medical help in the hope of being able to meet subsequent bills through their own resources. When these expectations were frustrated we detect a fifth type of cash allowance: the substitute payment to replenish resources intended for other things. December 1816 brought a letter to Garstang parish from Edward Keighley of Lancaster saying that prolonged sickness had left him behind in the rent and that 'his landlord feeling the pressure of the times' was threatening to distrain for 50s. Keighley now requested his rent in addition to the 5s a week he had had from the town during his sickness. In November 1817 Thomas Greenwood wanted 25s towards his rent, he having been sick and 'unable to work for some time'. The Garstang vestry was sceptical, sending Greenwood only 15s 'with a recommendation to employ it towards his rent' and forwarding to Keighley a note with half of the requested amount to say that he must find the rest himself.[70] This was also a more general attitude. Sophia Curchin's undated (but certainly 1829) letter from Wisbech (Cambridgeshire) to Thrapston noted that Dr Stuart had taken Sophia and her husband to court for his unpaid

bill and that the court had levied a weekly arrears payment of 2s 6d. She asked the parish for help to prevent the family of seven being sold up to pay the debt. The Thrapston overseer responded with a letter which suggested her to be a bad manager of the family affairs.[71] Yet paupers who claimed that their clothing had been compromised by the expenses associated with prolonged illness, who had pawned their goods to pay bills and now asked for help in retrieving their possessions or who had rested during sickness on the goodwill and resources of neighbours all tended to get a favourable hearing in their quest for cash allowances. Nowhere was this clearer than in Leicestershire. When Jonathan Hargreaves approached the overseer of Walton-on-the-Wolds to seek help with clothing and apprenticeship fees, having had to break into sums put aside for these purposes because of extended illness in the family, the official response – 'that in respect of the good conduct of Jno Hargreaves he trying not to rest on the parish the overseer to afford him 30s' – spoke to a much wider culture of support across the county.[72]

Understanding what role the constellation of these cash payment types played in the surging importance of the medical welfare component of parochial spending from the mid-1810s, and in the spatial patterning of such spending, is clearly complex. The sheer scale and fluidity of the data make anything other than broad generalisations unsupportable. Three broad observations are, however, important. Firstly, across all county and typological subsets there was an increased tendency by the early 1800s to give both the in-parish and out-parish poor cash resources from which to pay for various aspects of medical welfare rather than providing residual cash once the parish itself had provided such medical support directly. Secondly, in almost all parishes the number of recipients of cash allowances increased. This was felt most keenly in Berkshire and Wiltshire but also in West Yorkshire, and on one reading might be seen to be related to the increasing scale of sickness traced in Chapter 2. Finally, it is possible to trace a subtle change over time in the constellation of the spending types outlined above towards those that imply the greatest longevity or intensity of payment.

Table 6.1 outlines the matrix of experience for the different county samples from 1800 to 1834, though it is important to remember that the situational nature of much cash relief results in significant short-term

Table 6.1 The incidence of cash allowances in seven counties, 1800–34

Place	Transient	Time-limited	Open-ended	Crisis/packaged	Substitution
West Yorkshire	Medium	High	Medium	Low	Medium
Leicestershire	Low	High	Medium	Low	High
Northamptonshire	High	Medium	Medium	High	Low
Lancashire	High	High	Medium	Low	High
Berkshire	Medium	Low	High	High	Medium
Norfolk	High	Low	Medium	Medium	Low
Wiltshire	High	High	Low	Medium	High

Sources: 117-parish sample.

volatility within these samples. The representation is of course crude, but it captures the idea that similar quantitative trends in the provision of cash allowances mask very important differences in the complexion and intent of the policy. Wiltshire and Berkshire parishes collectively saw a very significant increase in the importance of cash allowances, absolutely and in relation to other elements of medical welfare. Yet as Table 6.1 suggests, Wiltshire overseers sought to impose strict time limitations to their allowances and to reward prior efforts at self-help, whereas those in Berkshire provided a more holistic and open-ended set of cash benefits. At the opposite end of the spectrum, Leicestershire and Norfolk saw little growth in the importance of cash allowances. Nonetheless the emphasis of Norfolk overseers was, Table 6.1 suggests, firmly on the provision of transient allowances, whereas officials in Leicestershire sought to impose strict time or other limitations on payment. These important differences speak to very different cultures of medical welfare from an experiential and sentimental perspective, matters to which we return ultimately in Chapter 10.

Payments in kind

A careful reading of the figures in Chapter 4 suggests that payments in kind – discrete and packaged with other benefits – absorbed a roughly constant 6–9 per cent of medical welfare resources across the period. Interpreting this picture is again far from easy. Many parishes gave cash allowances for paupers themselves to purchase food, clothing and bedding, and to pay rents. Where the reason for payment was noted the cost can be ascribed to the 'kind' envelope of medical welfare. Where it was not, we introduce a cash bias into the analysis. Thus in 1785 the vestry of Woodford Halse (Northamptonshire) granted Thomas Meacock the classifiable sum of 6s 'for stuff for his wife's eyes'. Later in that year the overseer gave an unexplained cash payment of 4s to the same family. We know it to have been for clothing only because a separate bill of supply survives.[73] More relief in kind goes unaccounted for because it is indivisible from cash relief. Hence at Easington in 1753 John Wilson was paid 18s 6d, presumably in cash, 'inn his illness and towards fire'.[74] And some provision goes unrecorded (or at least uncounted) because it had no present monetary value. At Warham the overseer noted in 1814 that Isaack Secker was '75 years next

Michaelmas in a poor shabby state & gave him a short Duffield jacket made by Platfoot'.[75] Several Lancashire and West Yorkshire communities granted turves and peat blocks as fuel. The only reason we know that such provision was made is because the overseers were obliged to meet the cost of carting such material from the moors. Similarly, in Leicestershire the great storm of 1813 led overseers to stock up the wood piles of sick paupers, the aged and (above all) pest-houses, with only the small cost of carriage recorded. Across all parishes, these issues are magnified by the payment of undifferentiated bills to suppliers of food, clothing and coals, and (where they existed) uncosted allowances of clothing and fuel out of stocks held at the workhouse. Even if accounting entries are seemingly clear we must be cautious in their interpretation. In particular, where clothing, fuel or food was given as part of a package with the costs of nursing, it is not always clear whether payment in kind was for the nurse or the patient!

Many of these potential problems can be ameliorated through careful record linkage, yielding a baseline impression of the nature and broad distribution of payment in kind. Two other interpretive issues are rather more intractable: the first is pricing trends in cloth, clothing, fuel and food, given distinctive regional experiences of inflation. In West Yorkshire, for instance, woollen cloth tended to fall in price over the period 1790–1820 while ready-made worsted, wool and cotton clothing increased in price. The majority of parishes in our West Yorkshire sample thus moved subtly away from the provision of ready-made clothing and towards cloth and the cash to make it up. This process capped the costs of clothing provision for the sick even as inflation rose, but it was not duplicated in places like Berkshire. Clothing provision to the sick in these two counties thus signifies very different things. A second issue is that end-of-process overseer accounts record what was given, not what was requested. Yet we know from pauper letters and recorded appearances of claimants before vestries that requests for unspecified support or just what officials thought appropriate to the case were the rhetorical staple of approaches to negotiation. William Lacy's letter from Hull to Beverley on 11 January 1815 said that Mary Wray 'appears to be in a dying State'. Lacy noted that 'she cannot do any longer without a woman to attend her her [sic] friends is qu[ite] tired out in doing for her & she is almost lost', and asked for an unspecified package of support.[76] Similarly, when George Barber, the overseer

of Thrapston, wrote to a fellow overseer on 9 January 1833, he said that 'medicines being very expensive' he expected a liberal (but unspecified) treatment of the pauper concerned.[77] Such requests might be systematically transformed into cash payments in some parishes and places, and payment in kind in others.

If we bear these caveats in mind, three forms of payment in kind dominate this category of medical welfare spending.[78] First in order of scale were cloth, clothing and bedding. Occasionally doctors themselves ordered cloth and clothing as part of their treatment regime, and this remains true even at the end of the difficult task of distinguishing cloth for clothing from that intended for bandages, dressings and compresses. Thus in 1765 the overseer of Forncett St Peter paid William Harvey 6s in cash because of his wife's illness, 2s for a nurse and 3s 6d 'for a yard of bays ordered by the doctor for her'.[79] In most places, however, clothing and related items were given in response to pauper requests or overseer and vestry initiative. Aside from the 'normal' regional and typological variation one that might find in any list of clothing types,[80] the range of provision was remarkably uniform. For sick women the category was dominated by shifts, petticoats, stockings, stays and handkerchiefs,[81] while for men shirts, breeches, aprons, hats and jackets were the most common spending points. There was a tendency, already noted above, for some counties to swing distinctly to the ready-made end of the clothing spectrum, but in the sample as a whole cloth and the costs of making it into clothing remained important even in the 1830s. Children, either when they were sick in their own right or because their parents were sick and thus unable to put money aside, were the most regular recipients. Few adults were incrementally given a whole change of wardrobe over a period of months or years, but this was relatively common for sick children and children in sick households.[82] In all counties there were surprisingly few instances in which the sick poor were provided with shoes, often in contradistinction to other pauper groups. This presumably reflects the fact that sickness was and was expected to be something that kept people from going out and about, a familiar rhetorical refrain in the letters of paupers themselves.[83]

In turn, clothing and bedding came to the sick poor through three sorts of parochial decision-making: as discrete provision, either episodic or (for children) regular;[84] as part of a wider package of support, both time-limited and ongoing; or coincident with parishes sending

paupers to institutions. The latter was particularly important in some counties. When George Langstaff, house surgeon and apothecary for the Salisbury Infirmary, wrote to the overseers of Longbridge Deverill (Wiltshire) on 24 July 1819, he pointed out that their pauper Noah Butcher was 'much distressed for a pair of Shoes and a round frock'. Langstaff assumed that a remedy to the situation would be automatic and 'shall thank you to send it to him as soon as possible'.[85] More widely, paupers entering institutions had to do so clean and decently clothed, sometimes requiring provision of a whole new outfit, while those returning from institutions usually received further clothing and bedding as part of their ongoing care. Such provision is unsurprising. Parochial officers were extremely sensitive to charges that they had allowed pauper clothing and bedding to deteriorate and to related rhetorical suggestions of female and child nakedness. Equally, arguments that compromised clothing prevented paupers from showing themselves in the locality or working could have significant purchase. Such rhetoric is emblematised by Frances Soundy, who on 18 February 1824 would 'Entreet the gentillmen' of Pangbourne (Berkshire) 'to remit to Battersea oversears our rant and a pair of shoes for my husband as he can not go to work without danger of having nales run in to his feet'. She renewed this rhetorical line two years later, noting that her son could get work to help alleviate the burden on the parish 'if he ad deasent things to put on but he can not put a foot out doors for he have not a shoe to his feet and he must apeer tidy be fore the gentillman [employers]'. And in February 1827, as she sought to make a case for ongoing relief, Soundy noted to her parish that 'I have distreesed my salf so that I can not go out of dores for want of things to keep me warm.'[86] She was drawing upon an understanding of clothing as a negotiating tool which was shared with officials and advocates. Thus George Elliott, overseer of Longtown (Cumberland), wrote to his counterpart in Hayton (Westmorland) on 7 February 1825 to inform him that his pauper George Peel 'is in great distress and confined to his bed'. Noting that he had survived for more than a year on the charity of neighbours, Elliott observed that 'his present distressed situation calls loudly for your assistance'. Peel's bedding was simply 'filthy raggs not fit for a dog kennel', and Elliott supposed the Carlisle ratepayers to be a 'very hardened set of people' to allow their pauper to get into such a state during his sickness.[87]

A second type of payment in kind – food – was less contentious. Paupers sometimes claimed they were starving and cold, and doctors occasionally ordered food for eating as part of their curative plans. Most provision, however, was generated independently by officials as part of a specific relief package, as an annual or seasonal response to old age and disability or in the form of casual relief. In terms of food, paupers and officials shared a language of 'necessary nourishment' during sickness and recuperation. The range of such 'necessaries' varied strongly by county and hardly at all by typological subset. Norfolk parishes purchased almost no bread for paupers to eat (as opposed to its use for poultices) but did buy cakes to help recuperation.[88] There is little evidence for sustained purchases of mutton, but beef and above all fish were common additions to Norfolk relief packages. By contrast there is only one example of a Berkshire community acquiring fish (Shellingford purchased a barrel of white herring in 1801), and yet the provision of pease and prunes was ubiquitous. For the eighteenth century, Wiltshire could boast a particularly diverse food response to sickness. Upavon St Mary's treatment of Francis Tuck in 1763 is emblematic: Betty Usher was paid 9s for 'looking after' him, while Tuck also had during the year 48s of cash, bushels of wheat and barley and three and a half pounds of cheese.[89] By the 1800s, and broadly coincident with increasing institutional engagement, food supplements to Wiltshire care packages had become rather rarer. It was, however, parishes in the Midland and northern counties which did most to continue eighteenth-century traditions of providing 'necessary nourishment'. This remains true even when we allow for the distorting influence of pest-houses, which absorbed significant quantities of food-related medical welfare. In these places, bread, cheese, milk (particularly for those with smallpox), wheat, barley, malt and above all mutton were clearly seen by officials as an integral part of both treatment and recuperation.

A third type of kind-payment – fuel provision – also had distinctive regional formats. Parishes in Berkshire, Wiltshire,[90] Norfolk and Northamptonshire spent their resources largely on wood, turf, furze, faggots and more rarely compacted straw 'bricks' or peat. Those in Lancashire, West Yorkshire and Leicestershire, by contrast, purchased more coal, right across the typological subsets of parishes.[91] Fuel purchases for pest-houses, particularly during outbreaks of smallpox, were ubiquitous, and more widely we can see clearly that fuel was added to

packages of support involving nursing or pregnant women 'lying in'. These provisions were consistent across time. Thus care for William Money's widow at Scottow (Norfolk) in November 1760 involved 19s of cash, 1s 6d towards nursing and a rug, sheet and blanket (14s), as well as an unspecified amount for wood.[92] The Leicestershire parishes of Syston and Gilmorton added 'coals' or 'firing' to 40 per cent of relief packages from the early 1780s, while in the West Yorkshire townships of Morley, Bingley and Mirfield almost all sickness responses involved coal, turf or (for smallpox cases) wood. Outside these broad packages discrete deliveries of fuel for those in prolonged illness, those with physical or mental impairment and old people on long-term relief because of 'decline' were episodic in the southern and Midland counties but rather more regular in Lancashire and West Yorkshire. Indeed, the sense that fuel was an integral part of the response to illness in all of its forms in the north can be seen in vestry entries like that for Halliwell (Lancashire) on 27 March 1790, when the ratepayers noted with disquiet that Old William Morris 'has been provided with coals but he has been so negligent of taking care of them that the last load lay in the lane' and promptly resolved to supply no more fuel.[93]

These examples point to considerable range and depth of payment in kind. Yet the difference in emphasis on welfare packages highlighted in Table 6.1, allied with the spatial nuances revealed in Figure 4.8, suggests that there were variations in the scale, longevity, constellation and meaning of in-kind payments at regional and local level. Thus in Lancashire, Norfolk and Wiltshire, such provision declined in relative importance as an element of medical welfare. This is particularly true after 1800 and (for Norfolk and Wiltshire) becomes especially marked where we strip out the support packages offered to paupers prior to and after attendance at an institution or when smallpox was being treated. At the very least, then, we see a downturn in the resources devoted to *ad hoc* and discrete in-kind payments to the sick poor. By contrast, spending on in-kind payments relative to other aspects of medical welfare rose over the same period for Leicestershire, West Yorkshire and Northamptonshire, reaching levels not seen since the 1750s. A similar trend, however, masks very different causation. In Northamptonshire the growth of in-kind allowances reflects the presence and value of food, fuel, clothing and other material relief in broad care packages offered to the sick poor. Meanwhile, in West Yorkshire and Leicestershire, and as

Table 6.1 implies, fewer welfare resources were packaged in this way so that growing provision in kind reflected a multiplication of *ad hoc* or regular seasonal events. Finally, Berkshire demonstrates an unusually stable pattern of spending on material support for the sick. To some extent this experience is illusory, a function of counterbalancing trends at parochial level. Caversham in the 1810s and Englefield in the 1820s witnessed a determined move away from cash allowances to payment in kind, whereas Thatcham and Bradfield moved in exactly the opposite direction. These experiences point to the contingent nature of in-kind payments, something that also applies to the more residual envelopes of medical welfare.

Other health

There was little systematic spatial, chronological or typological patterning in the 'other health' element of medical welfare, a spending category which was broadly orientated towards maintaining and establishing the independence of the sick poor. The volatility of this area apparent in Figure 4.8 reflects the fact that while all parishes sought to invest in this way, often expending very significant resources, they did so inconsistently. In part this fluidity embodies ideological differences associated with the turnover of vestries and officials. There were, however, also highly situational drivers to such spending: Whether money was needed for apprenticing children with impairments, for instance, depended upon their prior life chances in each locality, and also on the migratory patterns of their parents. Nonetheless, it is arguably in the detail of this category of medical welfare that we can garner the clearest sense of the importance that parochial officials attached to meeting the needs of the sick in all their guises.

The range of spending represented under this heading is startling. On 22 October 1784, the Halliwell vestry noted that Widow Cunliff had been 'much hurt by one Thomason violently riding a horse over her'. She was given 3s of cash relief 'for the present' but the overseer was to 'apply to Mr Rathbone and order him to give notice in writing to the said Thomason that if he will not make proper satisfaction for the offence that Mr Rathbone do prosecute him at the expense of the township'.[94] The cost of the subsequent prosecution falls into the 'other health' category. In Norfolk the parish of Holme Next the Sea

paid John Ringwood in May 1775 to teach 'the idiot Matthew Dix' to play the violin, presumably by way of finding him future employment.[95] And almost all Norfolk parishes paid extra for a parishioner to accompany a sick pauper when they had to travel. In the Lancashire parish of Chorley, the perennially sick Elizabeth Vaughan and her children were given £2 plus expenses in March 1811 to catch the Dublin packet at Liverpool so that she could go in search of her errant Irish husband.[96] Across that county, Clitheroe organised a special vestry on 26 June 1833 in order to agree £2 for Oliver Whittaker 'to bear his expences to Blackpool. He being in a very precarious state of health and from the certificate he has produced from the surgeon he recommends him to go here for the purpose of recovering his health.'[97] In Leicestershire the overseer of Anstey paid in June 1802 for the child John Bridge to go to Brighton and be accommodated there for one month in a last-ditch (and ultimately failed) attempt to preserve his life after a series of illnesses. His counterpart at Walton-on-the-Wolds boarded out eight of Samuel Parker's children when his wife was in a 'melancholic state' after a recent pregnancy.[98] And in West Yorkshire the overseers of Tong and Thornton both sent paupers to Harrogate to take the waters, at a combined cost of £17.[99]

Judged by simple magnitudes, however, three forms of support for the sick poor dominate this spending category. The first was apprenticeship and other forms of occupational training. While our understanding of the nature and outcomes of pauper apprenticeship has recently become more nuanced and arguably less severe, there has been very little consideration of the conundrum that sick children or the offspring of sick or dead parents posed to parochial officials.[100] Discussion of children with permanent physical impairments has been even more muted notwithstanding the scale of the potential problem. For instance, nine of the fifty-nine children apprenticed by Newchurch (Lancashire) between 1759 and 1774 had traceable impairments, and this must have been the tip of a considerable iceberg.[101] In practice, overseers went to notable trouble and expense in order to apprentice such children promptly. Some sense of what this might involve can be gained from a letter that the weaver John Ridge wrote from Wellingborough (Northamptonshire) to Thrapston on 8 April 1828. He informed the overseer that a Mr Ives had come to offer him a fee of £10 (paid by Thrapston parish) to take his son as an apprentice. However, 'I had a

trial of him and found he knew but little of the business and the lameness worse than expected therefore I cannot take him for less than £18.' Rather than abandoning the placement, James Benson, the Thrapston overseer, replied on 16 April 1828 'Respecting Wm Ives the lame boy' and invited Ridge to visit him 'the first opportunity you have the soon the better and should we not agree I will pay your expenses'. They eventually settled on a fee of £16, a significant portion of the medical welfare for the town in that year; this was one of eight similar children placed between 1810 and 1834.[102] Nor were efforts confined to children with impairments. The overseer of Horsforth (West Yorkshire) apprenticed four of Thomas Wade's children in 1808, 'he not being expected to live', with at least three apprenticeship fees paid to family members.[103]

Yet overseers did not always or perhaps usually resort to the permanent breaking of families where children or adults were sick. Instead, a second major form of spending in the 'other health' category was on temporary support through boarding, a practice which combined simultaneously aspects of nursing, lodging and recuperation. Such arrangements could be eye-wateringly expensive, enough in fact to influence the scale of total welfare spending for the period concerned. Thus Thomas Newcome of Shenley (Hertfordshire) recorded in 1822 the case of a pauper from Islington who 'who had his thigh broken on Ridge Hill'. The vestry 'passed a Bill for £33 for ten weeks Keep only … (& his nurse & her wages)'. Noting a doctoring charge of £7 and costs of removal, Newcome recorded mournfully that 'this accident to a mere Stranger of Islington cost this parish 40gs at least or about 3.5d per acre therein'.[104] The ratepayers of Spofforth (West Yorkshire) no doubt had similar feelings about equivalent instances which for 1816 and 1817 cost them £18 and £31 respectively.[105] In most cases, however, the costs of boarding were more reasonable, and the fact that overseers kept coming back to this mechanism as a way of dealing with adult and child illness, particularly in places like Lancashire, suggests that they constructed it as value for money. Moreover, paupers and their advocates actively sought such arrangements, or at least asked parishes to pay for those already put in place. James King's letter from Old Weston (Cambridgeshire) to his overseer counterpart in Thrapston is representative. Ann Marriott was 'a poor girl *residing with friends* at this place'. She had been unwell for a long time and 'laid upon them for support who are themselves supported by this parish'. Marriott

was, King assured his counterpart, 'so much a cripple as to incapacitate her from doing anything by which she can support herself', and he asked Thrapston to act.[106] These informal arrangements were supplemented by proactive approaches from those who wanted to generate an income from a type of boarding that combined nursing and custody. In December 1833, for instance, the vestry of Tarleton (Lancashire) agreed that Robert Hesketh's wife, who had applied to 'maintain Ellen Hunter, a poor delirious girl belonging to the township', should do so at a rate of 2s 6d per week.[107] And of course overseers themselves proactively sought out boarding opportunities, particularly seeking to bargain with kin over their sick relatives. Thus James Benson, the overseer of Thrapston, wrote to Mrs Morton in Northampton on 18 June 1827 to say that he had 'been informed by a Neighbour that you have expressed a desire to have under your care S Sanderson your relation'. Benson was, he informed Mrs Morton, happy to support this arrangement and to 'allow you with her 2/6 per week and some clothes'. Mary Morton replied on 21 June affirming the terms and asking for money to be remitted 'to us every two months as it will be a pound and will be giving you the least trouble'. So began a relationship that was to last eight years as Sanderson sank into the progressive decline associated with old age.[108] Not all boarding relationships were so stable and harmonious. William Grange wrote from Keswick (Cumberland) to Greystoke (Westmorland) in March 1823 to demand that the overseer make new arrangements for William Gash, 'for he has turned so dirty that I believe he is as disagreeable a Man as is living'.[109] Nonetheless, boarding was a persistent feature of parochial responses to sickness across the spatial and typological subsets.

Officers also had to field demands for help with a third major category of 'other health' spending, namely rents. A letter from Jonas Smith, assistant overseer of Burnley (Lancashire), to his counterpart John Seed in Billington embodies the conundrum facing officials. Recounting the history of the persistently sick Charlotte Eastwood, Smith was obliged 'to state that she is indebted to her landlord for Rent to the amount of 3.10.0 or thereabouts and if the same is not paid her goods will be sold, which will make very little although they are worth much more than the rent'. By way of economy and a promise that Eastwood would try and help herself, the overseer bargained that 'if you will send her 2.10.0 the landlord will not take her goods for

6 months to come and she will not trouble you again till after that time'.[110] That requests for rent were more than mere rhetoric is well illustrated in a letter sent by Richard Slater of Clitheroe to his friend Isaac Sutcliffe at Lango Chapel (Lancashire) 'with speed'. Dripping breathless urgency, it asked:

> Mr Sutcliffe you must take this paper to James Seed the Overseer and get me the one pound that was granted at the last rent meeting for me and tell him he [Slater's landlord] has some money to pay and he will not look of it any longer so you must not fail in getting me it of the overseer and either send it or bring it me As I am in such a poor state for walking at the present and tell him it is for my landlord James Thompson and you can tell him you have seen me and I desired you to get it for me or anything you think best to tell him.[111]

How Seed received this letter is unclear, but for officials across the sample obvious irritation at frequent appeals for help with the rent had to be balanced pragmatically with the practical and reputational consequences of sick paupers being thrown onto the street. Thus rents were paid, and with surprising regularity. Few paupers were as lucky as John Flowers of Bradden (Northamptonshire), who had thirty months of rent arrears paid in October 1775.[112] Equally, few parishes followed the example of Chilton Foliat (Wiltshire), which calibrated sickness and rent contributions on a daily or weekly basis. Rather, overseers trod a delicate path between the interests of ratepayers and sick paupers, seeking solutions which were fair and just. Across all of the county samples, requests from women were treated more favourably than those from men, and approaches from advocates (other than landlords) more favourably than those made directly by sick paupers. In turn, rent was a more pronounced and frequent category in the 'other health' spending envelope for parishes in West Yorkshire and Lancashire than it was for those in Midland and southern counties. While there are many potential readings of this observation, the one preferred here is that officials, paupers and advocates in these counties had a shared understanding that sickness, where accompanied by every effort to otherwise make do, created a moral right to support with lump-sum-type payments. Thus, although there are no consistent typological or spatial patterns to the 'other health' category, broad spending trends still mask the insistent presence of strong localised cultures of medical welfare.

Conclusion

A surge in the importance of medical welfare spending apparent in most counties from the 1810s was driven primarily by an expansion in the number, duration and intensity of cash allowances. Exploring this trend yields unending colourful stories like that of the 'company of comedians who were sent here [Stilton] from Cambridge by an order of the Vice Chancellor'. Suffering from cholera, they had 'left 2 or 3 ill of that disease at Pomersham'. The overseer of Stilton (Huntingdonshire) thus wrote asking his counterparts at Peterborough to give them some cash to help them reach their ultimate destination at Lincoln, 'where they will have their vans &c cleansed and purified'. The overseer assured his counterpart that they had no choice in this matter given the Vice Chancellor's interest in the comedians and that 'There is none of the present party infected.'[113] Yet cash was only one element of a suite of responses to sickness. At times of cholera, smallpox and other epidemic disease, parishes acted decisively and often expensively, in simultaneous acts of containment, confinement and treatment. In other cases of sickness there is considerable evidence to suggest that parochial officials went out of their way to support paupers and return them to a semblance of independence. Indeed, the notion of what was fair and proportionate in cases of sickness seems to have been elastic. For counties such as Wiltshire, institutional treatment increasingly took centre stage (something to which we return in Chapter 8), and this had a muting effect on the range and depth of parochial responses. Communities in other counties developed a fluid envelope of medical welfare often, and in many places increasingly, constellated in the form of overarching care packages which included doctors, nurses, payment in kind, cash and other support payments. This picture varies remarkably little across the typological subsets. By the 1790s, then, pauper lives were becoming increasingly medicalised, but these conclusions do not do justice to the sheer intensity of spending at parochial level. In the space of five months between September 1795 and February 1796, the wife of William Tindham from Stratford-sub-Castle St Lawrence was given cash and nursing help during a difficult pregnancy, the cost of burying the infant, 12s to go to Salisbury for the amputation of her leg, crutches, a wooden leg, cash support on her return and a funeral when she died. The subsequent apprenticeship of her children cost the parish

more than £40.[114] There is much here, then, to support Joan Lane's view that the Old Poor Law provided a comprehensive medical service from the cradle to the grave. And it is to the grave part of this equation that we turn to in the next chapter.

Notes

1 NORO, PD 552/78, vouchers. On trusses see L. Hilaire-Pérez and C. Rabier, 'Self-machinery? Steel trusses and the management of ruptures in eighteenth-century Europe', *Technology and Culture*, 53 (2013), 460–502.

2 See D. Turner and A. Withey, 'Technologies of the body: Polite consumption and the correction of deformity in eighteenth-century England', *History*, 99 (2014), 775–96.

3 NORO, PD 136/65, overseers' accounts.

4 NORO, PD 421/132, overseers' accounts.

5 NORO, PD 374/56, overseers' accounts.

6 NORO, PD 145/47, overseers' accounts. Parochial officials were certainly attuned to wider developments in the medical market. See S. Reiser, *Medicine and the Reign of Technology* (Cambridge: Cambridge University Press, 1978).

7 Crowther, 'Health care and poor relief', p. 206.

8 WRO, 811/126, overseers' accounts.

9 WRO, 206/62–4, overseers' accounts.

10 WRO, 871/180, overseers' accounts, particularly entries in 1798 and 1799. For types of trusses see Turner and Withey, 'Technologies of the body', pp. 782–83.

11 WRO, 1228/29, overseers' accounts.

12 See A. Cooper, *The Anatomy and Surgical Treatment of Abdominal Hernia* (London: Green, 1827). Borsay warns against overstating the degree to which intervention was targeted at improving function. See A. Borsay, 'Disciplining disabled bodies: The development of orthopaedic medicine in Britain c.1800–1939', in D. Turner and K. Stagg (eds), *Social Histories of Disability and Deformity* (London: Routledge, 2006), pp. 97–116.

13 Something also highlighted by Langton, 'The geography of poor relief'.

14 For context see K. Timmermann and J. Anderson, 'Devices, designs and the history of technology in medicine', in J. Anderson and K. Timmermann (eds), *Devices and Designs: Medical Technologies in Historical Perspective* (Basingstoke: Palgrave, 2006), pp. 1–16.

15 NORO, PD 502/64, overseers' accounts; PD 629/50–1, overseers' accounts; PD 145/47, overseers' accounts.
16 See J. Reinarz and R. Wynter, 'The spirit of medicine: The use of alcohol in nineteenth-century medical practice', in S. Schmid and B. Schmidt-Haberkamp (eds), *Drink in the Eighteenth and Nineteenth Centuries* (London: Pickering and Chatto, 2014), pp. 127–39.
17 LCRO, DE 57/4, overseers' accounts.
18 It is also important to note the overlap between alcohol for consumption by the sick and that for other purposes. In 1787, for instance, it becomes clear from entries in the accounts of Stanford-in-the-Vale (Berkshire) that much prior beer purchase had been for poultices rather than inward consumption. See BRO, D/P 118/12/1, overseers' accounts. In Reading, detailed accounting entries for 1757 indicate that brandy was purchased for curing eye complaints rather than drinking. BRO, DP 98/12/130a, overseers' accounts.
19 The overseer of Chilton Foliat, for instance, paid 10d in 1801 for 'Bread & lard for poultices', showing how easy it is to misattribute payment entries. See WRO, 735/32, overseer's notebook. On food as medicine see: E. Leong and S. Pennell, 'Recipe collections and the currency of medical knowledge in the early modern medical marketplace', in Jenner and Wallis (eds), *Medicine and the Market*, pp. 133–52. For a good modern account see N. Etkin, *Edible Medicines: An Ethnopharmacology of Food* (Tucson: University of Arizona Press, 2006).
20 H. Marland, 'The medical activities of mid-nineteenth century chemists and druggists, with special reference to Wakefield and Huddersfield', *Medical History*, 31 (1987), 415–39.
21 For explanations of the making, purpose and effect of these medicines see the excellent compendium kept by Rowland Morris Fawcett. RSCE, M50040/1/5, Rowland Morris Fawcett miscellaneous notes.
22 NORO, uncatalogued, overseers' accounts 1762–81; NRO, 284p/189, vestry minutes.
23 BRO, D/P 109/12/2, overseers' accounts; D/P 109/12/3/22, voucher.
24 S. King, *A Fylde Country Practice: Medicine and Society in Lancashire 1760–1840* (Lancaster: Centre for Northwest Regional Studies, 2001).
25 See R. Porter and D. Porter, *In Sickness and in Health*, p. 271, and Lane, '"The doctor scolds me"'.
26 J. Reinarz, 'Introduction', in J. Reinarz (ed.), *Medicine and Society in the Midlands, 1750–1950* (Birmingham: Midland History Publications, 2007), p. 3.
27 NORO, PD 421/132, overseers' accounts.

28 The 'standard repertoire of therapeutic interventions'. See R. Porter and
   D. Porter, *In Sickness and in Health*, p. 265; NORO, 553/109, outdoor
   relief accounts.
29 BRO, D/P 162/12/5, overseers' accounts.
30 BRO, D/P 162/12/12, overseers' accounts.
31 There are no systematic differences in the range and scale of local supply
   between urban and rural parochial subsets, for instance.
32 Parishes across the sample also purchased stays. For context see
   L. Sorge-English, *Stays and Body Image in London: The Staymaking Trade,
   1680–1810* (London: Pickering and Chatto, 2011).
33 CPL, vestry minutes.
34 BRO, D/P 52/12/1–4, overseers' accounts.
35 BRO, D/P 162/12/9, overseers' accounts.
36 We will again undercount such engagement. Chippenham in 1758 paid
   'Mr Johnson for J Collar, 11s.', and we only know that Johnson was a
   druggist because he supplied another nearby parish in that guise at the
   same time. See WRO, 811/126, overseers' accounts. On the concept of
   regional medical markets see P. Wallis, 'Exotic drugs and English medicine: England's drug trade, c.1550–c. 1800', *Social History of Medicine*, 25
   (2012), 20–46.
37 WRO, 1076/39, overseers' accounts.
38 NORO, PD 625/25, overseers' accounts.
39 See K. Carter, 'Nineteenth-century treatments for rabies as reported
   in the *Lancet*', *Medical History*, 26 (1982), 67–78; N. Pemberton and
   M. Worboys, *Mad Dogs and Englishmen: Rabies in Britain, 1830–2000*
   (Basingstoke: Palgrave, 2007).
40 NRO, 356p/7, Welton poor book. These seem to be the lower end of the
   cost spectrum if the 10s 3d rate for wooden legs at Ardleigh in Essex is a
   yardstick. R. Wall, 'Families in crisis and the English poor law as exemplified by the relief programme in the Essex parish of Ardleigh 1795–7', in
   E. Ochiai (ed.), *The Logic of Female Succession: Rethinking Patriarchy and
   Patrinlineality in Global and Historical Perspective* (Kyoto: International
   Research Centre for Japanese Studies, 2002), p. 118.
41 WRO, 206/69, 80 and 81, overseers' accounts.
42 BRO, D/P 70/12/1, overseers' accounts. This tendency to turn to
   regional suppliers mirrors the development of an increasingly sophisticated and specialised market in medical devices for the middling orders.
   See Turner and Withey, 'Technologies of the body', pp. 784–6.
43 D. Haycock and P. Wallis, *Quackery and Commerce in Seventeenth-Century
   London: The Proprietary Medicine Business of Anthony Daffy* (London:
   Wellcome Trust, 2005). See also H. Barker, 'Medical advertising

and trust in late Georgian England', *Urban History*, 36 (2009), 376–98.

44 On these national proprietary medicines see R. Davies, 'Dr Richard Stoughton and his great cordial elixir', *Pharmaceutical Journal*, 240 (1988), 377–87; M. Brown, 'Medicine, quackery'; W. Helfand, 'Samuel Solomon and the cordial balm of Gilead', *Pharmacy in History*, 31 (1989), 151–9; and J. Stead, *The Diary of a Quack Doctor: Being the Last Diary of John Swift, Aurist, of Newsome, Huddersfield, 1784–1851* (Huddersfield: Huddersfield Local History Society, 2002). For a more general overview, see M. Weatherall, 'Making medicine scientific: Empiricism, rationality, and quackery in mid-Victorian Britain', *Social History of Medicine*, 9 (1996), 175–94, and R. Porter, *Health for Sale: Quackery in England, 1660–1850* (Manchester: Manchester University Press, 1989).

45 Turner and Withey, 'Technologies of the body'.

46 BRO, D/P 118/12/1, overseers' accounts.

47 While medicinal, surgical and corrective advances seem to have percolated to the poor, some lacunae are obvious. There is not a single example of parishes purchasing false eyes and little evidence to support Corlett's assertion that eye complaints and their remedy were a mainstay of eighteenth-century medical welfare: H. Corlett, '"No small uncertainty": Eye treatments in eighteenth-century England France', *Medical History*, 42 (1998), 217–34. Dentistry in any form also has a very slight presence in the underlying data despite wider middling engagement with dentists: N. Richards, 'Dentistry in England in the 1840s: The first indications of a movement towards professionalization', *Medical History*, 12 (1968), 137–52; H. Forbes, 'The professionalization of dentistry in the United Kingdom', *Medical History*, 29 (1985), 169–81; A. Hargreaves, 'Dentistry in the British Isles', in C. Hillam (ed.), *Dental Practice in Europe at the End of the Eighteenth Century* (Amsterdam: Rodopi, 2003), pp. 171–282.

48 The term 'cash' is potentially misleading. It is not clear that recipients received cash with the regularity suggested in overseers' accounts, since amounts might be folded up into larger lump-sum payments, especially given a shortage of small change in the later eighteenth century. See C. Muldrew and S. King, 'Cash, wages and the economy of makeshifts in England, 1650–1800', in P. Scholliers and L. Schwarz (eds), *Experiencing Wages: Social and Cultural Aspects of Wage Forms in Europe since 1500* (Oxford: Berghahn, 2003), pp. 155–82.

49 Payments could be in compensation for prior spending on drugs, clothing, devices and doctors, or be granted specifically for that immediate purpose. In this sense, they were not 'cash' allowances at all.

50 Sokoll, 'Families, wheat prices'.
51 LRO, PR 2995/1/11, overseers' accounts.
52 S. King, 'Constructing the disabled child'.
53 LRO, PR 3168/5/1, vestry minutes.
54 LRO, DDX 386/3, vestry minutes. Both examples confirm observations earlier in this study that paupers themselves preferred the flexibility of cash when making applications.
55 Paupers might also fuse together different typologies of payment over a sickness life-cycle.
56 CPL, vestry minutes; LRO, PR 2995/1/9, 11, 13, 15, 18–19 and 22–5, overseers' accounts; LRO, DDX 386/3, vestry minutes.
57 Though Wiltshire paupers were often given small cash allowances for being 'hindered in their work' by sickness.
58 Marshall, *The English Poor*, p. 101; BRO, D/P 109/12/2, overseers' accounts.
59 LRO, DDX 386/3, vestry minutes.
60 BALS, PHA 1-3, Halliwell township books.
61 CPL, vestry minutes.
62 See S. King, *Poverty and Welfare*.
63 BRO, D/P 70/12/1, overseers' accounts.
64 'Open-ended' in this sense might mean chronologically continuous or episodically frequent and ongoing.
65 LRO, 386/3, vestry minutes.
66 S. King, 'Negotiating the law'.
67 BRO, D/P 162/12/5, overseers' accounts.
68 CRO, PR 5-67-5, letter, dated '1822'.
69 NRO, 133p/111, accounts.
70 LRO, DDX 386/3, vestry minutes.
71 NRO, 325p/194/162, letter.
72 LCRO, DE 2934/44, overseers' accounts.
73 NRO, 372p/11/A/S, Woodford Halse overseers' accounts.
74 LRO, PR 2995/1/9, overseers' accounts.
75 NORO, uncatalogued, overseers' accounts 1800–27.
76 EYRO, PE1-702-30, letter.
77 NRO, 216p/244/9, letter, 9 January 1833.
78 Each county could of course boast colourful examples of other forms of payment in kind, as for instance when Stanford-in-the-Vale (Berkshire) paid for the expenses of moving and resettling Sarah Pinnell 'when the house fell down' in 1773. BRO, D/P 118/12/1, overseers' accounts.
79 NORO, PD 421/132, overseers' accounts.

80 Smocks, for instance, tended to be a feature mainly of the rural south while aprons were disproportionately concentrated in northern industrial areas.

81 These were more akin to aprons and bibs than to modern handkerchiefs.

82 S. King, 'Re-clothing the English poor 1750–1840', *Textile History*, 33 (2002), 37–47.

83 S. King, '"I fear you will think me too presumtuous in my demands but necessity has no law": Clothing in English pauper letters 1800–1834', *International Review of Social History*, 54 (2009), 207–36.

84 Purchase of clothing sometimes overlapped strongly with medical treatment, as for instance where twenty-three parishes in our sample purchased or renewed straitjackets for the insane and idiot poor.

85 Hurley, *Longbridge Deverill Poor*, p. 1.

86 BRO, D/P 91/18, Pangbourne correspondence.

87 CURO, WPR 102-116-10, letter, 7 February 1825.

88 Lancashire and Leicestershire parishes purchased biscuits.

89 WRO, 1834/11, overseers' accounts.

90 It is difficult to determine in places like Malmsbury what fuel the term 'flaming' refers to. See WRO, 1589/34, overseers' accounts. For context on Essex see French, 'An irrevocable shift'.

91 On regional fuel types: C. Muldrew, *Food, Energy and the Creation of Industriousness: Work and Material Culture in Agrarian England 1550–1780* (Cambridge: Cambridge University Press, 2011).

92 NORO, PD 145/47, overseers' accounts.

93 BALS, PHA 1-3, Halliwell township books.

94 BALS, PHA 1-3, Halliwell township books.

95 NORO, PD 629/50, overseers' accounts.

96 CPL, vestry minutes.

97 LRO, DDX 28/257, vestry minutes.

98 LCRO, DE 199/2–4, overseers' accounts, and DE 2934/44, overseers' accounts.

99 WYRO, DB 17/C13/5, overseers' accounts, and Tong 12h/1–5, overseers' accounts; 15D74/10/2/3, overseers' accounts.

100 K. Honeyman, *Child Workers in England, 1780–1820: Parish Apprentices and the Making of the Early Industrial Labour Force* (Aldershot: Ashgate, 2007); J. Humphries, *Childhood and Child Labour in the British Industrial Revolution* (Cambridge: Cambridge University Press, 2010); A. Levene, 'Parish apprenticeship and the Old Poor Law in London', *Economic History Review*, 63 (2010), 915–41; and M. Rose, 'Social policy and business: Parish apprenticeship and the early factory system 1780–1834', *Business History*, 31 (1989), 5–32.

101 RL, RC 331.55 Ros, indentures for Newchurch 1759–74. See also RC 331.55 Lov, apprenticeship indentures for print works.
102 NRO, 325p/193 and 194, Thrapston copy letter books.
103 WYRO, RDP 43/163–70, overseers' accounts.
104 F. Kilvington and S. Flood, 'Diary of Thomas Newcome Rector of Shenley 1822–1849', in J. Knight and S. Flood (eds), *Two Nineteenth Century Hertfordshire Diaries* (St Albans: Hertfordshire Record Society, 2002), p. 116.
105 WYRO, RDP 96/76, overseers' accounts.
106 NRO, 325p/194/161, letter (my italics).
107 LRO, PR 3168/5/1, vestry minutes.
108 NRO, 325p/193/77 and 78, Thrapston copy letter books.
109 CURO, WPR5-67/2, letter, 4 March 1823.
110 LRO, PR 2391/16, letter, 29 January 1827.
111 LRO, PR 2391/37, letter, 7 July 1832.
112 NRO, 43p/14, overseers' accounts.
113 NRO, 216p/242/42, letter, 24 June 1832.
114 WRO, 1076/39, overseers' accounts.

7

Dying, being buried and leaving people behind

Introduction

On 14 October 1829, Frances Soundy, a familiar figure from earlier chapters, wrote from Battersea (London) to Pangbourne (Berkshire) seeking assistance with her rent. She claimed to have been unable to save for this expense because

> wan my dear child died i was in hopes that battesea parrish would have assisted me in buring her *as thay did all others* but they refused me and sayd as i found a home for my chilldren and kept them from the parrish i mite do as i could and gentillmen wen i ad got a *undertaker* to barer her and to taik [illegible] so that *my poor child was a fortnight before she was buried* and than i want to them a gain and i told them i would go to a Magastreat and then thay granted it to me so gentellmen it took me 4 months to pay the undertaker ... [1]

Soundy had buried her daughter after two weeks of putrefaction on the credit of the undertaker and without any assurance of reimbursement.[2] She felt that her treatment had been harsh and that the Battersea parish officers treated their own poor differently from those settled elsewhere. Pangbourne duly paid, and this was one of more than 5,000 parish-supported funerals referenced in the dataset. Indeed, payments for or towards funerals were, along with cash payments, the most chronologically, spatially and typologically constant element to the complexion of medical welfare as revealed in Figure 4.5.

Historiographical views on the character of such provision have been almost entirely negative. Established research suggests that Soundy's daughter (like most other, particularly urban, paupers in death) would have been interred in a mass ('pit' burial) or common grave without

any monument to her life and with equally little ceremony.[3] For Julie Rugg eighteenth-century pauper funerals 'bore some resemblance to the rituals attending other members of the community'.[4] Thereafter – and broadly consonant with the so-called 'crisis of the Old Poor Law'[5] – experiences changed. By the 1830s, Ruth Richardson argues, 'working-class lives were cheap and expendable',[6] while Thomas Laqueur has suggested that after 1750 'the funerals of the poor became pauper funerals and pauper funerals became occasions both terrifying to contemplate oneself and profoundly degrading to one's survivors'.[7] Julian Litten notes that it was not just the form and parsimony of such funerals that worried contemporaries, but the sense of 'one's failure to maintain a position, however lowly, in contemporary society'.[8] In turn, the dependent and marginal poor are seen to have abhorred the very idea of pauper funerals.[9] They 'signified poverty, suggested insufficient grief and condemned the dead to obscurity', such that any attempt to fashion a respectable funeral would be seen 'to claim for the dead an identity and a modicum of dignity'.[10] While Julie-Marie Strange has done much to problematise the emotional responses of the labouring poor to death for the later nineteenth century,[11] the sense that at earlier dates the final months, weeks or days of the dying poor were infused with an absolute fear of the parish has been a constant.[12]

This is a compelling picture, and there can be no doubt that in the most rapidly growing and densely packed urban areas the shortages of burial space and associated mass graves, highlighted for London by G. A. Walker in the 1840s, were very much a reality.[13] Alexander Somerville likened pauper funeral experiences to prisoners being buried in the prison grounds, while Robert Southey claimed that the poor dreaded 'the disrespectful and careless funeral' which was the best the parish offered.[14] The poet Charlotte Smith stumbled across a parish funeral in 1792 and thought she saw 'cold, reluctant parish charity', having four years previously put to poem an unseemly tug of war between a parish and house of industry over the cost of burying a pauper corpse.[15] And William Blake could see the workhouse from his own home, noting that 'the Grave Digger neglects to cover the Coffins of the Dead with Earth when buried, which occasions a very offensive smell to the Neighbourhood and Persons in the workhouse'.[16] Indeed, for the most overcrowded cities, the coffins of all classes 'were by necessity stacked rather than interred, since there was no longer sufficient

fresh earth for burial'.[17] Yet moving from totemic stories to broader generalisation about sentiment is not easy. There were real problems of logistics – what to do with a dying or dead pauper who had no legal settlement in a place – and of basic law. In terms of the latter, it was not always clear that officials had the power to bury the dead. Nineteenth-century guidance manuals for overseers differed considerably in their rendering of this matter. One handbook in multiple editions spanning the Old and New Poor Laws reminded officials that save for bodies washed ashore or otherwise abandoned 'overseers have no power to bury the bodies of persons at the cost of the poor rate', instead suggesting that the 'occupier of the house in which a death has occurred is under an obligation at common law to bury the body, and to defray the expenses'.[18]

Ambiguities like this are important. They stand alongside extensive evidence in my data for an alternative rendering of the fate of people like Frances Soundy's daughter. Accounts and bills often recorded a final illness, burial and relief for those left behind as one expenditure event, one seamless whole of medical welfare. This is simultaneously justification for the inclusion of burial costs in the definition of medical spending but also indicative of a rather more concerned attitude on the part of overseers than is sometimes allowed. Keith Snell's large-scale survey of gravestones suggests that commemorative inscriptions could, even for the very poorest, be instituted so as to confirm their membership of a local community.[19] And where stone memorials were not feasible wooden grave-boards might be purchased so as to provide a focal point for bereaved families.[20] The unceremonious dumping of pauper bodies could certainly be avoided.[21] More positive attitudes are perhaps masked by the fact that we generally obtain the richest perspectives on the form, content and extent of pauper funerals when something went wrong or neglect took place. There is not a single letter in the data used for this study which thanks the overseer for a timely and sensitive parish funeral even though (as we shall see below) officials would often go to considerable expense. Moreover, the number and scope of pauper burials is certainly under-accounted in the parish archives, leading us to underplay their very ubiquity. Fees for coffins and other funeral-related services were sometimes hidden within general payments to tradesmen. Moreover, as the case of Frances Soundy suggests, paupers might secure an 'independent' funeral but then apply

for consequential relief to cover rent, food or other expenses that could not be paid because of meeting funeral costs. Conceptually, the distinction between the two forms of spending is a fragile one. Overseers themselves also masked expenditure, as for instance when they paid (unspecified) 'relief' to other paupers for duties connected to the care of the dead and dying. Consequently, we probably miss some of the ritual that might still be associated with pauper funerals, such as washing and dressing the body. The experience of Frances Soundy – actively seeking support from Battersea parish to bury her daughter 'as thay did all others' – begins to suggest that pauper attitudes towards, and experiences of, parish burial were more variegated than much of the literature would show. There is even evidence that some paupers saw a parish funeral as a basic right, one actively to be sought out.[22]

This chapter, then, is informed by a sense that historians have been too ready to generalise particular scandals and transpose attitudes formed in the immediate aftermath of the New Poor Law onto parish officials under the Old. We have been unimaginative in setting the yardsticks against which the form, scope and meaning of the pauper funeral might be judged, losing sight of the fact that the funerals of the independent labouring poor might be no better than those afforded by the parish, particularly for children.[23] And there has been an unfortunate tendency to consider the issue of pauper funerals in isolation, as discrete events removed from their context. In reality, however, and as I have already suggested, overseers were often intimately involved in the process of dying and were often called to pick up the pieces of a death for bereaved family and kin. Understanding this process, as well as its particular focal points such as the interment, is vital if we are to understand the meaning and experience of 'the pauper funeral'.[24] The chapter will thus explore four key stages in the process of dying: the ways in which paupers and officials came to recognise and respond rhetorically and practically to a final illness; the spectrum of pauper burial experiences; the nature of the negotiation process between pauper families and officials over burial; and the relationships between officials and paupers' residual families. It will suggest that variations of experience and provision were greater within parishes than between them; that the nature of the pauper funeral was an acceptable ground of contestation between paupers and officials; and that parishes tended towards the more generous and elaborate end of the spectrum of

funeral provision, implicitly or explicitly recognising an obligation in
this area.

Recognising and treating impending death

As Chapter 2 suggested, it was officials rather than doctors who ultimately judged the seriousness of a medical condition and the relief
that should be attached to it. Unsurprisingly, they struggled with the
identification of a potentially 'mortal' illness.[25] This was especially the
case for infants and young children, for whom payment of costs associated with a pauper funeral were infrequently preceded by extensive
supplementary resources related to a final illness.[26] Even among adults
and older children, however, the likely outcome of an illness was often
difficult to gauge.[27] This partly reflected imperfect understanding of
disease aetiology but also two other problems, the first of which was
how to reconcile the multiple voices which described and characterised the illness. For the out-parish poor, the intensity and likely consequences of an illness had to be judged at a distance, via second-hand
reporting, the prognosis of doctors conveyed in letters or the opinions
of other overseers. The language used in such reporting was colourful
and powerful. Letters received by parishes in Northamptonshire and
Oxfordshire employed rhetoric like: 'he cannot continue much longer';
'in a 'very poor state'; 'to all human probability [he] will not recover';
'She cant – in the Course of things – be long troublesome to you';
'I am every week – expecting to hear that she is removed from her
present state of pain & infirmity'; '[she] wishes for Death with seeming
vehemence'; '[she] is not likely to be any long Time a Burthen to you';
'a miserable appearance of death'; 'going dead'; and 'to all appearances
in a dying state'. How to interpret such language was a task that vexed
officials. The situation was just as complex for sick paupers living within
their parish of settlement, where multiple voices might be supplemented by hearsay. A second and related problem was that paupers
depicting their illnesses invariably melded together the reporting of
fact with the colour needed to secure relief. How, for instance, should
the overseer of Colchester (Essex) have read William James's assertion
of 13 September 1827 that 'Neither of us [he referred to his sick daugh-
ter], according to the Course of Nature, are not likely to Live long'?[28]
Or how might the Rothersthorpe (Northamptonshire) overseer have

received Amy Hardwick's undated (but probably 1812) letter which opened 'The Vale of Tears comes now to me and this is the Last I shall Ever Rite to you'?[29] The problem of assessing the seriousness of illnesses remained even where the person could (like the in-parish poor) be inspected on a daily basis. This is well demonstrated with an example from the Midlands: when faced with a request from the parish of Wing (Rutland) to be allowed to pay relief to Elizabeth Watson, the overseer of her 'home' parish of Oundle (Northamptonshire) wrote candidly that

> Eliz Watson was in our workhouse some short time ago & derived great benefit from the treatment. Indeed got as she herself said quite well & left it. She has been for some years constantly on our Parish Books & we were much astonished at her very quick recovery from her treatment at the workhouse and my orders were not to allow her any more money or relief out of the house but from your own signatures which tell me that it is right. I am willing to allow what you ask.

> PS We considered that she came the old soldier over us to use a Common phrase for the last year or more.[30]

However we interpret their meaning, claims and observations of final illnesses are common in the underlying data. Paupers like Elizabeth Watson experienced miraculous recoveries. Yet some two thirds of all seemingly mortal cases recorded in pauper letters and vestry minutes resulted either in rapid death or the onset of a series of sickness episodes that would eventually prove fatal. John Gunnell, the cholera sufferer already encountered in Chapter 2, is emblematic of paupers in this category. Writing from Manchester on 6 January 1834 he noted:

> I wrote to you some time ago requesting your Assistance but have not had any answer I therefore once more Repeat my Request nothing Doubting but it will be my last. I have for a long time been very ill, not able to do anything at all, and for a considerable time confined to my Bed with not the last hope or expectation of ever leaving it in this Vale of Tears but the Lord's will be Done I am Resigned to it and it alone for he alone knoweth best what to Do with his Children.[31]

This reference to the Bible and to the text of the common funeral ceremony was clearly requisitioned to emphasise the seriousness of the case and to give credibility to a claim that this was going to be his 'last'

illness. By 22 January (when his widow wrote), and before a letter
from the parish containing £3 had arrived, John Gunnell was dead. The
fact that Oxendon parish appears to have dispatched a substantial sum
of money begins to suggest that officials and vestries recognised the
spectre of mortal illness as requiring a response, even if this was not
legally mandated. Indeed, officials often berated one another where
action on potentially mortal illness was seen to be insufficient. Thus a
letter from York to the overseer of Woodmansey (West Yorkshire) in
July 1808 urged a faster response to an earlier request to help Emma
Binnington 'in her last extremity'. The clock 'was ticking away on her
life and she in such abject need as to bring shame on the payers of
Mansey [Woodmansey] in the eyes of his neighbours'.[32]

While my data contains spectacular examples of neglect, disinterest,
delay and cruelty, this was not the representative experience. Whether
out of humanity, custom or concerns for economy (it was cheaper
to treat paupers than to pay for funerals and the support of bereaved
relatives), officials in the later decades of the Old Poor Law seem to
have recognised an obligation not just to respond to life-threatening
illness, but to do so relatively generously. For the earlier part of our
period the responses largely coalesced around the provision of food,
fuel, cash allowances, casual nursing and consequential payments such
as rent arrears. By the 1790s the attention of doctors had become more
important in stock responses to potentially mortal illnesses. So had
sustained nursing, as the Old Poor Law increasingly came to pay for
nursing and support services that might previously have been provided
gratis by friends and neighbours. Indeed, over time and in almost all
parishes, we see the development of multi-faceted and at times very
expensive relief packages attached to final illnesses as the whole process
of dying came increasingly firmly within the ambit of the overseer and
his purse.

For the in-parish poor, the nature and scope of these packages is relatively easy to reconstruct from vestry minutes and overseers' accounts.
In Culcheth (Lancashire), for instance, William Richardson saw his
allowance doubled during a final illness from December 1815 to March
1816, in addition to receiving rent payments, clothing, and nursing and
funeral costs. Thomas Catton was given 17s per month during his final
illness from April to November 1818, as well as two rent payments
totalling £11 8s 1d. Thomas Jenkinson was paid between 1s and 10s 7d

per month (plus two rent payments totalling £9 1s and clothing allowances) during his wife's final illness, which stretched out from April to December 1818.[33] Comprehensive support packages were likewise to be found in the Midlands. Thus at Stoke Mandeville (Buckinghamshire) in April 1829, Sarah Smith was paid 5s for nursing the dying Richard Thorne, almost the final act in a year of increasing cash payments, rent support, food and clothing allowances for this pauper. On the night of his death, the parish in addition paid Mrs Ryman 3s for sitting up with Thorne, while she and Mary Flitney were paid 6s for laying out the body and making the shroud.[34] At Thurcaston (Leicestershire) twenty-two final illnesses between 1804 and 1810 involved an average of sixteen different payments, with Jonathan Scott's protracted death and subsequent funeral between 1808 and 1809 absorbing 6 per cent of the total welfare resources of the parish on its own.[35] In Berkshire, Stanford-in-the-Vale seems to have been particularly attentive to the in-parish poor in the last throes of life. Robert Betts's funeral (17s 6d) in 1765 was preceded by nursing (£2), cash allowances (£5 19s), fuel and 'putting up bed' (15s 7d). The death and funeral of Henry Griffin in 1787 were preceded by payments for vinegar (to wash the bed chamber), shirts, wood, the costs of men and women 'sitting up' and 'waiting', cash relief and food.[36] While epidemic diseases or the question of what to do with travelling folk may have undermined the 'normal' parish response to potentially mortal illness, there is strong evidence that officials acted quickly and comprehensively when informed of a really serious illness of a settled pauper.

Bills transmitted between officials for the out-parish poor suggest that a comprehensive approach is generalisable to this group as well. Thus on 28 January 1834 the overseer of Hammersmith (London) wrote to his counterpart in Pangbourne (Berkshire) to inform him of the death of John Hope, who had been ill since 16 December 1833. He enclosed a bill for the funeral and for cash relief given to Hope, but the two together were only just greater than the £3 1s 6d costs of medical attendance by John Bosoling and son. Their detailed bill was enclosed and suggests that either father or son attended the pauper every day between 16 December 1833 and 14 January 1834, the day of Hope's death. They provided twenty-four doses of 'mixture', five boxes of pills or powders, a bolus, two 'injections' and a 'pipe' (presumably a catheter) as well as bleeding and generalised services.[37] A bill for the last

illness of Thomas Wood sent from Trowbridge (Wiltshire) to Chard (Somerset) in 1802 had rather less doctoring but fully £5 of cash payments and £2 worth of drugs to be administered by paid nurses.[38] Much further north, the overseer of the small rural community of Stanhope (West Yorkshire) wrote to the overseer of Dent (Westmorland) to explain that his bill of £8 for the six-month illness, death and funeral of Margaret Webb reflected his attempts to exercise 'the most economy consistent with my duty to our poor'.[39] This is eloquent testimony to a perceived obligation to act and to act well which was shared across the spatial and typological boundaries inherent in our extensive corpus of overseers' correspondence.[40] An implicit assumption in some of the historiography that end-of-life care was a matter of nursing, acceptance and patience is wide of the mark.[41]

The pauper burial experience

Where the accumulated resources of the parish were insufficient to preserve life, the pauper funeral beckoned. How common this event was is unclear given the accounting lacunae confronted throughout this study and the mass burials at times of epidemic. The very definition of a pauper funeral is also complicated by the fact that relatives might raise part of the funeral costs and then seek a parish supplement. Hence, Lovell Squire, the overseer of Bluntisham-cum-Erith (Cambridgeshire), wrote to his counterpart in Peterborough (Northamptonshire) on 15 May 1834 about the recently deceased Margaret Searson, asking him to pay £4 10s for 'the expenses incurred in her maintenance, nursing & burial expenses'. He noted, '(her mother having paid a part) otherwise it would have been more'.[42] James Sanderson, the overseer of Higher Booth (Lancashire), wrote to his counterpart in Billington (Lancashire) to say that 'The bearer [of this letter] James Driver has had the misfortune to have a child burned to death he has an annuity and is entitled to your consideration for something to bury it'.[43] Communities and occupational colleagues might also step in. Thus, Jonathan Lawrence, the overseer of Colnbrook (Staffordshire), wrote to his counterpart in Tilehurst (Berkshire) on 4 February 1830 about the eldest daughter of Widow Wiggens, 'who died after six weeks of illness during which time her mother was obliged to be at home to attend her'. In asking for a small allowance to support Wiggens, he

noted, 'The Burial Expences was Rec'd by a Subscription Raised at the mill ware she work'd'.[44] Moreover, self-help via burial clubs (often lodged with undertakers[45]) and friendly societies could also forestall or supplement pauper funerals. We should, however, beware of overstating such mechanisms. Less than 5 per cent of the paupers who wrote to parishes requesting help with funerals in the underlying letter corpus mentioned alternative sources of funding. Rather, they usually stated that the burial costs were beyond them, in effect asking for a parish funeral.

Set against this backdrop, reconstructing the character and scope of pauper funerals is complex. While, as we have seen, many commentators have suggested that this prospect was met with dread – that the request itself embodied the final descent of the pauper family into degradation – there is no evidence whatsoever in the underlying data of this sort of feeling being elaborated, or of dogged resistance to the involvement of poor law officials. This observation perhaps reflects the fact that the label 'pauper funeral' could mask a spectrum of spending, sentiment and experience. For Essex, the inter-parish spectrum was relatively narrow throughout the period. Thomas Sokoll shows that £1 was a standard allowance for funerals, with some evidence that paupers saw such a sum as a 'going rate'.[46] Even in Essex, however, it is possible to find extraordinary parish generosity, as in the case of David Rivenhall, whose letter of May 1826 contained a bill (subsequently met by his parish) for two child funerals which encompassed coffins, pillows, mattresses for the bodies, hoods and scarves.[47] West Yorkshire also displays a relatively narrow inter-parish spectrum, one end of which is located in the woollen town of Dewsbury. Its overseer James Burnley wrote to his counterpart in Market Harborough (Leicestershire) to contest a bill for the final illness and burial of Rebecca Hazelgreave. Burnley noted that the Dewsbury vestry thought the bill 'most enormous' and offered only a partial payment. He particularly disputed the burial costs, noting that 'nor do we pay any funeral expenses except for workhouse people', and offered 14s for a coffin with 5s 6d for burial fees.[48] The average cost of a pauper funeral within the parish was £1, and even in an area well known for its parsimony in poor relief Dewsbury stands out.[49] The other end of the spectrum is represented by Horsforth, where average pauper burial costs exclusive of partial contributions reached £1 11s by the 1810s.[50]

For other counties, the range of parochial experience could be very wide indeed. In Lancashire, Kirkham parish paid for sixty-one funerals between 1804 and 1816 at an average cost of just over £1 each. This low figure – broadly on a par with Essex – is partly explained by the presence of babies and children (who were relatively cheap to bury) in the list of funerals, but excluding this group would still only give a figure of £1 5s.[51] By contrast, Culcheth paid 14s and 18s for the funeral expenses of unidentified children in 1815 as well as £1 10s for the funeral of the aged William Richardson. By December 1818 costs had clearly risen, with the overseer paying £2 8s 9d for the funeral of Thomas Jenkinson's wife, while by 1820 the overseers of Culcheth were paying £1 1s 4d for the coffin alone when Thomas Coleshill was buried, and £2 14s for the combined funeral expenses of Thomas Yates by 1821.[52] Other places encompassed a similar range. When Sarah Foster died in September 1823 the Stoke Mandeville overseer paid 5s for laying-out of the body, 4s for new calico and its making up into a shroud, and 5s 2d for the bread, cheese and beer consumed by mourners at the funeral. This was in addition to a coffin, a service, a plot and the ringing of bells. In addition, the parish paid for the washing and boarding of the six orphaned children and kept them all in clothing for five years. In total, the death episode cost the parish a minimum of £11 in terms of immediate and deferred expenditure.[53] Nowhere, however, was the range of pauper funeral costs as varied as in Wiltshire. Here, vagrants and wandering strangers who happened to die were usually treated with parsimony, as for instance in the case of the 6s expended on the funeral of 'the woman that was frozen to death' at Trowbridge in 1794.[54] Controlling for this group, however, does little to narrow the spectrum of experience. One end is located by funerary culture in the parish of Kintbury (Berkshire), where officials tended to spend less than 3s on the funerals of children and £1 or less for adults.[55] At the other extreme, Hardenhuish was spending 15s on child funerals as early as the 1760s, while adult funerals in Malmesbury and Chippenham were costing £2 by the early 1800s. Even in Trowbridge the cost of pauper coffins in 1813 was sufficient to absorb 6 per cent of all poor law resources for the parish during that year.[56]

Some of the obvious explanations for this sort of inter-parochial variation – urban–rural, rural–industrial or rich–poor dichotomies – have little traction. Poor rural communities in Oxfordshire or

Northamptonshire generally spent more on parish funerals than richer proto-industrial parishes in West Yorkshire. Lancashire industrial and proto-industrial parishes spent more than West Yorkshire communities with a similar socio-economic complexion. Parsimony was to be found in some urban areas. Reading, for instance, paid an average of only 15s for the funerals of its in-parish poor.[57] On the other hand, Oxford spent an average of £1 8s on funerals, somewhat above the normal level for places like Henley-on-Thames.[58] Moreover, even in the largest urban areas, it was possible for a pauper to garner a relatively expensive funeral. Nicholas Robinson, assistant vestry clerk for Bloomsbury (London), wrote to his counterpart in Market Harborough on 29 September 1828 to thank him for sending the costs of attending one John Lamb in his final illness and of the subsequent funeral. The Harborough overseer had, on learning of Lamb's death, dispatched a note asking his London counterpart to deal with the funeral 'as you would one of your own paupers'. The sum charged – £4 3s – is both substantial and a reflection of the fact that Bloomsbury seems to have funded 'decent' pauper funerals.[59] In similar fashion, when Edward Buckeridge wrote on 7 October 1828 from Lambeth (London) to Pangbourne about a funeral for his mother he 'would wish to Remind the Gentlemen that the expences of the funeral when all is paid will not be a farthing less than six pounds and that will not amount to a years Money [i.e. his mother's previous allowance] at three shillings per week'. The vestry subsequently paid the enormous sum of £10 for the funeral.[60]

Other explanatory variables have more potential. In Leicestershire communities that came under the ambit of an undertaker funded fewer and cheaper funerals than those that did not. This may reflect the fact that the provision of credit kept families from full dependence upon the parish, rather than merely substituting for the lack of parochial action. Some of the variation between parishes may also reflect differences in the background understanding of what made a 'respectable' funeral. Overseers in most English counties would have had a keen appreciation of funerary standards for the different social groups in their locality, not least because they attended so many. They also had some independent yardsticks of quality in the sense, for instance, of funeral allowances made by burial clubs and friendly societies. While such information is not always easy to find, Shaun Morley's remarkable study of more than 700 Oxfordshire friendly societies suggests that funeral allowances

could vary between £2 and £4 while the more widely defined death benefits (which might also include a widow's pension, for instance) varied
between £2 and £11. Here, and also in Lancashire, 'club benefits' drove
down the absolute number of funerals that the parish had to support,
but the average cost of the remaining pauper funerals in such parishes
tended to be significant because background expectations were also
higher.[61] Meanwhile, at least some of the variation between parishes
must reflect ingrained local and religious customs. Thus it matters that
the Northamptonshire parish of Braybrooke tended to buy funeral
clothes for mourners whereas most other Northamptonshire parishes
did not; that the Berkshire parish of Thatcham always purchased beer
for funerals but never paid for people to bear the coffin; that Englefield
(Berkshire) paid the expenses of mourners; and that Mawnan Smith
(Cornwall) paid the smoking and drinking expenses of mourners,
funded candlelit processions and provided the wood for bonfires after
parish funerals.[62] When places like Blackburn (Lancashire) petitioned
against the passage of the Anatomy Act in the 1830s, they did so precisely because their tradition of burying with dignity was so ingrained
in the very expectational fabric of the town.[63]

There is much more to be written about the essential localism of
funerary practices to counter the stark and urban-centred generalisations that have come to dominate the historiography. Meanwhile,
moving further than broad-brush explanations involves an acknowledgement that individual communities could also evidence (both
over time and in any single year) a wide spectrum of costs and thus
variation in the character and content of pauper funerals.[64] Indeed, variations were often more marked within parishes than between them. A
detailed case study allows us to explore this experiential spectrum. Thus
in Hulme, by the early nineteenth century witnessing the inexorable
encroachment of Manchester, a particularly fine collection of pauper
letters, overseers' correspondence and bills provides extensive detail
on the conduct and composition of the pauper funeral.[65] The parish
received literally hundreds of hastily written notes from overseers in
other parishes informing them of the deaths of their out-parish paupers.
Invariably they asked the Hulme overseer to treat the deceased 'as you
would your own' such that subsequent funeral bills probably reflect
normative standards. The Hulme overseer likewise wrote to other parishes with the same instructions when dealing with his extensive list of

out-parish poor. Normative yardsticks can also be understood from the bills of tradesmen. Some give only the very broadest indication, such as bills submitted by makers for 'large and small coffins'. Other coffin makers were more specific. An unnamed supplier in January 1834 sent a bill for three sizes of 'small' coffin for deceased children (ranging from 2s 6d to 3s 9d) and for a series of 'large coffins' at around 10s apiece. John Hazelhurst's collective 1834 bill for supplying thirty-eight coffins to Hulme parish specified eleven different grades and sizes. The parish also paid rather higher bills, including 19s for 'a coffin with full lining' for (the presumably adult) Catherine Blake and a coffin with brass nails and a silver plaque for the child Sarah Burgess at a cost of 8s. Julian Litten traces at least thirty different coffin types available to over-seers, arguing that 17s 'got a good inch elm coffin, smoothed, oiled' and finished with decorative nails, while shrouds 'of common quality were to be had at 2s 8d for 6 feet and 3s 8d for middling quality'.[66] These, however, were London rather than provincial benchmarks, and an 1832 bill to Hulme from John Singer specifying 'good elm coffins' places an adult size at between 8s and 12s in this area of Lancashire. For Hulme at least, the generalisation that the coffins of the poor were 'cheap and flimsy' does not seem an adequate representation of the range of experiences, though identifying a 'typical' pauper coffin is probably beyond the data.

Coffins were just one element of the pauper funeral. Many of the scribbled notes from overseers just refer to their willingness to pay the 'dues' associated with burial. By the 1830s St George's Church in Hulme had a pre-printed bill-head for all burials which provides more detail. The dues for interring a child stood at a relatively uniform 3s 6d, while the interment of those found dead – such as the 'late female found drowned in the Medlock river' on 1 August 1834 – were charged at a standard 7s 6d. For others, however, there was rather more variation. The proforma for Esta Burgess's funeral (12 January 1833) entailed the burial itself (5s), church fees (1s 4d), fees for the clerk (1s), fees for the sexton (2s 6d) and ringing of a bell (1s), with a total bill of 10s 10d not including the coffin or food and drink for mourners, which were the subject of a separate account. For John Taylor's funeral a year later the costs were: burial (7s 6d), dues (1s 10d), clerk (1s), sexton (3s), bier (6d), bell (1s) and an unspecified extra (1s). In general, interments for adults varied between 9s and 19s, with a mean coalescing around

11s, all excluding supplementary costs such as entertaining mourners. Total costs ranged widely. Samuel Smith's burial on 31 March 1834 comprised a coffin (15s), dues (7s), pall and cloak (4s), funeral bread (18s), meat and drink (12s 2d) and mourning gloves (4s), or £2 15s 3d in total. The consolidated bill for the funeral of Thomas Brownhill one week later was just 24s. As the comparison between Burgess and Taylor begins to suggest, however, there was a tendency for some elements of the fee structure, particularly the costs of digging the grave and the church dues, to increase significantly over time. Notices like that of 14 August 1834, stating that gravestones might be purchased and palls and cloaks 'had' from the clerk, also became more common from the late 1820s, suggesting some increase in expectations of the 'normal' pauper funeral.[67]

If the Hulme collection is particularly fine, the core lessons from the parish – that the pauper funeral could be respectable and in some cases elaborate, that there was some tendency for aggregate costs per funeral to increase over time and that there was a wide spectrum of experience – is duplicated for this and earlier periods in other parishes across the country. Explaining such intra-parochial variation is challenging. Indeed, some things were so situational as to defy explanation. An unexplained 1784 decision by the Brimpton (Berkshire) vestry to replace entertainment for mourners with more elaborate ceremonials for the body, including coffin bearers, had a significant impact on the character of pauper funerals. The fact of the change speaks to Keith Snell's sense that funerals and memorials could be used to signal the embeddedness of paupers in their community rather than their exclusion, but the reason for the changed policy is unclear.[68] We can, however, begin to discern some more general explanatory variables. While there is no sense from the underlying data that women were treated more or less favourably than men, or that the aged were invariably regarded as more deserving than other groups, it is clear that Welsh, Scottish and Irish migrants got short shrift in terms of pauper funerals.[69] More generally, while we lack the family reconstitutions with which to pinpoint the migratory status and family situations of dead paupers, there is a broad sense in which these variables mattered. Children whose parents were already dead generally had more expensive funerals than those whose parents were alive and might be expected to organise a familial contribution. Belonging also mattered. In all of the sample parishes the

dead poor from long-resident families seem to have warranted more expensive funerals than the newly migrant.[70] Indeed paupers traded on their long residence in a place when trying to secure funerary resources. Such considerations were, though, sometimes outweighed by the nature of the death involved. The funerals of adults and children whose deaths were attributable to horrific accidents in the domestic or work environment seem to have occasioned particularly generous responses from officials. At the opposite extreme, cholera patients were treated perfunctorily in funerary terms. A bill from the Manchester Board of Health to Hulme on 6 October 1834 charged just £5 14s 6d for burying more than forty victims.[71]

These are important observations. They suggest that we have too readily adopted a negative perspective on the pauper funeral under the Old Poor Law. It is certainly true that some pauper funerals were more important than others and some obligations were felt more keenly than others. Nonetheless, most places most of the time tended towards the more generous and elaborate end of the spectrum of provision. In this sense, pauper resistance to parish funerals may have been muted because many officials were highly sensitive – not to say empathetic – to the need to deal 'well' with the dead poor. And if most parishes sat towards the more generous end of provision and the average cost of funerals was rising over time as in Hulme, it is entirely possible that pauper funerals were not very different from, and in many places may have been rather better than, those afforded to the independent labour-ing poor via familial, community or workplace provision. This is not to say, of course, that funeral provision was always given as of right, and it is to the agency of the poor and their advocates in negotiating funeral provision that we now turn.

Negotiating a place on the spectrum

In thinking about the process of dying there has been a tendency in the secondary literature to focus on an end point – the recording of what was spent on funerals. Yet few places followed the example of some Essex parishes and adopted a well-known 'tariff' for funerals. Rather, these matters had to be negotiated by the families of the deceased, whether they were in- or out-parish paupers. Those entering this arena seem to have employed both the rhetorical strategies adopted by the

sick poor more generally and some that were specific to obtaining resources for burial and associated costs. The former encompassed notions of economy, respectability and contribution. Thus Joseph Yates wrote from Huntingdon to Peterborough on 12 September 1799 to say that unless the parish met the expenses of his daughter's funeral (37s) the overseer of Huntingdon would remove him. This, he reminded his settlement parish, would mean 'I can't get my bread' and he might thus cost rather more than 37s to maintain.[72] Other paupers grasped the concept of economy in the funeral itself. James House, in an undated letter to Pangbourne on the occasion of the death of one of his children, asked for assistance with funeral expenses, 'which I will endeavour shall be done in the cheapest manner'.[73] The in-parish poor were equally likely to deploy this device. For some writers, economy had to be balanced by contribution to, and standing in, the community. At its broadest, such contribution was implied simply by noting long residence or connection with a place, but some of those seeking funerary support made more direct claims. Elizabeth Firth had attended the vestry at Downham Market (Norfolk) on 6 July 1802 to pick up a cash allowance. She wrote from Shelton three weeks later seeking support for the burial of her dead daughter, claiming that 'all hereabout think it a scandal that you do not act I am known here Gentlemen and your neglect shall not go unspoken'.[74] Even if others did not go this far, the provision of testimonials from those of higher social status, claiming the friendship and protection of the overseer, and observations on the prior respectability and self-reliance of families and individuals all implied that officials should act to protect the reputation of the parish and the dignity of the dead.

Other strategies were more explicitly tailored to securing acceptable funerary provision. The first, as we have already seen, was to request a contribution to supplement the resources of the community or the family. This strategy influenced both the cost of parish provision and its character and range, and might run from specific requests for instance for a coffin or internment dues, and specific sums through to requests like that of William Martin to the overseer of Leeds for 'a small trifle' to bury his newborn child.[75] An analogous approach was to emphasise the limited pool of kinship and its poverty when trying to secure substitution for personal resources. Edward Buckeridge of Lambeth, a pauper familiar from earlier analysis in this chapter, wanted to bury

his mother but 'I have not got one belonging to me that is able to give me a sixpence towards the burying of her. My Brother Charles I cannot expect any thing from him he as enough to do he as got a wife and 7 children my other two Brothers is out of employ.'[76] The sense that parishes ought to step in and provide what an otherwise willing kinship group could not is repeated consistently.

Whatever the exact constellation and wealth of kin, a second specific strategy was for bereaved families and their advocates to inscribe appeals into structures of local custom. Some paupers sought in effect to create custom: John Thorpe's central argument when he applied to the Oakham (Rutland) vestry for the costs of burying his wife was that 'as you had the support of her in life so you must have the burying of her in death'. While few paupers or advocates were as direct as this in their letters, the implication that prior support created obligation is latent in many letters.[77] Other paupers drew explicitly on customary practice. When John and Elizabeth Mason wrote from Crays Hill (Essex) to Rochford (Essex) in April of an unspecified year seeking payment of a funerary bill for their recently deceased daughter they explained the size of the bill with reference to local custom: 'the form that the poor is Buried Some times there is Six to Carry and Some times there is Eight to Carry and the Custom is to give Each man one shilling a Peace'.[78] Custom carried even more force for the relatives of dead paupers who were in their settlement parish because local practice was simply more transparent. In Stoke Mandeville, Joseph Charge received a pension of 8s plus food, clothing, extra payments during sickness and fuel between 1826 and 1831. At the latter date the vestry, clearly irritated by his continued dependence and fecundity (the family had borne eleven children), reduced his allowance to 6s per week as he was 'to take his chance'. Despite his status as a pensioner, on 15 May 1829 the vestry refused both relief and a coffin on the occasion of the death of one of his recently born children. Three days later, however, the overseer had ridden roughshod over the wishes of the vestry, granting relief, a shroud and a coffin, citing 'custom'.[79] This sense that overseers had a keen appreciation of, and were susceptible to, claims framed in terms of local custom can be seen in their own correspondence. Thus, when the Oundle (Northamptonshire) overseer wrote to his counterpart in Peterborough in March 1833 about the death of Widow Gladhall he noted that 'We generally allow £1 towards the funeral', but

not knowing local custom, he deferred to his counterpart and 'would feel obliged by your doing the same as if she belonged to you and if you will add the acct to the other and let me have it'.[80] While the variety of pauper funeral experiences within most parishes would suggest the absence of a single knowable 'custom', past practice clearly did shape the outlook of officials.[81]

A third tailored rhetorical device was for writers to call on the essential humanity and empathy of the overseer or vestry. The aptly named Hannah Death wrote from hospital in London to Chelmsford on 8 July 1824 on the occasion of the death of her son Thomas. Asking for 'a little money to help to bury him', she enjoined her correspondent Dr Prichard to 'have Compassion and lay it before the Gentlemen he is dead and must be buried'.[82] That this was a shared rhetorical landscape is revealed by extensive references in overseers' correspondence to the need for parishes to act with humanity in relation to cases where particularly horrible deaths or a persistent run of illnesses or deaths had overwhelmed a family. And while the language of appeal for the in-parish poor is more difficult to discern, there is some evidence at least that such paupers also used the rhetoric of humanity. Robert Hargreaves, for instance, attended the Calverley vestry in April 1814 and asked the ratepayers to 'consider in your own breasts what it must be for a father to bury his son'.[83]

Of course, none of these rhetorical and strategic devices were necessarily discrete. Harriet Hughes, writing from London to Pangbourne on 29 July 1827, was one of more than 200 paupers who used a suite of the approaches outlined here. Her letter was to

> let you know my baby is dead and hope you will be so Good as to assist me in putting it under the ground as is am very much distressed on account of her being ill so long my mother is likewise very ill and not near able to help herself for some time so hope you will take it into consideration to send us some money to relieve us as soon as you can as it is time my baby was in the ground as soon as possible you can ... [84]

Here the inability of Hughes to act as a mother should was inscribed into a framework of appeals to the basic humanity of the officers ('it is time my baby was in the ground'), promises of economy (she wanted assistance and not the whole bill), respectability and the favourable track record of the family (she had looked after her mother and daughter

without recourse to the parish). The success, partial success or failure of strategies like these, duplicated as they were for the in-parish poor, located dead paupers on the spectrum of recorded parish funerary provision, and while that spectrum could be wide, officials found it hard to ultimately refuse bills for pauper funerals when they were presented to them. Even where they had discretion – as for instance when relatives or advocates asked vestries for unspecified help with funerals – officials more often than not responded with relative generosity. In turn, that generosity extended in most places and at most times to ongoing support for relatives left behind, and it is to this issue that the chapter finally turns.

Relatives left behind

As I have observed, little work has been done for this period on the way in which the poor experienced grief and loss. Yet the sources are redolent with sentiment and emotion. There are plenty of examples of families for whom death continued in the early nineteenth century to be understood in terms of Godly will. For many, however, the deaths of children, partners and other relatives were met with more than just resigned acceptance. Some paupers nodded obliquely to their feeling, referring to 'untimely' death, 'my poor' husband, wife or child, or 'sudden loss'. Others were much more direct in their elaboration of grief, worry, depression and familial stress. William James of Colchester wrote to James Allen of the same town on 26 February 1823 to say that his wife had died. He 'did not expect her to have gone so soon' and asked for a further allowance to bury her, explaining his multiple requests with reference to 'Grief and Confusion'.[85] Richard Porter, writing to Rayliegh (Essex) from Ashby-de-la-Zouch (Leicestershire) on 10 March 1826 concerning the death of his wife, was even more direct. He was experiencing 'most pitiable distress' having 'suffer'd a severe loss in the death of my poor wife'. Her death, his own illness and the recent death of his father-in-law had reduced him 'to the lowest Ebb'.[86] Perhaps unsurprisingly when we consider recent attempts to rethink the emotional relationship between parents and offspring, the deaths of children could be met with considerable turmoil.[87] Jonathan Peaks, for instance, wrote to Rothersthorpe from Norwich (Norfolk) to say that he 'was threwn to the laste eextreemety' by the loss of his

last surviving child.[88] Where parents, husbands and wives were unable to linguistically frame their emotions, epistolary advocates and even officials themselves might step in. James Wilson, overseer of Otley (West Yorkshire), thus wrote to his counterpart in Hulme on 14 June 1804 to say that Jane Pimm had 'sunk into a deathly melancholy' after the recent death of her husband.[89]

For many, death in the family prompted the threat of financial ruin as well as emotional pain. In turn, local policy on this issue varied considerably and with no sustained spatial or typological patterning. In the Lancashire parish of Kirkham officials paid out only £2 8s 6d of consequential relief to bereaved families between 1804 and 1816.[90] The parish of Calverley paid an average 2s per week to bereaved families and for less than three months, a similar sum and duration to that offered in rural Welton (Northamptonshire).[91] Hatfield parish (Hertfordshire) was equally restrictive. An 1820 set of 'Regulations for the Management of the Poor' allowed that 'Widows or families may, at the discretion of the select vestry, receive relief out of the workhouse, for one month after the death of the master of the family, but no longer.'[92] Culcheth represents the other end of the spectrum of engagement. Here deaths of adults in particular occasioned considerable consequential expenditure and related orders that officials regularly 'attend' bereaved families.[93] In turn, the nature of the support given was multi-faceted. Where bereavement was of a mother or father, the consequential relief might extend to apprenticeship or boarding of children, as we saw in Chapter 6. In Cliviger (Lancashire), for instance, the vestry minutes for 19 November 1829 record an agreement that the four youngest children of the recently deceased weaver James Holt were to be put to the care of Thomas Marshall for one year at a combined cost of more than £18.[94] The provision of clothing for bereaved relatives was also part of the 'normal' response to death on the parish. Moreover, officials could provide less tangible, but no less important, support. Out-parish families frequently requested that the overseer inform relations and acquaintances of a death, while of their own accord officials often sought to rally wider kinship groups.

Nonetheless, it was cash allowances that dominated the landscape of engagement between officials and bereaved families. Three types of payment are found in the underlying sample. The first and least frequent consisted of loans, often in cases where insurances or legacies would

eventually be paid, where relatives had pledged help but it had not arrived, or where money was needed to build a viable alternative business in the event of the death of the breadwinner. The Chorley vestry on 3 October 1810 ordered the overseer to help Betty Hodgkinson in pursuit of property taken from her 'and take such measures to recover it as may be found'.[95] In Caton (Lancashire), for instance, an 1810 vestry resolved that 'John Mays to have money lent by the overseer and give him a promissory note for the same to be paid again when he receives his wife's legacy'.[96] Similar payments can be seen in the eighteenth century; in 1790, for instance, officials at Worle St Martin (Somerset) lent money to the Wilkins family on the basis of an agreement by their son to pay for the funeral of his father.[97] A second and more numerous form of cash payment comprised incidental or customary support. Thus on 5 August 1835 the overseer of Bury (Lancashire) wrote to his counterpart in Hulme asking him to inter Sidney Crompton 'same as your own poor providing he is in no Searciety but if they have provided a coffin and etc themselves you may allow it to them in money'.[98] This commitment to paying a contribution to the bereaved family in whatever form reflects the sense outlined earlier in this chapter that officials felt an implicit obligation. Immediate rent payments, meeting the bills of doctors and short-term cash allowances to stabilise the situation of the family also fall into this category. Culcheth parish in 1815, for instance, paid for the burial of Moscrop's child (18s), a one-off allowance (5s 6d), part of his rent (£3 3s) and an allowance of 1s 6d for a year. Such payments could legitimately be made irrespective of the immediate earning capacity of the bereaved family. Thus the Chorley vestry of May 1817 resolved that the recently widowed Jane Allinson was to 'be allowed 10s temporary relief' even though her two eldest children were bringing home 10s per week between them.[99] A final type of cash payment – 'ongoing support' – ran rather further than simply stabilising the finances of bereaved families or (as was often the case where children died) beginning to mend family finances drained by the nursing of the bereaved. George Little wrote from Rayleigh to Colchester on 26 July 1826 asking for money to bury his wife and to support his two small children. Subsequently the grocer Thomas Bishop wrote requesting a regular pension to reflect Little's inability to earn.[100] In Culcheth Thomas Unsworth's death in 1819 occasioned payment of an immediate 8s to his wife and children for support and

then monthly payments of 5–8s for almost a year, while his widow was assigned £2 12s for rent.[101] At the opposite end of the chronological spectrum covered by this study, Ann Lapworth wrote from Caversham (Berkshire) to Oxford St Martin on 17 August 1754 noting that a letter from the overseer had arrived for her husband but had been passed to her, 'he laying then dead'. She requested that the parish 'allow me 4s a week for the support of myself and Children I will do the utmost to breed them up'.[102] The latent sense of this letter – a need to avoid the sickness and death of an individual feeding into lifelong or inherited dependence for other family members – is something that we also detect in the correspondence of overseers and pauper advocates and points again to a flexible and pragmatic Old Poor Law in the run-up to 1834.

Conclusion

Parochial expenditure on the last illnesses and funerals of paupers varied significantly between and, particularly, within parishes. Yet, and acknowledging breathtaking examples of neglect, officials seem to have recognised an implicit duty to act, to act quickly and to act well in the process of dying. The 'medicalisation' of poverty clearly extended into and beyond death. For those who did not experience miraculous recovery the question of what constituted 'the pauper funeral' is complex. To be sure, one can trace examples of mass graves, while counties such as Essex or West Yorkshire seem to have adopted a *de facto* (and minimal) tariff for burials. Even in these counties, however, one can trace examples of considerable generosity, and across the country it is clear that parishes were willing to contribute to hybrid funerals in which relatives, friends or insurance paid part of the cost of obtaining a rather better funeral than a parish allowance alone would have paid for. For most parishes a spectrum of experience and expenditure makes it hard to identify a singular type of 'pauper funeral'. What we can see is a gradual increase in funeral costs over time and a tendency for most places at most times to be orientated towards the more generous end of the funeral spectrum. Collectively payments for final illnesses, funerals and allowances for bereaved dependents could be extremely expensive. In Culcheth Thomas Yates, whose wife's funeral had cost £2 in 1820, was given cash and clothing totalling £3 10s in

1821; Thomas Marsh senior received £11 2s 6d in cash relief between April 1818 and his funeral (for which the parish paid for a coffin at £1 2s and drink and other expenses of 7s) in March 1821. In addition to these sums the parish had spent £6 8s 4d on clothes, 19s 6d on supplementary food and 19s 6d on rent in addition to unspecified sums for nursing and doctoring. These micro-examples point to the need for a more holistic view of the process of dying. We see little abhorrence of the pauper funeral precisely because there was no single or dominant funerary experience and because the funeral itself was usually wrapped up in a longer and larger package of support for sick families and bereaved relatives. Explaining this flexible parochial attitude towards the dying and dead poor is not easy, particularly in the sense that the usual dichotomies – between urban and rural or rural and industrial places, between regions, between rich and poor places or between men and women – have little purchase. Rather, variables such as custom, normative experiences in the wider community, the strength of pauper agency, belonging, migratory status, the presence or absence of kinship and the strength of humanitarian sentiment exhibited by individual officers and ratepayers determined where individuals fell on the parochial support spectrum, and thus where parishes sat within the quantitative spending categories outlined in Figure 4.5. These variables have equal purchase on the likelihood that parishes would turn to institutions to support the sick poor, and it is to this theme that the next chapter turns.

Notes

1 BRO, D/P 91/18, Pangbourne correspondence (my italics).
2 On undertakers see J. Litten, 'The English funeral 1700–1850', in M. Cox (ed.), *Grave Concerns: Death and Burial in England, 1700–1850* (York: Council for British Archaeology, 1998), pp. 7–9.
3 For more on the different character of these two forms and the assertion that they were the norm 'all over London, and in inner city areas of provincial cities throughout Britain', see R. Richardson, *Death, Dissection and the Destitute* (London: Phoenix Press, 2001), p. 60. Also J. Litten, *The English Way of Death: The Common Funeral since 1450* (London: Robert Hale, 1991), and J. Rugg, 'Constructing the grave: Competing burial ideals in nineteenth century England', *Social History*, 38 (2013), 328–45, at pp. 328–30.

4 J. Rugg, 'From reason to regulation, 1760–1850', in P. Jupp and C. Gittings (eds), *Death in England: An Illustrated History* (Manchester: Manchester University Press, 1999), p. 224.

5 Lees, *Solidarities of Strangers*.

6 Richardson, *Death, Dissection*, p. 213.

7 T. Laqueur, 'Bodies, death and pauper funerals', *Representations*, 1 (1983), 109–31, at p. 116.

8 Litten, 'The English funeral', p. 16.

9 See C. Gittings, *Death, Burial and the Individual in Early Modern England* (London: Croom Helm, 1998), p. 98; Laqueur, 'Bodies, death', p. 109.

10 J.-M. Strange, 'Death and dying: Old themes and new directions', *Journal of Contemporary History*, 35 (2000), 497.

11 J.-M. Strange, *Death, Grief and Poverty in Britain, 1870–1914* (Cambridge: Cambridge University Press, 2005).

12 For re-interpretation of the Act see E. Hurren, *Dying for Victorian Medicine: English Anatomy and its Trade in the Dead Poor, c.1834–1929* (Basingstoke: Palgrave, 2011).

13 Walker's activities were intensively reported – see for instance 'Burial in towns', *The Times*, 5 April 1849, p. 5 – and he himself published extensively. See G. Walker, *Gatherings from Graveyards* (London: Longman, 1839). The reported problems in London had considerable longevity. See V. Harding, 'Burial on the margin: Distance and discrimination in early modern London', in Cox (ed.), *Grave Concerns*, pp. 54–64; V. Harding, *The Dead and the Living in Paris and London 1500–1670* (Cambridge: Cambridge University Press, 2002). See also P. Jupp, *From Dust to Ashes: Cremation and the British Way of Death* (Basingstoke: Palgrave, 2006).

14 K. Snell (ed.), *The Whistler at the Plough* (London: The Merlin Press, 1989), p. xiv; J. Simmons (ed.), *Letters from England: Robert Southey* (Stroud: Alan Sutton, 1984), p. 145.

15 C. Smith, 'Elegy', *London Review*, 22 (1792), 382. On the underlying dispute for the 1788 episode between Toftrees and the Norfolk house of industry, see NORO, PD 618/1, Town Book.

16 P. Ackroyd, *Blake* (London: Vintage, 1999), p. 18.

17 J. Rugg, 'A new burial form and its meanings: Cemetery establishment in the first half of the 19th century', in Cox (ed.), *Grave Concerns*, p. 45.

18 Anon., *The Overseers' Handbook* (London, 1851), p. 453.

19 K. Snell, 'Gravestones, belonging and local attachment in England, 1700–2000', *Past and Present*, 134 (2003), 47–73.

20 G. Jekyll, *Old West Surrey: Some Notes and Memories* (Chichester: Phillimore, 1999), pp. 235–6.

21 R. Houlbrooke, *Death, Religion and the Family in England, 1480–1750* (Oxford: Oxford University Press, 1998), p. 366.

22 E. Hurren and S. King, 'Begging for a burial: Death and the poor law in eighteenth and nineteenth century England', *Social History*, 30 (2005), 321–41.

23 For a particularly good example, though rather late for this book, see 'The hideous outrage to public decency', *The Times*, 28 August 1883, p. 9.

24 Conceived in this way, the spending category 'Funerals' traced in Figure 4.5 would be more important, as cash allowances, payment in kind and 'other' payments accrete to individual funerals.

25 Some perhaps more than others: John Jones was both a doctor and overseer of Luckington (Wiltshire) in the 1780s and recorded his own doctoring expenses! WRO, 1108/11, overseers' accounts.

26 Rather, I have argued elsewhere that the Old Poor Law in particular tended to intervene in precautionary ways to preserve infant and child life. See S. King, 'Pauvreté et assistance'.

27 In some cases (for instance when John Moxon of Hull was writing to his fellow overseer in Beverley in July 1832) a pauper literally died during the course of constructing the correspondence. See EYRO, PE1-702-53, letter, 6 July 1832.

28 Sokoll, *Essex Pauper Letters*, p. 481.

29 RPC, letter.

30 NRO, 249p/216, letter (underlining in the original).

31 NRO, 251p/98/5, letter.

32 WYRO, DB 3/C56/A/96, letter. Urban areas are under-represented in our evidence but letters like this written from such communities point to a shared rural-urban understanding of obligations to the dying poor. For wider context in Leeds, see J. Morgan, 'The burial question in Leeds in the eighteenth and nineteenth centuries', in R. Houlbrooke (ed.), *Death, Ritual and Bereavement* (London: Routledge, 1989), pp. 95–104.

33 LRO, PR 2853/1/2 and PR 2853/1/5, overseers' accounts.

34 BURO, PR 196/12/1Q-8Q, overseers' accounts.

35 LCRO, DE 157/1–3, overseers' accounts.

36 BRO, D/P 118/12/2, overseers' accounts.

37 BRO, D/P 91/18, letter and bill.

38 SRO, D/P/Chard/13/7/1, complaints of the poor, and D/P/Chard/13/2/14, vouchers.

39 CURO, WPR 70/7/3/1/31, overseers' accounts.

40 One might expect that the presence of a workhouse would cut down the expense of doctoring in a final illness. In fact exactly the opposite is true.

41 M. Wheeler, *Heaven, Hell and the Victorians* (Cambridge: Cambridge University Press, 1994); E. Schor, *Bearing the Dead: The British Culture of Mourning from the Enlightenment to Victoria* (Princeton: Princeton University Press, 1994).

42 NRO, 216p/243/6, letter.

43 LRO, PR 2391/4, letter (my italics).

44 BRO, D/P 132/18/15/5, letter.

45 See Litten, 'The English funeral', p. 15.

46 Sokoll, *Essex Pauper Letters*, pp. 189–91, 221. In East Yorkshire, by contrast, average funeral costs were £1 in the decade 1760–70, rising to £2 by 1810 and £3 by 1830. See Hopkin, 'The Old and New Poor Law', p. 291.

47 Ibid, p. 232.

48 LCRO, DE 1587/156/24, letter.

49 S. King, 'Reconstructing lives'.

50 WYRO, RDP 43/160–63, overseers' accounts.

51 LRO, PR 806 and 810, overseers' accounts.

52 LRO, PR 2853/1/2 and PR 2853/1/5, overseers' accounts.

53 BURO, PR 196/12/1Q–8Q, overseers' accounts.

54 WRO, 206/71, overseers' accounts.

55 BRO, D/P 78/12/1–11, overseers' accounts.

56 WRO, 1186/18, overseers' accounts; 1589/35–8, overseers' accounts; 811/129 and 194, accounts and orders; 206/78–9, overseers' accounts.

57 BRO, D/P 98/12/1–226, overseers' accounts.

58 Anon., *Henley-on-Thames Poor Relief 1822–1835* (Oxford: Oxfordshire Family History Society, 1987).

59 LCRO, DE/1587/156/20, letter.

60 BRO, D/P 91/18, letter.

61 Morley, *Oxfordshire Friendly Societies*. Lancashire boasted the densest male and female membership network for friendly societies in the nineteenth century, and so the impact of benefits from such societies was likely to be disproportionately felt. See M. Gorsky, 'The growth and distribution of English friendly societies in the early nineteenth century', *Economic History Review*, 51 (1998), 489–511.

62 NRO, 47p/91–4, overseers' accounts; BRO, D/P 130/12/1–4, overseers' accounts; BRO, D/P 52/12/1–4, overseers' accounts; Anon., *Some Particulars of Mawnan Church and its Rectors* (Falmouth: Falmouth Printing, undated).

63 See Richardson, *Death, Dissection*, pp. 187–8.

64 Though there was remarkable consistency in the treatment of stillborn children, for whom burial costs of 1–3s were common throughout the country.

65 See MCL, M10/808–14, letter books.

66 Litten, 'The English funeral', pp. 9 and 13.

67 For further elaboration see Hurren and King, 'Begging for a burial'.

68 Snell, 'Gravestones, belonging'.

69 The proportion of child burials influences the average cost of a funeral and absolute level of expenditure in a parish. Where, as in Thatcham (Berkshire) or Marlbrough (Wiltshire), the proportion was 50 per cent or more the effect could be marked.

70 Communities with very high migrant populations, such as those close to major transport routes, tended to spend less for funerals than did more remote communities.

71 MCL, M10/813, bill.

72 NRO, 261p/242/9, letter.

73 BRO, D/P 91/18, letter.

74 NORO, PD 358/50/6, letter.

75 EYRO, PE1-702-114, letter, 25 August 1834.

76 BRO, D/P 91/18, letter.

77 LCRO, DE 2694/610, vestry minutes, and DE 3178/12, letter, 16 June 1820.

78 Sokoll, *Essex Pauper Letters*, p. 598.

79 BURO, PR 196/12/1Q–8Q, overseers' accounts.

80 NRO, 249p/216/50, letter.

81 For consequent disputes over customary burial rights in the first decade of the New Poor Law, see S. King, 'Rights, duties and practice in the transition between the Old and New Poor Laws 1820–1860s', in Jones and King (eds), *Obligation, Entitlement and Dispute*, pp. 263–91.

82 Sokoll, *Essex Pauper Letters*, p. 189.

83 S. King, 'Reconstructing Lives'.

84 BRO, D/P 91/18, letter.

85 Sokoll, *Essex Pauper Letters*, pp. 424–5.

86 Ibid., p. 568.

87 J. Bailey, *Parenting in England, 1760–1830: Emotion, Identity, and Generation* (Oxford: Oxford University Press, 2012).

88 RPC, letter, 12 June 1794.

89 MCL, M10/814, letter.

90 Ramsbottom, 'Christopher Waddington's peers', p. 137.

91 S. King, 'Reconstructing lives'; NRO, 356p/16, overseers' accounts.

92 W. Sturges Bourne, *Report from His Majesty's Commissioners for Inquiring into the Administration and Practical Operation of the Poor Laws*, vol. 1 (London: B. Fellowes, 1834), pp. 299–301.

93 LRO, PR 2853/1/5, overseers' accounts.

94 LRO, DDX 1822/1, Cliviger order book.
95 CPL, vestry minutes.
96 LRO, PR 501, vestry minutes.
97 SRO, DP/wor/13/10/1, inventory.
98 MCL, M10/809, letter.
99 CPL, vestry minutes.
100 Sokoll, *Essex Pauper Letters*, p. 322.
101 LRO, PR 2853/1/2 and PR 2853/1/5, overseers' accounts.
102 ORO, PAR 207/5/A2/7, letter.

Part III
Parochial medical welfare in context

8

Institutions and the sick poor

Introduction

On 18 February 1812, John Mitchel, vicar of Iselworth (Hertfordshire), wrote to the overseer of Rotherfield Greys (Oxfordshire) concerning Anthony Harris, who 'became deranged in his Intellect some months ago, & it is now no longer safe to himself & others'. Unfortunately Harris 'On Thursday morning left his Home again, & has not since been heard of – His poor Wife is half distracted, & after walking yesterday 30 Miles, & making every Inquiry where there was a chance of any Intelligence, is very ill from Anxiety, Fatigue & Distress'. Mitchel suggested that

> If he should return to this place, it will be necessary to place him somewhere in confinement – Indeed it ought to have been done long ago – I will undertake through the Medium of some Friends to procure his admission into St Luke's Hospital [Holloway, London[1]], provided you are disposed to indemnify me for the Expence – There must be a Deposit of Six Pounds in the Hands of the Treasurer on his Admission, & 2 Housekeepers must enter into a Bond of 100£ to remove him from the Hospital at the Expiration of the 12 Months, provided he should be deemed incurable.[2]

By 2 March Harris had been found and admitted but 'this Object could not be effected without some Expence – I have deposited with the Committee 6 pounds, & the contingent Expences of Removal amount to £3 4s 8d – the former sum will be returned in case the patient dies or should be discharged <u>cured</u> within the Space of one Month'.[3] Mitchel's initial intervention in the case was underpinned by an assumption that the parish would want to leave 'no human Means … unattempted to

restore his Reason'. Hope of a cure dwindled rapidly.[4] Harris was still
in an institution by December 1830.[5]

As Chapter 1 suggested, the conundrum of what to do with the
insane[6] has fostered a considerable literature.[7] It is now clear that in my
period familial and communal care of the insane, and those with mental
or physical impairments with which this group is often confused, was
the norm. The loss or absence of family, deteriorating familial circumstances or a pronounced change in the tenor of the insanity, as was
the case for instance with Anthony Harris, could propel individuals
out of their domestic context.[8] For some this meant residence in the
workhouse or long-term boarding arrangements. Others, like Harris,
ended up rather further removed from their communities, committed to private madhouses (often around London) or sent to public or
charitable lunatic asylums from the 1820s.[9] Indeed, it has been argued
that over time more parishes accepted that institutions were 'the best,
if expensive, solution to the problem of lunatics'.[10]

Asylums were just one element of a patchwork of institutional provision that parochial officials, families and paupers themselves turned to
at times of sickness. The spectrum ranged from workhouses and charitably funded voluntary hospitals on the one hand, through pest-houses, to
specialist institutions for particular conditions. Once parochial officers
had decided that a case required institutional care, they rarely stinted
on the costs of sending paupers to distant and expensive facilities.[11] Yet
for the pre-1834 period our understanding of how and when the sick
poor utilised the medical functions of most institutions is surprisingly
thin. Medical historians have done much to improve our picture of the
funding, staffing, policies and broad role of hospitals and (to an extent)
dispensaries.[12] There has been rather less work on where hospital care
fitted into the medley of responses to ill-health by parishes. In turn,
our understanding of the medical functions of the Old Poor Law workhouse remains, as Chapter 1 suggested, superficial.[13] Questions about
the access of the sick poor to other institutional contexts – almshouses,
isolation cottages or specialist providers – are less frequently addressed
still.[14] Consequently the constellation and complexion of the institutional treatment regimes afforded to the dependent sick poor, the triggers for seeking institutional sojourns, pauper and parochial attitudes
towards such care and its place in a life-cycle of responses to illness,
remain issues in need of substantial empirical exploration.

This chapter will thus provide an overview of the constellation of institutional engagement, drawing on key lessons from Figures 4.5 and 4.8. It will contend that for the period as a whole the workhouse was the single most important form of institutional provision, albeit with distinct county-level features. Over time the frequency of interactions with non-workhouse institutions such as asylums, voluntary hospitals and homes for the blind increased in most places. To borrow a phrase from the opening of an earlier chapter, what was right, proper and fair in terms of parochial responses to sickness clearly involved by the 1820s the potential for an institutional sojourn. Such observations, this chapter argues, must be placed alongside the intertwining facts that even by the 1830s most sick paupers in most parishes spent no time in institutions of any sort, and that the proportion of medical welfare resources spent on non-workhouse institutions was relatively small. Regional differences in this picture and deeply ingrained variations in parochial practice highlight the need to step beyond conventional ana-lytical frames. In particular, the chapter turns to the subtle influences shaping whether parishes turned to institutional provision at all and, within this context, what made some paupers more likely to end up in institutions than others. We turn first to the question of the constella-tion of institutional provision.

Constellating institutions

Four issues influence how we can analyse the frequency and com-plexion of parochial engagements with institutions. Two of them – the fact that cash payments to individuals might mask spending on institutions; and the sometimes poor survival of records for transient institutions – will be familiar from earlier chapters. A third centres on how to conceptualise 'institutions'. It is easy to define and locate voluntary hospitals. The fact that they needed to raise charitable funds for initial building and ongoing costs from individuals ensured that they were firmly implanted in the public mind and public record.[15] By contrast, defining what a 'workhouse' was remains highly problematic. In Northamptonshire, for instance, while towns like Kettering were relatively consistent in identifying buildings as a 'workhouse', other places were certainly not.[16] Welton experimented with a 'workhouse' on five separate occasions between 1729 and 1834, but the vestry

also made reference variously to 'the poorshouse', 'the almshouses', 'Mr Sheltons house' (Shelton was the farmer of the poorhouse), 'house of industry' and (in a doctor's contract from 1804) 'the old people's hospital'.[17] Such variation in terminology related to more or less the same set of buildings throughout the period. This sort of ambiguity can be seen in all of the counties analysed here and helps to explain why, in 1777 parliamentary returns, a county like Leicestershire acknowledged nineteen 'workhouses' (ranging in size from two inmates at Burbage to ninety in Hinckley) but a survey of parochial accounts suggests the existence of at least double that number.[18] More widely, distinctions between isolation houses, workhouses, houses of industry, poorhouses, nursing and convalescent homes, and even the private residences of doctors and apothecaries appear to have been extraordinarily fluid. A related and fourth problem is that some institutions were not just transient, but 'phantom'. Vestrymen at Swanage (Dorset) tried to rent, buy or build a workhouse on numerous occasions between June 1788 and November 1816, claiming that such an institution was operating on five separate dates when it never did.[19]

Set against these caveats, Figures 4.5 and 4.8 offer more precision on the scale of institutional welfare for the sick poor than there was. There are broad lessons, however. For all of the 117-community sample the workhouse (widely defined to include buildings with associated labels such as poorhouse or house of industry) was a consistent but – excepting the 1790s – relatively small element of medical welfare. The aggregate picture, however, obscures divergent county experiences. In Norfolk, for instance, workhouses absorbed a steadily rising proportion of medical welfare, reaching over 20 per cent by the 1820s. This contrasts with the much more episodic and lower level engagement of parishes in Northamptonshire, Lancashire (with the exception of the 1790s) and West Yorkshire. A sharp fall in workhouse spending in Berkshire from the mid-1820s does much to explain the plateau in the importance of overall medical welfare spending seen for that county in Figure 4.6. In typological terms, urban and industrial areas seem to have made greater use of workhouses than arable or pastoral areas, but the differences are small. Switching our attention to other forms of medical institution, we can see a significant chronological increase in the absolute number of places accessed by parish officers.[20] Hospitals and specialist institutions began to make a particularly strong

appearance after 1800, in part coinciding with the wave of such places founded or re-founded after this date. While there are many potential readings of this observation, the one preferred here is that parochial officials were more likely to commission, or agree to pauper requests for, medical care in institutions of all sorts in the 1830s than was the case in the 1750s. Yet if, as Chapter 4 suggested, absolute spending on such places increased over time, there was still a slight fall in the proportion of medical welfare absorbed by non-workhouse institutions, to just over 3 per cent. To some extent, and as with other spending categories analysed earlier in the study, this is a statistical artefact, a reflection of the strong growth in cash payments in most parishes after 1800. Nonetheless, the fact that there was also a flattening of volatility in the cost of institutional engagement in most parishes and counties over time also suggests substantive developments.

Some of this patterning is explained by the declining frequency and intensity of epidemic disease, allowing officials to spend the same or increased absolute amounts on institutions for more sick paupers and in a considered rather than reactive crisis mode. Nowhere is this clearer than in Northamptonshire, where in the eighteenth century recourse to pest-houses (for smallpox) and fever houses (for ague) periodically drove spending to what must have been painful levels. Another factor helping us to reconcile a falling proportion of medical welfare spending devoted to non-workhouse institutions with an increase in the range and number of such parochial engagements is the practice of subscription to voluntary hospitals. Sending someone to hospital was never a casual decision. The attendant costs (of transport, caution money, clothing and cash relief to families left behind) could be considerable. Yet such visits also potentially saved money,[21] while undertaking or maintaining a subscription seems to have signified a move in some parishes to earlier and more comprehensive (and perhaps ultimately less costly) intervention in the process of the descent of the sick poor into long-term dependency. Certainly this sense that institutional subscription might mute spending in the category as a whole, both directly and by shifting money that might previously have been spent on engaging institutions to other categories of medical welfare spending, would seem to fit with the experiences of Wiltshire, as Chapter 6 suggested. Even after controlling for parochial typologies and wealth, communities here were much more likely to use and subscribe to

voluntary hospitals than in any other county and yet the institutional spending category is the smallest of any of the seven counties by the early nineteenth century.

These are broad influences on the whole sample. They are of course imprinted upon the uneven spatial distribution of non-workhouse institutions, particularly voluntary hospitals, and of the scale of poverty, both of which help to explain some of the spending patterns observed in Figures 4.5 and 4.8.[22] Ingrained parochial variation in both the scale and complexion of institutional engagement at the intra-county level also shaped attitudes to institutional provision. Indeed, perhaps the most important feature of the underlying data is how proximate communities with similar poverty problems, wealth and options could nonetheless exhibit different attitudes towards institutional sojourns. This situation encompassed subscriptions to hospitals and dispensaries, sending those with physical impairments to specialist institutions of treatment and confinement, and above all insane paupers like Anthony Harris ending up at (or remaining long-term in) asylums. Local variation was partly a reflection of the personality of officers, but other factors were also at work. One was the existence and evolution of local traditions of engagement. Thus for some parishes, in places as early as the 1770s, it became 'normal' for officials to see an institutional sojourn as desirable or inevitable. Over time, the flattening of spending patterns in this area at county level might be read as pointing to the generalisation of this view – an invention or extension of tradition – and coincident with rising background expectations of access to institutional medicine among the wider labouring orders.

As with workhouse care, however, the data also suggests a more subtle situational picture. Anthony Harris ended up in an institution as a last parochial response to chronic illness. He shared this experience with more than 800 insane individuals, some of whom lived in parishes where institutions were only ever seen as a last resort and some in communities where officials made less transparent decisions about when and whether to intervene with an institutional engagement. In turn, Harris was to spend the rest of his life in an asylum, an extreme point on a spectrum of intensity for the sick more generally which might at the other end stretch to a day trip to the dispensary in Norwich. Yet, and notwithstanding some eye-watering figures on the number of discrete

cases treated by institutions such as voluntary hospitals,[23] only a small proportion of paupers and a smaller proportion of all sickness episodes experienced by those paupers were likely to have been encompassed by treatment in medical institutions. Even workhouse medicine probably played a very limited part in most of the ill-health life-cycle of the dependent poor, except perhaps in Norfolk. Against this backdrop making sense of broad trends in the scale and complexion of spending on institutions requires further work on the factors shaping why parochial officers saw institutional sojourns as an appropriate response to sickness, the point in the sickness story at which they intervened and the durations of the engagements that emerged. It is to these themes that the rest of the chapter turns.

Workhouses

Spending on workhouses constituted the single biggest institutional engagement for the parishes which had or used them. As we have already seen in Chapter 2, during normal times workhouses disproportionately housed the aged, decrepit and sick.[24] The comprehensive records of Warham (Norfolk) workhouse suggest that over 75 per cent of inmates in most years were sick, unable to work or 'Not capacitated to do much'.[25] At Blackley (Lancashire) a census of 1820 recorded 43 per cent of workhouse inmates as sick or the children of sick parents, while almost all the rest were either aged or maternity cases.[26] The master's admissions book for Bath Abbey (Somerset) workhouse in 1822 suggests that the 'afflicted' must have comprised 50 per cent of the institutional population, with the aged and children dominating the rest.[27] Such provincial perspectives have resonance with the situation in London. Tim Hitchcock, for instance, notes that more than half of those admitted to the workhouse in St Luke's, Chelsea, were in some form sick by the mid eighteenth century,[28] while an 1822 census of Finchley workhouse reveals eight of the fifteen inhabitants to have been over sixty.[29] Lynn Mackay similarly argues that almost a third of female admissions to the St Martin's workhouse were sick.[30]

   Against this backdrop our understanding of workhouses as medical institutions is surprisingly thin. In part this reflects the fact that so many workhouses were farmed to private contractors for fixed fees (with devastating consequences for recordkeeping), particularly in Norfolk.

Even where records do exist, detailed information on what was actually wrong with inmates is sometimes absent because most poorhouses and workhouses lacked any dedicated accommodation for the sick of the sort that might have led to the keeping of discrete records for this group. In London, workhouses and hospitals increasingly came to cater for mutually exclusive patient groups, with workhouses having an implicit obligation to treat paupers – such as those with syphilis – who could not access other forms of medical care.[31] Outside London the picture is more complex, but 'The Poorhouse Surgeon's Day Book', kept for Reigate (Surrey) by Drs Thomas Martin and Thomas Steele between 1805 and 1815, provides vital detail.[32] The book records both annual summative abstracts on the nature of ill-health in the workhouse and more detailed notes on individual cases. Considered in the round, the surgeons at Reigate poorhouse treated a similar range of complaints to William Stutter in his time at the Suffolk General Hospital in the 1830s.[33] This spectrum included infectious diseases (measles, chicken pox, fevers – themselves divided into five different categories – and smallpox), venereal disease, a full range of chest complaints, rheumatism, accidents, cancers, ringworm and a considerable number of intestinal problems. The exact character of ailments changed from year to year, while the number of cases ranged between forty and sixty. That some of these medical conditions were generated within the poorhouse rather than paupers being admitted with them is testified by a note on 21 March 1809 stating that 'The general state of health of the house is improved, the cases of fever and cold having for the most part recovered.' A sense that both the summative figures and detailed case notes still provide perspective on only a subset of those with ill-health is revealed by caveats appended to each annual report. That for 1807–8 notes: 'Many trifling complaints, as chilblains, slight colds & etc are not reported.' Nonetheless, the clear lesson from the day book is that sickness across a spectrum from trifling to mortal shaped the very character of the institution.[34] Indeed, we can discern five typologies of the sick poor confined in workhouse-like institutions: the aged with chronic conditions; those with sudden and severe ailments, particularly infectious diseases and injuries from accidents; paupers with multiple health problems or from families where other illnesses were already in play; paupers in need of respite or convalescent nursing; and maternity cases for women on long-term relief.

This picture is perhaps not unexpected. Nonetheless, vestries which had workhouses still sent only a subset of people there for treatment or to die. The rest of the sick poor remained on various forms of outdoor support including sojourns in non-workhouse institutions. Four variables seem to have played an important part in this decision and thus shaped the particular role for workhouses in the delivery and organisation of local medical welfare. The first was the nature and policy of institutions themselves. Many parish workhouses were simply too small to cope with the sorts of sickness traced in Chapter 2. Others were too transient to put into effect the long-term planning that caring for chronic sickness required. In Syston (Leicestershire), for instance, the workhouse was closed before an order of 1804 for the creation of a lunatic cell could be carried out. The data is also littered with examples of workhouses routinely refusing to take some categories of the sick poor. On 21 July 1768 Hannah Weston, 'she being infected with the itch was not fit to lodge in the [Market Harborough work] house', becoming one of twenty cases of refused admittance for this single town.[35] In nearby Oxenden (Leicestershire) on 5 February 1781 the child Ellen Hodgkinson was only to 'be admitted into the workhouse as soon as it is cured of the present disorder'.[36] At Lutterworth (Leicestershire) the workhouse rarely took in the sick poor and broke this rule only in the aftermath of smallpox and other epidemics.[37] These unwritten conventions – akin to the rules governing who could be admitted to most voluntary hospitals – have an important bearing on the complexion of county spending on workhouses as a component of medical welfare. Thus not only did Norfolk and Wiltshire have more and less transient workhouses than other counties in the sample, but we rarely see the informal rationing of places through a framework of exclusion.[38] It was in this sense easier for parochial authorities in these two counties to use the workhouse as a feature of their response to sickness.

A second and related factor shaping how parochial officers used the workhouse was the constellation of alternative parochial provision. Specialist pest-houses, fever 'hospitals' or smallpox cottages could depress the number of admissions to the house or even negate the need for one.[39] This was particularly true for instance in eighteenth-century Northamptonshire, where workhouse provision and use played the most minor part in medical welfare. And as we saw in earlier chapters, the presence or absence of nursing homes and boarding houses was

also an important determinant of the complexion of local policy. Thus the virtual disappearance of the workhouse as a spending category in Berkshire from the mid-1820s was at least partly related to the expansion of domestic nursing as a stock response to sickness in the county. More widely of course the propensity of officials to turn to the workhouse was in part influenced by their connectedness to a wider network of extra-parochial medical care from regional and national doctors. While we should be wary of assuming that the presence of a workhouse inevitably suppressed parochial willingness to turn to provision at distance – after all, parishes like Warham spent considerable sums on both avenues – the data suggest that at the margins the workhouse was a substitute for sending paupers away.

Such observations should not lead us to view the workhouse as merely a residualist institution. Indeed, a third factor shaping local decisions seems to have been a genuine belief on the part of some parochial officers that the workhouse was the best place to deal with chronic sickness. This view would have been problematic to some contemporaries. George Crabbe's 1783 poem *The Village* was scathing of the workhouse:

> Here too the sick their final doom receive
> Here brought, amid the scenes of grief, to grieve
> Where the loud groans from some sad chamber flow
> Mixed with the clamours of the crowd below
> Here sorrowing, they each kindred sorrow scan
> And the cold charities of man to man.[40]

Nineteen years later Ann Candler's 'Reflections on My Situation' was equally condemnatory:

> Within these dreary walls confin'd/\
> A lone recluse I live/
> And, with the dregs of human kind
> A niggard alms receive
> Uncultivated, void of sense/Unsocial, insincere
> Their rude behaviour gives offence
> Their language wounds the ear.[41]

These portrayals fit well with the negative perceptions of the parochial workhouse that have dominated the historiography,[42] and find

resonance with some pauper attitudes when faced by the prospect of admission. An order to Shocklack Oviatt (Cheshire) from the Hulme overseer on 2 January 1836 that Phoebe Rowland be sent to the workhouse for her confinement, for instance, occasioned an extreme reaction. Rowland 'begged so much not to be sent' that the Shocklack overseer gave her outdoor relief.[43] At the opposite end of the country, Henrietta Carritt, writing from Cheapside to Chelmsford (Essex) in the persona of her husband Thomas on 10 June 1829, told the overseer that 'on my own account I have a great dread as to going in the House ... if I must go to the House I must sink under the punishment I could not survive it ... my horror of the House is as great as a man can have of Death and I am confident will be the Death of me, and in a short time'.[44] While there is no patterning to such sentiments across space or community typology, paupers seem to have particularly resisted forced or voluntary admission to workhouses and /poorhouses which were subject to farming contracts. These sentiments are understandable when juxtaposed with the conditions revealed by surveys of some workhouses.[45]

Yet while such attitudes were common they were not, particularly from the 1810s, without contradiction. Some commentators have used the autobiographies of those who spent time in workhouses to suggest a more positive picture of attitudes towards care.[46] This alternative reading sits well with cases where workhouse admission was actively sought. Frances Soundy wrote from Battersea to Pangbourne (Berkshire) on 3 June 1827 to say that her daughter-in-law, who was approaching a confinement, 'must go to workhouse for i can not bare to see her lay on the ground at sush time'. She used reference to the workhouse as a rhetorical strategy to obtain extra relief. Others applied for such admission where alternative avenues had been exhausted. Charlotte Dummett of Twerton, for instance, wrote to Bradford-on-Avon (Wiltshire) on 3 July 1834 to say that she had 'no Peace' with her husband, who was insane. She would be 'thankfull to you sir if you will be so kind to send after him immediately and fetch him to the Poorhouse'.[47] More common than both cases were those in which workhouse admission was seen as one of the normal responses to sickness. Indeed, the vestry of Garstang (Lancashire) had to prohibit admissions to the workhouse 'unless by order'.[48] None of this is to suggest that paupers had any affection for the institution, but rather

to highlight the sense that workhouse residents, particularly the sick, were not always incarcerated against their will. The view of one Leeds pauper that it was 'better for a sick Man to Be in the Poorhouse than a Hovel' has traction here.[49] The idea that workhouses might have a more positive role as a site of sustained and intensive support was also played out in places like St Marylebone, for which Alysa Levene argues that officials were 'progressively-minded … especially in the field of medical care.'[50]

A final influence on who ended up in the workhouse was the 'normal' timing of official interventions in sickness histories. Anthony Harris was ultimately constructed as a hopeless case, and vestry minutes, pauper letters and overseers' correspondence are redolent with similar examples of late intervention and lost hope. Workhouses might also be used as places of confinement or 'dwindling' where treatment in other institutions had failed or, as in Luckington (Wiltshire), where another institution such as a pest-house had done its job. In parishes like Warham or Trowbridge (Wiltshire), however, the workhouse seems to have played a more positive role in a patchwork of early intervention by parochial officials to try and head off lost hope. This theme is developed further below in the context of non-parochial institutions.

Figures 4.5 and 4.8 are hence underpinned by substantial differences between places in the likelihood of founding or keeping workhouse-like institutions. Local policy in this area was driven by example, cost, panic, exasperation, parish size and local understandings of the nature of the poverty problem. In our sample, parishes in Norfolk were more likely than elsewhere to commission workhouse space. They were also more likely to use such space for the treatment or confinement of the sick poor. It remains the case, however, that parochial engagement with workhouses in most places and at most times was small, episodic or partial and that the complexion of local, regional and national institutional provision for some paupers was richer than a focus simply on workhouses allows.

Other institutions

The sheer range of engagement between parishes, paupers and non-workhouse institutions by the early 1800s is impressive.[51] Overseers' accounts show that our sample parishes subscribed

regularly to twenty-two voluntary hospitals and dispensaries and in places appear to have demonstrated more enthusiasm for these institutions than has been suggested by Alannah Tomkins or Amanda Berry.[52] Use by Wiltshire parishes in particular of proximate hospitals was consistent, but even communities that did not subscribe to voluntary hospitals nonetheless appear to have kept the matter under review.[53] The overseer of Chard (Somerset), for instance, kept the rules for sending patients to Bath Infirmary and the printed subscription leaflet (dated 1815) for the Somerset Hospital.[54] He was one of thirty overseers, with significant concentrations in Leicestershire, Wiltshire and West Yorkshire, to retain such documents. These actions support several readings, but one is that the option of institutional treatment had a firm presence in the suite of potential responses to claims for medical welfare.

Sending parishioners to hospitals could be costly. Market Harborough stood equidistant between institutions in Leicester and Northampton, and periodically used both, though it subscribed to neither. Admission involved transport, someone to accompany the sick pauper, admission fees of 15s, caution money, the provision of decent clothing where the pauper did not already possess it, laundry costs, repatriation once treatment was finished and then convalescence or outpatient costs. In 1766 individual cases like that of Widow Bradfield drew bills of £4. By 1802 the average bill had risen to £6, and from the early 1820s the figure was nearer £8.[55] In Wiltshire, parishes such as Cricklade and Marlborough paid between £5 and £6 for voluntary hospital cases, and such sums were magnified considerably where the duration of treatment was extended. Edward Wilkes of Cricklade, for instance, wrote from the men's ward at Bristol Infirmary on 2 February 1811 to ask for provision of a full outfit of clothes. He was laid 'up with two Bad leags and have be so for several Months', but 'I have nothing scarse for to hide my Nackedness If the Infirmary Releaves the Poor with Medicall and shurgry assistance thay will not find Close on less I have the above mention articuls I shall be dismissed from the house to my Parish'.[56] Per capita admission and treatment costs tended to be lower for northern communities: Calverley (West Yorkshire) paid bills averaging just £3 in the 1820s while in Pennington (Lancashire), the figure was £4. Nonetheless, the tendency for officers in some northern parishes to seek multiple sequential institutional solutions for the

chronic sickness of individual paupers, in contrast to southern England, where institutional treatment outside the workhouse was more often one-off, raised aggregate bills.[57] One of the key conundrums of the underlying data – evidence of increasing institutional engagement at the same time as this spending category dwindled in importance for overall medical welfare – is thus to be explained in part by the longevity or renewability of institutional sojourns.

As the case of Anthony Harris shows, asylum care was potentially the most expensive form of institutional engagement. The underlying dataset references directly eighteen different asylums, as well as implying the existence and use of others. Certainly by the 1810s there is clear evidence of an increase in the use of such institutions across the sample. Aggregate figures, however, mask considerable spatial (though little typological) variation. Thus Norfolk parishes appear to have made less use of asylums than their Wiltshire, Warwickshire and Leicestershire counterparts. Even within counties, however, individual parishes demonstrated ingrained differences in attitude towards funding asylum treatment. In Northamptonshire, for instance, the parish of Rothwell used four different asylums – at Huntingdon, Leicester, St Luke's in Chelsea and the White House in Bethnal Green – but sent most of its long-term patients to London. Between 1823 and 1834, sixteen lunatics were processed through these channels. By contrast, the nearby (and in most respects similar) town of Wellingborough rarely sent its insane paupers to extra-parochial institutions.[58] Equally stark differences are to be found elsewhere: Robert Willett wrote to Bradford-on-Avon from Lavington (Suffolk) on 9 December 1833 to make arrangements for the return of the lunatic Mr Cleveland 'Agreeable to your request'. But, he warned, 'I doubt whether he has sufficient government of himself to prevent your having trouble with him.'[59] Cleveland was one of seven lunatics from Bradford-on-Avon in this single institution by the 1830s. On the other hand, the parish of Box (Wiltshire) consciously tried to keep insane paupers in the domestic or workhouse context.[60] Such differences do not reflect the presence or absence of workhouses as an alternative custodial venue. Nor do they map easily onto per capita poor law expenditure or other proxies for the relative wealth of communities. Rather, one can observe ingrained parochial policies with considerable longevity, a matter to which we return below.[61]

Voluntary hospitals and asylums are, of course, well-known facets of the institutional patchwork for the poor. Parochial officers were also willing to try more specialist institutional solutions. Eleven parishes (two from outside Yorkshire) sent paupers to the Leeds Eye Dispensary. Across the Pennines, Thomas Jump of Oldham (Lancashire) asked his parish to send him to 'the [Manchester] eye institution to try if they can do any for me'[62] and was one of forty-three paupers sent by twenty-seven parishes to this institution. On the south coast, the Swanage vestry determined in 1816 that the blind child Elizabeth Rawles should 'be sent to the Asylum for the indigent blind, Callowhill Street Bath'.[63] It was one of six parishes to seek treatment for paupers in this institution, the most distant being Lancaster (Lancashire). The Somerset parish of Twerton sent (or agreed to the requests of other parishes to send) paupers to five specialist institutions including the Hadland Hospital (Gloucester; a surgical institution for cripples), the Bristol Eye Hospital and the Manchester Children's Dispensary.[64] This appetite for exploring the curative potential of often distant specialist institutions expanded noticeably in the early nineteenth-century and coincided chronologically with increased spending on therapies such as sea and spring water bathing and drinking, which are explored in the next chapter. Closer to home, almost all communities at one time or another discussed or commissioned isolation buildings for everything from smallpox to putrid fever. In late eighteenth-century Chippenham smallpox patients were sent to one of four isolation cottages staffed by parish nurses and supplied regularly with ashes and lime as disinfectants.[65] Such buildings occasionally melded seamlessly with the nursing homes explored in Chapter 5.

Parishes and their sick paupers could thus be enmeshed into a complex patchwork of local, regional and even national institutional provision. Bradford-on-Avon, as well as using workhouses had (at various times) paupers in Bristol Infirmary, Lavington (Suffolk) lunatic asylum, Southampton Infirmary, Southampton Dispensary, Swindon Dispensary, Bath Hospital, Reading Infirmary, Kendal (Cumbria) Dispensary, St Peter's Hospital in Bristol, St George's Hospital in London and Melksham Asylum. The mining and industrial town of Chorley (Lancashire) sent sick paupers to various workhouses, a nursing home, Liverpool Infirmary and the Manchester Eye Hospital. Thrapston likewise used the Manchester Eye Hospital but also had

paupers in seven different workhouses and four asylums and paid for paupers at the Peterborough Dispensary, Leicester Infirmary, Northampton General Hospital and Reading Infirmary. These examples are important, and no parish in the sample failed to have at least some engagement with non-workhouse institutions. Plenty, however, were like Buckland (Berkshire), where officials drew on this avenue of medical care only once every five years on average. As with workhouses, then, we need a better understanding of why parochial officers in some places were more inclined to institutional provision than others and why in all parishes some paupers were sent to institutions and others with similar conditions were not.

Variables with explanatory power, some of which are familiar from the discussion of workhouses, include *inter alia*: long-term traditions and customs; local disease and impairment patterns; institutional reputation; ease and cost of access; advertising; and differences between parishes in the speed with which officials intervened in illness. Coronial records for Nottinghamshire, Wiltshire and Northamptonshire also suggest consistently that accident cases (and others with acute surgical needs) were transported to voluntary hospitals even if they were at some distance.[66] Several other factors, however, seem to have particularly shaped the frequency, timing and duration of institutional engagement at parish level. First, for the post-1800 period officials began to get a better sense of the nature of practice elsewhere and of the 'national' poor law system. Circulars, newspaper reporting, visits, guidance manuals and personal contacts allowed parishes to locate the expense and range of their practice within a broad local and regional hierarchy. And rather than a race to the bottom in terms of average costs there is evidence that parochial standing became more important to vestries as they discovered alternative models of action. At the same time, it is clear that early nineteenth-century officials were garnering a much better understanding of the economics of overseeing than their eighteenth-century counterparts.[67] For some parishes at least, such awareness translated into a rethinking of the ubiquitous policy concept of 'economy', the yardstick for which slipped subtly from minimising present costs to reducing the long-term impact of sickness on the rates. One can see this sort of transition played out in overseers' correspondence, where, by the early nineteenth century, officials dealing with out-parish paupers living in their communities

often simply assumed that institutional care would be the cheapest long-term option. Thus Thomas Haywood, overseer of the poor at St Chad, Lichfield (Staffordshire), wrote to his counterpart in Lilleshall (Shropshire) on 10 March 1817 in respect of 'poor old [Thomas] Dorling'. He had a 'very bad hand, which I fear must be Amputated', and Haywood had taken the decision to send 'him to the Infirmary so you will have no Doctor to pay'.[68] Similarly, the overseer of Kensington (London) wrote to his counterpart in Bradford-on-Avon on the subject of 'Webb's wife' on 9 February 1833. She

> is much worse both legs are bad now and our doctor is getting tired of giving his attendance it being rather a hopeless case he recommends St George's Hospital for her to go into and our Parish does subscribe in order to avail ourselves of the *Superior advice to be had there* that as soon as we have a vacancy I must give a Letter and they will Soon Settle it there one way or another.[69]

This is not to argue that officials suddenly became less interested in their annual poor relief bills. It is to suggest that many parishes came to employ a more variegated sense of value for money over time, particularly when it came to those with young families and the young in general, where future dependence was likely to be most costly. It is a short step from this point to an assertion that better comparative perspective led some parishes to increase institutional engagement, if only as a matter of civic pride.

A second factor shaping parochial attitudes was the growing number of doctors working with officials. Irrespective of geography or socio-economic typology, parishes which consistently contracted medical care were more likely than others also to turn to institutions. The marked increase in the practice of contracting traced in Chapter 5 was thus directly correlated with increasing institutional engagement at the aggregate level and with the particular spending profiles of counties such as Northamptonshire and West Yorkshire as well. The nature of this inter-correlation can be exemplified using overseers' correspondence. William Worlidge, who was 'received into this house [a workhouse in Birmingham] a fortnight ago on the commendation of Dr Dyson', was one of eleven Thrapston out-parish paupers sent to institutions by parish doctors in their host communities.[70] In turn, the doctors contracted to Thrapston itself recommended institutional

medical care some fourteen times between 1826 and 1831, on all occa-
sions having their directions taken up.[71] Similar observations might be
made for northern communities such as Hulme (Lancashire), where
J. G. Elkington's note to say that Mary Mooney was 'labouring under
Phillans Palmonati Succeeding of Pneumonia' and ought to be sent to
Manchester Infirmary was one of thirty-nine such recommendations.[72]

Exogenous influences such as these which shaped the likelihood of
officers turning to institutional provision at all were supplemented by
others that determined why some paupers were sent on institutional
sojourns while others were not. One of the most important was a growing nineteenth-century sense that certain forms of sickness among the
poor were, or might be, remediable. The early nineteenth century, medical historians have suggested, saw the decline of the patient narrative
as a diagnostic tool, the prescribing of more complex medicines, better
surgical practice and a more interventionist framework for medicine
inside and outside institutions. It was in this period too that doctors
began to seek normative benchmarks in terms of disease aetiology and
patient recovery and experience.[73] Such changes necessarily shaded
into the experience of the sick poor and the attitudes of officials. Yet
pauper patients were not simply dragged along by a background tide
of changed understanding of illness and curative practice. Many of the
medical welfare interventions traced already in this study balanced pre-
cariously on the fine line between acting out a duty to the poor and not
providing this group with standards of medical care somewhat above
the possibilities of independent members of the parish. In engaging
with specialist institutions officials arguably crossed this line, pointing
on one reading to a sense that parishes ought to push the limits of
the possible in medical terms. For some overseers and vestrymen such
sentiments were couched in terms of frustration or exasperation, particularly with chronic or sequential illnesses. They found themselves at
their wits' end and saw institutional care as a last straw to grasp. Thus
Robert Harris, the overseer of Rothersthorpe (Northamptonshire),
observed in a letter of 3 June 1818 about Margaret Eastwood that
'we have tried every chance with her and at no little cost but I am
informed [by the parish doctor] of a place at Bath that might promise
hope. I propose Gentlmn to send her there for one month to try for a
cure at last.'[74] Sometimes the desperation of the officers literally drips
from the letters, as for instance when Thrapston sent Charlotte Fox

to Northampton Infirmary in September 1824 and simultaneously subscribed for the first time to the institution.[75] Many other officials, however, inscribed their sense of the remediability of sickness into a framework of decidedly humanitarian action. Thus in the late 1820s the small Oxfordshire parish of Wooton struggled with a solution to the periodic insanity of William Drinkwater. Eventually he was committed to the Radcliffe Asylum in Oxford, from where F. T. Wintle (the resident apothecary) wrote on 27 November 1828 to advise that Drinkwater was

> sufficiently recovered to return home. He has been working about the garden for the last week or two, & has, for the most part, discontinued his spiritual conversation, added to which he has a very great desire to see his family which he frequently expresses with tears. I trust you will not have any further trouble with him.[76]

The consequent bill – £6 6s – was not inconsiderable for a parish of this size and might be read as pointing to a degree of care over the case, notwithstanding perceptions of a dilution of humanitarian sentiment in the final three decades of the Old Poor Law.

This is not to argue that instances of the cynical manipulation of the sick poor disappeared. Indeed, there are numerous examples like that of John Strickland of Charmouth (Dorset), who died at the Bath General Hospital on 28 September 1823. His father applied to have his 'few cloaths mostly old things which may be worth 20 shillings'. Seeking permission to release the clothes, George Tap, the hospital clerk, received a short sharp letter on 9 November in which the overseer of Charmouth was 'directed to inform you that the Cloaths belonging to the late John Strickland must be sent to this parish and not delivered to his father', a clear indication that the officers were trying to recoup their costs.[77] Such instances are, however, much outweighed by stories like that of Thomas Cooper of Oundle. Having sent him variously to Bethlem and asylums in Peckham and Bethnal Green in the early 1830s, by 4 December 1833 the vestry had decided his affliction would be permanent. Rather than simply confining him in a cheaper asylum as a long-term solution, Cooper's father was sent to get him on 4 February 1834, but not before the overseer was ordered (on 4 September 1833) to 'Build a place in the workhouse for him'.[78] One can see a similar humanitarian sentiment in the case of Anne King of Swanage, who,

aged and sick, 'quitted her house for the accommodation of the Parish and is gone to reside in the Poor House'. Her possessions were taken to the poorhouse but the vestry resolution contained an important caveat that 'her goods will be restored to her son on her death'.[79] Rather than absorb Anne King's possessions into the 'parish stock' as per their legal rights, Swanage officials adopted a much more humanitarian position. Increasing recourse to institutions in the early nineteenth century, one might argue, reflected both a greater awareness of curative potential and a humanitarian imperative to explore it in chronic cases.

Meanwhile, and as Chapter 3 suggested, it is also necessary to factor pauper demands into an understanding of why certain people ended up in institutions. There was an undercurrent of resistance to the idea that institutional care could simply be imposed by officials. Alice Rogers of Melksham (Wiltshire) was told that her leg needed to be amputated but the doctor 'refused to do it himself'. Rather 'he said he would send her to the Hospital', which Rogers refused on the basis that 'when she was there some time ago they refused to do it, saying that she could not bear the operation'.[80] Henry Summerson refused a suggestion from the Rothersthorpe overseer that he attend the Northampton General Hospital because he did not want to be 'butchered like a pig'.[81] Paupers were less able to resist confinement in asylums, but they could protest once there. William Woodman escaped from the Lavington asylum on 30 May 1834 'notwithstanding He was chained hand & foot to his bedstead after releasing himself from these He contrived to make a hole through a Nine Inch brick partition into the Court Yard and scaled the wall ... and is gone'; he 'seems bent upon doing all possible mischief Knowingly He says to make us tired of Him'.[82] Yet on the whole non-workhouse institutions were regarded favourably by paupers, usually on the basis that an institutional sojourn would 'do them some good'. Some sick paupers were active in seeking out independent recommendations to hospitals and dispensaries.[83] Recommendation letters survive patchily,[84] but the fact that access often was, or became, a partnership with the parish means that one can trace this sort of independent activity in administrative and financial documents.[85]

Many more paupers approached their parishes of settlement directly to garner support for institutional treatment. Indeed, one might conceive that the persistently 'noisy' were among the subset of the sick poor most likely to be referred by parochial officers to hospitals. Ellen

Foster, writing from Hull to Rothersthorpe on 17 May 1784, had 'hurd of a New Hospittul at York of [her neighbour] Mrs Baines' and 'Wuld be Pleased to Try it for my Backe if the Gentlmn Shud think Proper of it'.[86] She was one of a mere handful of eighteenth-century pauper letter writers to reference institutional care outside the issue of madness.[87] By the 1810s the number had increased exponentially. While this trend certainly reflects a more complete corpus of correspondence, the sense that people simply knew – had 'hurd' – more about institutions is clear. Paupers particularly sought institutional admission in cases of accident and sudden and recurrent illness, an observation that applies irrespective of region or community typology. Thus in Oundle Mrs Timms attended the vestry on 3 December 1828 'and requested that the parish would endeavour to procure the admission of her daughter into some infirmary or dispensary', the daughter having been beset with chronic ague. Similarly Widow Wood applied on 16 June 1830 'for some allowance to convey her son ill with a rupture to Northampton Infirmary'.[88] Thomas Earl, a resident of Southampton, was determined in February 1833 that 'i must try to Get on the Despencery tomorrow'.[89] Nor did paupers always want to leave institutions once they got in. James Sykes wrote from London to Tilehurst (Berkshire) on 21 January 1830 to say that he 'was in the [Middlesex] hospital', and 'although I am turned out of the Hospital I am very far from being made a cure of and the Physician [Thomas Watson, in charge of out-patients] says that I must on no account attempt to do any Kind of work ... I still spit a great quantity of blood and in [obscured] a very weak and Imisciated [damaged]'.[90] The phrase 'turned out' might be read as signifying a perceived entitlement to institutional support until the medical problem was properly resolved.

Short-term, and sometimes extended, institutional care had thus become a potential and accepted part of the armoury of parish officers on the one hand and the expectations of paupers on the other. The advocates of the poor – men like John Mitchel in support of Anthony Harris – appear to have had an even stronger assumption of the necessity of institutional treatment and the obligations of parishes to provide it. Thus when the overseer of Gedney (Lincolnshire) requested information on his pauper Thomas Burning, then living in Oundle, the reply could not have been clearer: Burning had turned into a violent lunatic 'going into tradesmens shops insisting upon paper and ink

to write to the King, Duke of Wellington and many other noblemen
... Also driving his wife out of the house threatening to murder her
and her children.' The correspondent noted that he had been obliged
to have him chained to the bed in the workhouse with two men to
watch him. Hence, although 'now he is only mad on some points',
there was an absolute necessity of arranging temporary institutional
confinement.[91] It follows then that communities and counties with
particularly large or active advocate groups would have both a greater
engagement with institutions in general and a propensity to send those
paupers with advocate support to those institutions. This is certainly
a significant part of the explanation for the wide range of institutions
tried by Leicestershire parishes. For West Yorkshire and Lancashire it
also meant sustained pressure on officials to seek multiple institutional
solutions to the cases of particular paupers, rather than seeing an institutional sojourn as a singular event.

Locating institutional medicine

Where institutional sojourns fitted into a life-cycle of sickness, cure and
parochial medical welfare is a complex question. Voluntary hospitals
and, in particular, specialist institutions such as eye hospitals offered
more advanced surgical procedures than were to be had at the parochial level.[92] Fever cottages and pest-houses probably offered more
expert and regular nursing than was to be found in the workhouse.
And all institutions offered more regular treatment and better diet than
was likely to have been afforded to the sick poor living at home.[93] We
should beware, however, of overstating the novelty and effectiveness
of institutional interventions, even if paupers and officials framed their
expectations of such treatment differently from those they had when
simply consulting the parish doctor. At the very end of the period
covered by this study, William Stutter's patient case records from the
Suffolk General Hospital detail, as we have already seen, a forbidding
array of purges, infusions, syrups, digitalis, tinctures, lineaments, poultices, emulsions, vomits, blisters, juleps, mercury and composite medicines, alongside dietary improvements and supplements and surgical
interventions.[94] The case records span the ordinary labouring classes,
and it is impossible to discern whether the treatment of the dependent
poor was in some way 'different'. However, the range of prescriptions

recorded by Stutter closely mirrored those to be found in the case-books relating to Dr Loxham's practice in late eighteenth-century Lancashire.[95] This is perhaps not unexpected, given that the same medical men often simultaneously held positions both at parochial level and in institutions. The limitations of institutional treatment are also clear. Stutter recorded nine different outcomes to his cases – relieved or somewhat relieved, discharged herself or himself, out-patient, no outcome, dead, discharged, 'go on', incurable, transferred to surgeon – but barely a majority were 'cured'.[96] Even the word 'cured' is ambiguous. In the underlying dataset the vast majority of those who attended hospitals continued to need medical or consequential relief whether 'cured' or not. Thus in Oundle 'The mother of Elizabeth Hutchinson living at Elton applied for relief for her she having returned from the Infirmary Northampton, incurable.'[97] Nearby, Thrapston received a letter from Joseph Richards on 28 December 1825 asking for an extra allowance because

> my complaint that I have on me is so bad in my right arm that I cannot do any sort of work at all and likewise the complaint which I went into the infirmary at Leicester [with] is almost as bad as ever that it comes down as bad as ever and I cannot keep it up.[98]

The same picture might be drawn for northern England. At Malton (North Yorkshire), for instance, John Lightfoot attended the 'York Infirmry and has returned home incurable'.[99] And the child William Spacey was returned from Leeds Infirmary to Spofforth (West Yorkshire) in 1817 with a six-month treatment plan to be effected by the overseers.[100] Similar perspectives can be taken on other institutions. The vast majority of parochially funded lunatics in asylums either remained in such institutions long-term or were discharged uncured, uncurable or simply 'improved'. For this group of sick paupers, the idea of 'cure' was a relative one, subsumed into the question of whether the individual could be safely inserted back into their familial or (in the case of workhouse accommodation or boarding out) settlement communities.[101]

It seems unlikely, then, that an institutional sojourn marked for many paupers a turning point in their life-cycle of illness and treatment. Where one can link together official correspondence or pauper letters and overseers' accounts it is possible to reconstruct, for a subset of the

sick poor, outline medical biographies or (as Kevin Siena styles them) the 'back-stories', so as to explore this point further.[102] Doing so suggests three typologies of institutional engagement over and above the aged poor long resident in the workhouse, who were ubiquitous. Thus for some paupers an initial engagement with institutional medicine built into a sequence of admissions into similar institutions. By definition, these paupers were experiencing chronic ill-health, but this aside, multiple sequential engagements were not confined to either gender or to particular life-cycle stages. Some of the conditions encompassed by this experience, lunacy for instance, are not unexpected. Mrs Simms was a long-term pauper lunatic settled in Oundle. She was placed in an asylum by the request of her family in 1828, and on 21 October 1830 the parish constable was sent to convey her from one lunatic asylum in Bethnal Green to another. She was still in this asylum on 29 June 1831 when a further bill was paid to the White House in Bethnal Green, and on 10 November 1831 when the surgeon at the White House provided an update on her continuing insanity. By 8 May 1833, when Mr Martin, the governor (farmer) of the workhouse, was granted an extra 2s per week a head for lunatics, Simms was in the workhouse. On 28 November 1835, parochial officials were bargaining for a place in the Peckham lunatic asylum.[103] Sequential admission to institutions was not, however, confined to the insane. Thus Widow Styrin wrote from Leeds on 2 August 1832. Noting her recovery from cholera, she told the overseer that 'My youngest Little Boy So Verrey Ill & he will I Expect Going to the Informery he as gone throe an Operation & is likely to go throo an other so I Leave you to Judge My Situation.' By the time Styrin's local vicar wrote on her behalf two weeks later, the boy had become a 'patient of the Leeds Infermory'. Over the course of four years between 1830 and 1834 the unnamed boy was to experience five infirmary admissions, a long period as an out-patient, visits to three other medical institutions, a brief sojourn in the Leeds workhouse and treatment by four different doctors in his own home.[104] This sort of multiple sequential admission, as we have seen, does much to explain the continued importance of non-workhouse institutions in the medical welfare spending profile of parishes in West Yorkshire.

Yet while multiple institutional engagements are striking they are by no means representative. A second life-cycle typology encompasses what one might broadly conceive as respite care. Workhouses dealt

disproportionately with those in the last hours or days of either sickness or old age, but there were plenty of other cases where residence was of a short-term duration. Indeed, the often muted death rates evident in provincial workhouses are suggestive of a more diversified respite role. Vestry minutes are thus replete with references to paupers sent to the workhouse 'until they get well', notwithstanding the importance of family as a central plank of the medical economy of makeshifts, which is explored further in the next chapter. This was most clearly the case in Norfolk, where parishes such as Warham or Scottow recruited nurses for the specific task of caring for individual paupers sent to workhouses and townhouses so as to 'get ahead'. The experience was part of a shared understanding between parishes, paupers and families about how that medical economy ought to operate. One also sees this sort of sentiment at play in relation to voluntary hospital admissions, where such sojourns were sometimes explicitly referred to as respite care. George Brown, for instance, wrote from Bristol to Bradford-on-Avon on 8 August 1834 asking for relief because 'my Little Boy his ordered out of the infirmary this three Weeks by the doctor and I canot have him out because I have no bead For him to Lay on and he his a compleat cripple'.[105] Similarly, Joseph Wilson actually wrote from his hospital bed at Nottingham, 'where I have my haide [aid] and Supporte for nothing and not only that I ham not fit to be removed at preasant if incase I have the good fortune to stay in the Hospitle until the Spring I may recover my health again'.[106] Nowhere is this practice clearer than in Leicestershire, where parishes like Monks Kirby entered into disputes with doctors in the Leicester Infirmary when they thought their recuperating paupers had been discharged too soon.[107]

Finally, and as one might expect from the foregoing discussion, a third typology was the single institutional experience. Some 86 per cent of all paupers sent to institutions, disproportionately concentrated in the Midlands and south, never repeated the experience. For some this reflected death.[108] In other cases the medical problem was so ingrained as to make the single institutional sojourn a last desperate throw of the die. The unnamed correspondent writing on behalf of Rosey Jones of Lancaster (Lancashire) some time around the end of 1834 observed that 'her youngist Boy is near Lost his Aie sight I have im in Dispensry and he gets no better he as been Bad this 6 weeks'.[109] A few paupers ended up in a particular institution by accident, as

for instance in the case of the unnamed lunatic about whom James Cowass wrote to Preston Brook in 1823: he was sorry to inform his counterpart that 'the Hospital in this Town [Manchester] Cannot take any more Lunatics in they have to send them to the Hospital at Lancaster'.[110] Yet for most places and people, certainly by the early 1800s, the sole institutional sojourn had simply become an accepted part of the life-cycle of responses to non-accidental illness. Thus when the Rothwell (Northamptonshire) vestry recorded in October 1829 that 'Wm Spitt's wife ['wishes to have' crossed out] is obliged to go to the infirmary', officials were quite literally confirming this changed landscape in their crossing-out.[111]

Conclusion

The scale and scope of potential institutional provision expanded inexorably across our period. While the workhouse dominated numerically, the singular feature of this institutional landscape was its growing complexity and multiplicity. Such expansion was shadowed by an increase in instances where parishes and paupers mulled over, sought or commissioned institutional care. The extent to which paupers embraced the potential of (non-workhouse) institutional care is striking, although not unexpected given the discussion of pauper agency in Chapter 3. For some, the institution represented hope, while for others it was the last chapter in a life-cycle of ill-health. Parish officers had an equally broad sweep of motivations, ranging on a spectrum from a resigned sense that institutional care was the last option available through to a distinct humanitarian desire to 'try anything'. Joan Lane's conclusion (itself a development of work by Dorothy George and Geoffrey Oxley) that pre-1834 officials were willing to go to very considerable lengths to contain, cure or ameliorate the condition of the sick poor clearly has purchase here. Institutional engagement became a decidedly more visible sign of such determination after 1800.[112] Nonetheless, it remains true that even in 1834 the two largest categories of sick paupers were those for whom one can trace just a single institutional engagement or none at all. In some respects, then, the issue is not why we see institutions playing more of a part in the life-cycles of sick paupers, but why we do not see more substantial care of this sort. The answer partly lies in the spatial patterning of institutional provision and the situational nature

of the sickness spectrum that officers faced. Yet there was also something more, as the tendency of Wiltshire parishes to send their leprosy
cases to hospitals, whereas parishes in other counties did not, begins to
suggest. The art of the possible and the desirable was expanding at the
same time as expensive crisis responses to epidemic disease were falling, something that we see played out in the willingness of parishes to
fund single institutional engagements. But the relative absence of multiple engagements in the south and Midlands in particular also points
to ingrained local traditions. When the overseer of Stratton Strawless
(Norfolk) recorded the costs of Mary Burrell attending the 'Ospettle'
in Norwich in June 1775 he noted cash relief, the cost of journeys,
visiting, clothing, lodging, 'Bringing her home' and twenty-six weeks
of recuperation at 2s per week.[113] He was in other words recording an
event of real significance both for the pauper and for parish finances.
Out of humanity, desperation or possibility or because of particular
triggers, a sense of the value of local care had been overridden. For
the insane poor that trigger was the ease of management, something
clearly set out in a case before the vestry at Bray (Berkshire) on 28
February 1797, where Mr Jennings was 'to inquire at St Luke's whether
& upon what terms they will admit Ann Link the Lunatic into their
Hospital; as from her appearing to grow mischievous it is not deemed
safe to keep her any longer in the workhouse'.[114] In cases of chronic or
other illnesses the collective triggers are rarely so clear, though they are
important for an understanding of the spatial dimensions of spending
on institutional care. One of them, however, was likely to have been the
capacity and extent of local and regional makeshift medical economies,
a matter to which we finally turn.

Notes

1 For more on St Luke's see *Report of the Metropolitan Commissioners
  in Lunacy to the Lord Chancellor 1844* (London: Bradbury and Evans,
  1844); The National Archives, HO 44/51, Minutes of the Visiting
  Commissioners; and reports to advocates preserved in NRO, F(M) G
  666, Reports on St Luke's Hospital Middlesex, 1751–85.
2 ORO, MSS D.D. Par. Rotherfield Greys c.11/1, letter.
3 ORO, MSS D.D. Par. Rotherfield Greys c.11/2, letter (underlining in the
  original).

4 ORO, MSS D. D. Par. Rotherfield Greys c.11/3, letter.
5 ORO, MSS D.D. Par. Rotherfield Greys c.11/24, letter.
6 The term 'insane' encompasses people on a spectrum from depression
   and puerperal fever through to violent lunacy. P. Rushton, 'Lunatics and
   idiots: Mental disability, the community and the poor law in north-east
   England, 1600–1800', *Medical History*, 32 (1988), 34–50, at pp. 36–8;
   Miller, 'English pauper lunatics', pp. 318–28.
7 For overviews see A. Scull, *The Most Solitary of Afflictions: Madness and
   Society in Britain 1700–1900* (New Haven: Yale University Press, 1993);
   S. Cherry, *Mental Health Care in Modern England: The Norfolk Lunatic
   Asylum, St Andrew's Hospital c.1810–1998* (Woodbridge: Boydell, 2003);
   L. Smith, *Lunatic Hospitals in Georgian England 1750–1830* (London:
   Routledge, 2007).
8 J. Melling, B. Forsythe and R. Adair, 'Families, communities and the
   legal regulation of lunacy in Victorian England: Assessments of crime,
   violence and welfare in admissions to the Devon asylum, 1845–1914',
   in P. Bartlett and D. Wright (eds), *Outside the Walls of the Asylum: The
   History of Care in the Community 1750–2000* (London: Athlone, 1999),
   pp. 153–80, and A. Suzuki, *Madness at Home: The Psychiatrist, the Patient
   and the Family in England, 1820–1860* (Los Angeles: University of
   California Press, 2006).
9 East Dereham (Norfolk) sent its first pauper to Bethlem in 1750. On
   private madhouses see W. Parry-Jones, *The Trade in Lunacy: A Study of
   Private Madhouses in England in the Eighteenth and Nineteenth Centuries*
   (London: Routledge, 1972) and L. Smith, *'Cure, Comfort'*.
10 Rushton, 'Lunatics and idiots', p. 49.
11 Something also observed by Thomas, 'The Old Poor Law', pp. 3–4.
12 As a small selection, see K. Waddington, *Charity and the London Hospitals
   1850–98* (Woodbridge: Boydell, 2000); I. Loudon, 'The origins and
   growth of the dispensary movement in England', *Bulletin of the History
   of Medicine*, 16 (1981), 322–42; A. Berry, 'Community sponsorship and
   the hospital patient in late eighteenth-century England', in P. Horden
   and R. Smith (eds), *The Locus of Care: Families, Communities, Institutions,
   and the Provision of Welfare since Antiquity* (London: Routledge, 1988),
   pp. 126–52; J. Reinarz, *Healthcare in Birmingham: A History of the
   Birmingham Teaching Hospitals, 1779–1939* (Woodbridge: Boydell,
   2009); Borsay, *Medicine and Charity*.
13 The London picture is increasingly rich. See Boulton and Schwarz, 'The
   medicalisation'; A. Levene, 'Children, childhood and the workhouse:
   St Marylebone, 1769–1781', *London Journal*, 33 (2008), 41–59; Green,
   Pauper Capital. For other areas see Hitchcock, 'The English workhouse'.

14 Though on permanent physical impairment see Phillips, *The Blind*, and Borsay, *Disability and Social Policy*. Specialist (mainly London) institutions dealing with sexual diseases have, by contrast, been well covered. See Siena, *Venereal Disease*. For almshouses see A. Tomkins, 'Retirement from the noise and hurry of the world: The experience of almshouse life', in J. McEwan and P. Sharpe (eds), *Accommodating Poverty: The Housing and Living Arrangements of the English Poor, c.1600–1850* (Basingstoke: Palgrave, 2011), pp. 263–83.

15 P. Elliott, 'Medical institutions, scientific culture and urban improvement in late Georgian England: The politics of the Derbyshire General Infirmary', in Reinarz (ed.), *Medicine and Society*, pp. 27–46, and D. Andrew, *Philanthropy and Police: London Charity in the Eighteenth Century* (Princeton: Princeton University Press, 1989).

16 Peyton, *Kettering Vestry Minutes*. For wider context see D. Green, 'Icons of the new system: Workhouse construction and relief practices in London under the Old and New Poor Law', *London Journal*, 34 (2009), 264–84.

17 NRO, 356p/7, vestry minutes.

18 T. Gilbert, *Report from the Committee Appointed to Inspect and Consider the Returns Made by the Overseers of the Poor, in Pursuance of Act of Last Session: Together with Abstracts of the Said Returns Relating to 16 Geo III, c.40* (London: Butterfield, 1777).

19 DRO, PE/SW/VE 1/1, vestry minutes.

20 If, as Chapter 2 suggests, sickness was increasing in frequency and intensity after 1800, then some of this increased engagement was merely a reflection of enhanced need.

21 Thus, the eleven-year-old Thomas Staples was sent to 'Bath Hospital' by officials in Englefield (Berkshire) but the parish paid only the cost of coach hire and an accompanied journey. BRO, D/P 52/12/3, overseers' accounts. When Ardington (Berkshire) stopped its subscription to Guy's Hospital in 1805, the scale of the bills for alternative provision convinced the overseers to restart by 1807 and to extend subscription to the Oxford Infirmary, where by 1811 they had an entitlement to send nine paupers per year. BRO, D/P 7/12/2, overseers' accounts.

22 Thomas, 'The treatment of poverty', p. 55. While the institutional patchwork available to urban parishes was numerically greater and more complex than that for their rural counterparts, an important feature of the increase in engagement was the periodic resolution of provincial and rural vestries to seek care for particular paupers in London or larger urban institutions. This blurs the urban–rural dichotomy that potentially emerges from a simple distribution analysis.

23 By 1827, Addenbrooke's Hospital (Cambridge) treated fifty in-patients and 400 out-patients per week. M. Murphy, *Cambridge Newspapers*, p. 50. See also Tomkins, '"The excellent example"' for a review of attempts to limit hospital access for the labouring classes even in an institution where they had an effective right to treatment by virtue of contribution.

24 This reading is broadly supported by Ottaway, *The Decline of Life*, pp. 250–1, and K. Siena, 'Hospitals for the excluded or convalescent homes? Workhouses, medicalization and the poor law in long eighteenth-century London and pre-confederation Toronto', *Canadian Bulletin of Medical History*, 27 (2010), 5–25.

25 NORO, uncatalogued, Warham overseers' accounts.

26 MCL, M10/4/2/1A-16, Blackley workhouse papers. By 1832 the nearby Manchester poorhouse had between 500 and 600 inmates but it was styled in the enquiries before the New Poor Law as 'an asylum for aged, infirm poor and children'. Redford, *The History of Local Government*, p. 107.

27 SRO, D/P/ba.ab/13/10/1, workhouse survey 1822.

28 Hitchcock, 'The English workhouse', pp. 194–202.

29 A. Collins, *Finchley Vestry Minutes 1768–1840* (London: Finchley Libraries Committee, 1957), p. 43.

30 L. Mackay, 'A culture of poverty? The St Martin's in the Fields workhouse 1817', *Journal of Interdisciplinary History*, 26 (1995), 209–32, at p. 221.

31 Siena, 'Contagion, exclusion', pp. 19–39. Tomkins, 'Paupers and the infirmary', p. 221, notices a similar dichotomy for Shrewsbury. See also W. Bynum, 'Treating the wages of sin: Venereal disease and specialism in eighteenth-century Britain', in W. Bynum and R. Porter (eds), *Medical Fringe and Medical Orthodoxy, 1750–1850* (London: Wellcome Trust, 1987), pp. 5–28.

32 RCSE, MS Add. 427, 3a, 'The Poorhouse Surgeon's Day Book' 1805–15. All succeeding discussion relates to this source.

33 Tomkins, 'Paupers and the infirmary', suggests little overlap between the patient groups of workhouses and hospitals in Shrewsbury.

34 Crowther nonetheless sees a key distinction between sickness played out in the workhouse and that played out in other institutions, arguing (largely for the post-1834 period) that people entering voluntary hospitals were patients whereas the sick pauper in a workhouse was still a pauper. M. Crowther, 'Paupers or patients? Obstacles to professionalization in the poor law medical service before 1914', *Journal of the History of Medicine and Allied Sciences*, 39 (1984), 33–54.

35 LCRO, DE/2132/2, overseers' accounts.

36 NRO, 251p/25, overseers' accounts.

37 LCRO, DE/2559/37–69, parish accounts, and DE 1463/6, town books.

38 On the spatial concentration of workhouse provision, see J. Taylor, 'The unreformed workhouse', pp. 62–4.

39 See G. Williams, *Angel of Death: The Story of Smallpox* (Basingstoke: Palgrave, 2011).

40 G. Crabbe, *The Village: A Poem in Two Books by the Rev. George Crabbe* (London: John Carr, 1783), pp. 15–17.

41 A. Candler, *Poetical Attempts by Ann Candler, a Suffolk Cottager with a Short Narrative of her Life* (Ipswich: T. Hurst, 1803), p. 53.

42 W. Bynum, *Science and the Practice of Medicine in the Nineteenth Century* (Cambridge: Cambridge University Press, 1994), p. 198, for instance, listed workhouses, hospitals and pauper burials among the 'Various fears [that] haunted working-class people in the [nineteenth] century'.

43 MCL, M10/815, letter.

44 Sokoll, *Essex Pauper Letters*, p. 288.

45 See for instance R. Lightning, *Ealing and the Poor: The Poor Law, the Workhouses and Poor Relief from 1722 to 1800* (Ealing: Ealing Local History Society, 1966), p. 47.

46 A. Tomkins, 'Workhouse medical care from working-class autobiographies, 1750–1834', in Reinarz and Schwarz (eds), *Medicine and the Workhouse*, pp. 86–102. For sceptical views of the life chances of the poor constructed through autobiographies, see S. Horrell, J. Humphries and H.-J. Voth, 'Destined for deprivation: Human capital formation and intergenerational poverty in nineteenth-century England', *Explorations in Economic History*, 38 (2001), 339–65.

47 B. Hurley, *Bradford on Avon Applications for Relief from Out of Town Strays* (Devizes: Wiltshire Family History Society, 2004), p. 14.

48 LRO, DDX 386/3, vestry minutes.

49 P. Stern, *Memorials of Leeds* (Leeds: Chadwick, 1828), p. 242.

50 Levene, 'Children, childhood', p. 43.

51 For a listing of available hospitals, see J. Woodward, *To Do the Sick No Harm: A Study of the British Voluntary Hospital System to 1875* (London: Routledge and Kegan Paul, 1974), pp. 147–8.

52 Berry, 'Community sponsorship'. Tomkins, 'Paupers and the infirmary', p. 217, suggests that Shropshire parishes 'remained largely impervious' to subscription for the Shrewsbury infirmary. By contrast Ashby sees dispensaries as a distinctive feature of medical welfare in Warwickshire. See Ashby, *One Hundred Years*, p. 129.

53 The status of 'subscriber' is by no means uncomplicated. Parishes accruing arrears were removed from the subscriber lists of some institutions,

while there are nine cases in the underlying data where parishes recorded authorisation to pay subscriptions in vestry minutes but there was no corresponding payment.

54 SRO, D/P/Chard/13/10/4, printed leaflets.

55 LCRO, DE 2132/5, overseers' accounts; DE 2132/2, overseers' accounts; DE 3074/2, vestry minutes. Contemporaries worried about these costs. See J. Aikin, *Thoughts on Hospitals* (London: Joseph Johnson, 1771), pp. 55–6.

56 B. Hurley, *Cricklade Absent Poor and Warrants for Reputed Fathers 1787–1837* (Devizes: Wiltshire Family History Society, 2005), p. 14 (my italics).

57 Even the contrast with Wiltshire is stark. In Chippenham, for instance, hospitals and dispensaries were used extensively, with four people sent in one month to Bath in 1765, but in the whole of the eighteenth century only one pauper went to hospital more than once.

58 NRO, 284p/189–90, vestry minutes, and 350p/161–75, overseers' accounts.

59 Hurley, *Bradford on Avon*, pp. 12–13.

60 WRO, 1789/27, vestry minutes, and 1719/4–32, overseers' accounts.

61 For an observation of equally strong intra-regional variation, see Rushton, 'Lunatics and idiots', p. 49.

62 King, Nutt and Tomkins, *Narratives of the Poor*, p. 231.

63 DRO, PE/SW/VE1/1, vestry minutes.

64 SRO, D/P/twn/9/1/1, vestry minutes.

65 Hinton, 'Notes on the records and accounts', p. 316.

66 As for instance on 20 December 1800: John Thompson was 'conveyed to the [Salisbury] infirmary' from Stratford-sub-Castle St Lawrence (Wiltshire) 'when the house fell on him'. WRO, 1076/39, overseers' accounts.

67 S. King, '"In these you may trust"', pp. 51–66.

68 King, Nutt and Tomkins, *Narratives of the Poor*, p. 293.

69 Hurley, *Bradford on Avon*, p. 34 (my italics).

70 NRO, 325p/193/136, letter, 29 March 1836.

71 NRO, 3250/194/1–78, letter book.

72 MCL, M10/815, letter, 30 November 1835.

73 This complex process is described by G. Risse and J. Warner, 'Reconstructing clinical activities: Patient records in medical history', *Social History of Medicine*, 5 (1992), 183–206, at pp. 191–2.

74 RPC, letter.

75 NRO, 325p/193/17, letter, 11 September 1824.

76 ORO, Wooton P.C. IX/iv/11b, letter (underlining in the original).

77 DRO, 15/PC/CMO/11/2/15 and 24, letters.

78 NRO, 249p/166, vestry minutes.

79 DRO, PE/SW/VE1/1, vestry minutes, 11 July 1810.

80 Hurley, *Bradford on Avon*, p. 22.

81 RPC, letter.

82 Hurley, *Bradford on Avon*, p. 52. See also L. Smith, '"The keeper must himself be kept": Visitation and the lunatic asylum in England, 1750–1850', in G. Mooney and J. Reinarz (eds), *Permeable Walls: Historical Perspectives on Hospital and Asylum Visiting* (Amsterdam: Rodopi, 2009), pp. 199–222.

83 Tomkins, 'Paupers and the infirmary', p. 217, notes that parishes themselves often put paupers in touch with independent subscribers.

84 Henry Tripp, overseer of Orchard Wyndham in Somerset, kept a stock of blank standard letters for admission to the Taunton and Somerset Hospital. See SRO, DD/WY/198, Bundle 29, blank letters. This sort of forethought reflected wider public debate. See A. Hutchinson, 'To the churchwardens and overseers of the poor, in and near London', *Gentleman's Magazine* (1824), 413–15. The Rothwell vestry recorded in January 1829 that Thomas Cross wanted travel costs 'to go seek a letter and to go to the Northampton infirmary'. NRO, 284p/190, vestry minutes.

85 See for instance LCRO, DE 1587/156/13, letter, 3 November 1828.

86 RPC, letter.

87 For context see R. Porter, 'Medical journalism in Britain to 1800', in W. Bynum, L. Stephen and R. Porter (eds), *Medical Journals and Medical Knowledge: Historical Essays* (London: Routledge, 1992), pp. 6–29.

88 NRO, 249p/164, vestry minutes.

89 Hurley, *Bradford on Avon*, p. 15.

90 BRO, D/P 132/18/15/2, letter.

91 NRO, 249p/216, letter 83.

92 Though see the discussion of the spread of surgical innovations in Stanley, *For Fear of Pain*.

93 On the treatment see J. Andrews, '"Hardly a hospital, but a charity for pauper lunatics?": Therapeutics at Bethlem in the 17th and 18th centuries', in J. Barry and C. Jones (eds), *Medicine and Charity before the Welfare State* (London: Routledge, 1991), pp. 63–81, and D. Wright, *Mental Disability in Victorian England: The Earlswood Asylum 1847–1901* (Oxford: Oxford University Press, 2001). See also P. Bartlett, 'The asylum, the workhouse and the voice of the insane poor in 19th century England', *International Journal of Law and Psychiatry*, 21 (1998), 421–32, at pp. 423–4, who argues that the insane received more personal

attention in the workhouse than the asylum and that workhouse 'cure' rates could be as good as, or exceed, specialist institutions.

94 E. Cockayne and N. Stow, *Stutter's Casebook: A Junior Hospital Doctor 1839–1841* (Woodbridge: Boydell, 2005), pp. xxxiii–xl and 129–59. For context on nineteenth-century 'cures' see Bynum, *Science and the Practice of Medicine*, pp. 17–19, and A.-H. Maehle, *Drugs on Trial: Experimental Pharmacology and Therapeutic Innovation in the Eighteenth Century* (Amsterdam: Rodopi, 1999).

95 S. King, *A Fylde Country Practice*, pp. 61–2.

96 For context see A. Borsay, 'An example of political arithmetic: The evaluation of spa therapy at the Georgian Bath Infirmary, 1742–1830', *Medical History*, 45 (2000), 149–72.

97 NRO, 249p/164, vestry minutes, 8 September 1831.

98 NRO, 325p/193, letter.

99 EYRO, PE1-702-88, letter, 30 October 1833.

100 WYRO, RDP 96/76, overseers' accounts.

101 BRO, D/P 132/18/12/19, letter. See also NORO, PD 553/64 for a Holkham example (1830) of Mr Bacon, who was 'not quite able to work, just returned from the asylum'.

102 Siena, 'Contagion, exclusion', pp. 19–39.

103 NRO, 249p/166, vestry minutes.

104 EYRO, PE1-702-43, letter, 2 August 1832; PE1-702-42, letter, 13 August 1832.

105 Hurley, *Bradford on Avon*, p. 10.

106 EYRO, PE1-702-93, letter, 20 January 1834.

107 LCRO, DE 13054/2/2, minute books of the Leicester Infirmary, 1811.

108 COWAC, B1344-32/St Clement Danes, letter, 12 December 1835.

109 EYRO, PE1-702-127, letter.

110 CRO, P120/4525/224/171, letter, 4 December 1823.

111 NRO, 284p/190, vestry minutes.

112 Lane, *A Social History of Medicine*.

113 NORO, PD/423, overseers' accounts.

114 BRO, D/P 23/18/1, workhouse accounts.

9

The medical economy of makeshifts

Introduction

Frances Soundy, a familiar figure already in this study, wrote to Pangbourne some time in January 1824. Building on an accumulating tale of misfortune, she was 'verry sorry to be under the Nessisety of trobelling you a gain but my husband as ad the misfortune of having his thumb smashed all to peases so that he can not work'. This misfortune compounded the problem of having a large family and herself having 'bene hill som time'. Soundy requested unspecified relief 'to assist us till he his able to work'. Lest the overseer

> have any doubt that I write to impose on your goodness the docter can satisfy you that he his not able to work the gentillman that attends him his Docter Mercally Battersea wich gentillman if you writ to battersay parrish offersears thay will Inquire for you tho gentillman I have not bene to them yet but if the honerable gentillman would writ as soon as possible thay can We shuld be vary thankfull if not my husband must go in to the Hospitall next Thursday.[1]

Though we must read these orthographic letters with caution, this appeal speaks directly to the dimensions of the wider medical economy of makeshifts within which parochial welfare must be located.[2] After James Soundy's injury, the family had turned to a doctor of their own accord.[3] In turn, Frances held out the prospect that her husband would, if not relieved, have to seek admittance to an unspecified hospital, presumably by petitioning a local subscriber.[4] The family were, in other words, shadowing some of the core medical solutions that the parish itself might have adopted in cases of sudden injury. Moreover, they did so without reference to the overseers of their host

or settlement communities, signalling the expectation that paupers could and ought to take control of their own health needs. They were not alone. The aged London pauper Mrs Turvey was in receipt of an allowance of 2s 6d per week from Tilehurst (Berkshire), and a letter of 31 July 1810 noted that she 'remains very Poorly and cant do without the Pothecary', a medical man who was called independently and paid for from her regular allowance.[5] And William King, another pauper encountered earlier in this study, writing in November 1828, trusted that the vestry would 'Behave with a feeling Spirit' when reading an account of his own illness and that of his wife, for whom 'I Yust Now Brought Medecine from Shordith for her from the Doctors'.[6] King did not seek reimbursement for medicines, simply buying them of his own accord. While these were discrete events, paupers like Walter Keeling of Hull were serially engaged in the wider medical economy, being 'Obliged to hire a Nurse as none of us could help another' (November 1786), soliciting treatment 'Which Cost me above 2 Ginnies for the Dockters' (July 1787), attending the noted East Yorkshire wise man William Cooks 'Where my Bowels was Lett out' (November 1795) and commissioning 'a nurse to the children I not being capable of that charge' (May 1829).[7]

The sense that paupers might take their own initiative in terms of healthcare should not surprise us. As Chapter 2 suggested, resignation is a feature of my material, but many claimants were rather less willing simply to accept and live with chronic or sudden illness. John Small, writing from Birmingham to Rothersthorpe (Northamptonshire), is representative of this group, telling the overseer in June 1817 that 'a poor man When Sick has the right to fight Adversity with every means he can'.[8] If parishes had, in the popular imagination, a duty to act at times of sickness, so paupers had a right, in a medical context where consumers purchased hope rather than cure, to pursue every ameliorative avenue.[9] They did so against the backdrop of a vibrant medical economy of makeshifts which for all social groups was peopled by doctors, quacks, apothecaries, druggists, hospital almoners, herbalists and considerable numbers of lay practitioners.[10] In a situation where the boundaries between different forms of medical knowledge and practice were 'fluid and contestable',[11] pluralism was a basic rule for navigating the market by individuals and, as we saw in Chapter 5, by parishes.[12]

How sick paupers fitted into this medical economy of makeshifts is the focus of the current chapter. This question is important. The complexion, extent, cost, availability and navigability of the economy of medical makeshifts potentially shaped who applied to the poor law for medical welfare, what they asked for and how long they remained dependent. And whether individuals and families accessed this wider palette of medical care simultaneously or sequentially, or indeed at all, coloured experiences of illness and recuperation. The chapter will thus explore four key themes: the range and depth of the 'shadow' medical economy of makeshifts, in which paupers sought independent solutions mirroring those of the parish itself; the outlines of the 'complementary' economy, in which paupers themselves might seek extra treatments at the same time as they were obtaining parochial resources; the extent and composition of the 'substitute' medical economy of makeshifts to which the poor had recourse instead of the Old Poor Law;[13] and the wider question of where parochial medical welfare fitted into a life-cycle of pauper responses to ill-health.

The shadow economy

Vestry minutes, pauper letters and official correspondence provide abundant evidence of sick paupers seeking independently the same sorts of treatment that parochial officials also provided. As Chapters 5 and 6 showed, they did so using cash allowances given by the parish, but also with their own or neighbourhood resources or simply by drawing on the charity of medical providers. This shadow economy is best explored by looking at the ways in which the poor accessed the services of doctors, some of whom were the very same medical men employed by the parish itself. The act of retaining doctors raised issues of the balance of authority, power and rights in a way that retaining nurses or buying drugs did not, and affords us a view of the process rather than simply the fact of the shadow medical economy. Whereas this phenomenon was rare in the 1750s, by the early nineteenth century vestries and officials often struggled with paupers who felt they had a right to consult doctors. Garstang (Lancashire) vestry addressed this matter in its June 1815 meeting, resolving that 'no doctors to be allowed for his trouble [doctoring the poor] unless directed by the overseer'. Periodic re-statement of this policy seems to have had little effect. A decade later

(21 June 1825) the vestry noted that a 'bill from Mr Rogerson [himself a member of the select vestry!] was presented for services and medicines to [the in-parish pauper] Jenny Witherington'. While ordering payment, the vestry added a blanket caveat: 'in order to prevent any misunderstandings and objections to the payment of bills incurred on account of paupers. That no accounts shall be paid unless a written order shall have been given by the overseer authorizing the same.'[14] Other communities were more direct. Welton (Northamptonshire), for instance, refused the bill of Dr Metcalf for treating William Pitt, 'this not being by order of the overseer and Dr Metcalf to desist from claiming again on this parish'.[15] The parish of Tarleton (Lancashire) provides a particularly rich sense of the complexity of this issue: Dr Burrell was retained on an *ad hoc* basis by the parish through the late 1820s and early 1830s and had his periodic bills paid. The parish also received bills from Drs Hunt, Barnes and Hesketh (all turned down) and from the apothecary William Baron. The latter was a particular thorn in the side of the vestry since he both supplied medicines under parish order and dealt directly with the poor. Thus while his bill of 7 April 1835 (10s 6d) was paid, that of 4 March 1834 'for medicines to sundry poor persons' was only partly met because some of the medicines had not been authorised. A bill for £2 on 2 June 1835 was turned down completely because it was 'not by order of the overseer', as was the bill of another apothecary (William Benson, for medicine given to the late John Fairclough's wife) on 5 January 1836.[16] More widely, all of the parishes used for this study provide direct or indirect evidence of paupers consulting doctors of their own accord. This is unsurprising given the assumed rights to medical relief and the increased medicalisation of poverty highlighted in Chapters 3 and 4 respectively.

A broad-brush observation of this sort, however, fails to do justice to the complexity of the motivations, expectations and experiences of any party to this aspect of the shadow medical economy. It is possible to discern at least three pauper mentalities. A first group – both those for whom the fact of a doctor's bill threatened independence and those already dependent – found the money to pay their doctors and never sought direct or compensating parochial welfare. We often discover such experiences by accident or have to imply them from second-hand evidence. Thus Mary Sawley of Bowling (West Yorkshire) sought to attest her previous good character in July 1803 by noting that she had

'scraped and sold all I had' to pay Mr Wade's medical bill.[17] While the size of this sub-group is unclear we find examples across the typological, spatial and chronological spectrums, suggesting a significant underbelly of unseen doctoring for the poor. They stand in contradistinction to another group of paupers (or their advocates), who wrote to settlement parishes explicitly acknowledging that they did not have the money to pay a doctor and asking for parish authority to do so. Edward Webster, writing from Wellingborough (Northamptonshire) to Market Harborough in the case of William Brown, noted that he 'has not yet Employed a medical man for he as not the means of paying one'.[18] The simultaneous existence of both rhetorics points to an ingrained sense among the sick poor that it was acceptable to commission doctors in a shadow economy.

A second group consulted doctors and clearly had an expectation that they would be able to pay the consequent bill. As Chapter 5 suggested, we encounter them in some numbers in cases when this expectation was frustrated, necessitating recourse to the parish either for help in paying the bill or for compensating payments where paying the doctor had eaten up other resources. Thus the servant Elizabeth Simmons wrote from Portman Square (London) to her settlement parish of Peterborough St John (Northamptonshire) on 2 May 1799 to say that she was in desperate need of relief. Simmons had 'paid my last quarter wage ser for the Docter threw the [clearly illegitimate] child ill health and the rest for the keep of the child as I have no assistants for us boath els I wuold not trouble you'. She had intended to pay the doctoring bill for her child and simply scrape by, but deterioration in the fortunes of relatives providing childcare had upset her calculations. 'My sister', she wrote, 'cannot afford to keep it [her niece] without the pay'.[19] Similarly, James Tomblin of Thrapston (Northamptonshire) wrote to a magistrate on 25 October 1833. He was labouring under

> a series of domestic affliction the latest and most considerable of which is that my wife has been very ill for nearly twelve months and is still unwell which together with former afflictions has incurred a doctors bill of more than £12. In consequence of the extra expense unavoidable during this affliction I have not been able to pay the last year's rent.[20]

Tomblin asked not for payment of his doctoring bill but for a parochial commitment to pay his rent and thus replenish the household

economy that had been depleted by the unavoidable decision to commission a doctor independently of the parish. Thomas Earl, writing
from Portsmouth to Bradford-on-Avon (Wiltshire), exemplifies this
group of paupers even more clearly. His letter of 19 January 1835 outlined a litany of sickness and noted that his wife, his daughter and he
himself were all under different local doctors. He did not seek to have
his parish pay the bills for these medical gentlemen, but rather enjoined
officials to 'help us through the winter ... at present we are in a starving state'.[21] Such examples were not simply confined to the out-parish
poor. George Pedder attended the Garstang vestry in August 1815
to say that his grandchild was 'lying ill' and that lack of employment
meant that the family could pay only part of the doctor's bill. His
request that the parish pay its share of the expense was turned down
but a repeat application in September, this time noting that Pedder was
both looking after his sick daughter and had an outstanding doctor's
bill, was favourably received.[22] It is easy to read these approaches to the
parish as mere rhetoric or indeed active dissembling, but this would be
inaccurate, not least because the majority of writers had already paid or
intended to pay part of their outstanding bills.

Moreover, the language and intent of this group must be set alongside a third subset of the sick poor, those who had no intention of trying
to meet the bills occasioned by their turning independently to doctors.
John Holt attended the Chorley vestry on 2 September 1805, asking
the parish to 'discharge a certain bill due to Mr Sharples of Ormskirk
for attending his wife when sick'. The vestry paid notwithstanding (or
perhaps because of) Holt's periodic absconding from his family when
there were bills to be paid.[23] He was one of more than 750 paupers who
wrote or attended vestries and simply assumed that their accumulated
bills would be met, the vast majority of whom were successful. Some
of this group rhetoricised a state of being overwhelmed by chronic and
multiple illnesses, employing the fact of their independent engagement
with doctors to try and establish long-term decline which might warrant
a parochial pension or its augmentation. The act of not paying was in
itself evidence of their hopeless position. Others did not even attempt
to dress up their purpose. Thomas Wheeler, writing from Halifax (West
Yorkshire) in August 1804, emphasised that the poor had the right to
mimic the actions of the parish in order to preserve life and health,
noting that 'urgent necessity compelled me to turn to Mr Alexander

in order that I might not be lost'. Situating his action within a wider
moral and expectational framework that justified agency in extremis,
Wheeler claimed to his correspondent that Mr Alexander 'concurs with
my action'.[24]

It would be unsurprising if, on the other side of the equation, doctors reacted to the clamorous calls of the poor with silence, delay or
refusal. Certainly coronial records provide a qualitative sense that doctors sometimes acted with caution, as for instance when the mother
of an illegitimate child from Sneinton (Nottinghamshire) overdosed
her child with laudanum on 29 January 1840. Four doctors 'had been
contacted but they would not come and the baby died on Wednesday
morning'.[25] Some doctors at least saw contracts with parochial authorities as themselves an act of charity, given the onerous duties imposed,
and saw little reason to extend such philanthropy further. Others
would become wary of forced charity during their training. Thus in
1776, Anthony Fothergill warned his young protégé James Woodforde
about engaging with paupers: 'If you set apart 2 hours every day in
prescribing for paupers', he noted, 'they will not fail to spread your
fame and bring in opulent farmers and by degrees the neighbouring
gentry.' Yet while this might be a good thing for a young doctor seeking
his way in the world, Fothergill warned that 'to do this [you] must sit
down resolutely bent to continue, for if the slightest hint escapes you of
a design to relinquish, it will at once destroy the interest you have made
and damp all future hopes of establishing amongst them'.[26] My data is
replete with doctors who did not heed this advice. Dr William Irving,
who sent an 'acct by Part' to the parish of Strickland (Cumberland) for
looking after William Gilpin and his family during a typhus outbreak in
Lancaster, is absolutely typical. He noted mournfully: 'Previous to the
date in acct. I attended W. Gilpin's family for five weeks, during which
time I had a claim against him, for eighteen journeys, and medicines,
not any of which are entered to your acct.; nor do I expect to be remunerated, unless by his Parish.'[27]

But not all charity was prised out of the grasp of the doctor, and
there are many examples of medical men intending to provide care
free of charge or on a subsidised basis.[28] Their range of motivations was
complex but three in particular loom large. First, some doctors clearly
responded to pauper appeals in the expectation that parishes would
eventually pay something, submitting bills as though they had been

commissioned to provide care by officers. The persistence and repetition of the practice could be remarkable. Between 1795 and 1825 the parish of Calverley (West Yorkshire), for instance, received forty-six unsolicited bills from doctors for independent treatment of the sick poor. Rather like settlement and removal cases, the consequent disputes seem to have ended up in court with some regularity, sometimes costing parishes rather more in legal expenses and restitution than the original disputed bill.[29] It would be wrong to imply, however, that all such bills represent the mercenary intent of the doctors themselves. Some sub-groups of the poor – such as vagrants and those passing through – held a liminal status when it came to treatment. Thus while Garstang parish persistently warned doctors not to treat the poor without authority from the overseer, Dr Graham's bill of £2 13s 2d for 'doctoring afforded to different vagrants' who fell sick was paid without question because failing to provide speedy remedy might incur long-term bills for the town.[30]

A second group of doctors appear not to have so readily assumed that their costs would be reimbursed, instead implicitly or explicitly viewing their attendance as an act of charity. William Howarth, curate of March (Cambridgeshire), wrote to Peterborough on 15 April 1833 about the Clarke family. Joseph Clarke was 'himself very ill and totally unable to work, and his wife has for some time been confined to her bed with inflamation on her lungs ... I found them and their four children without food, money, or a nurse and altogether in a most distressed and folorn condition.' Asking for a regular allowance, he added that 'the medical gentleman who is kindly [i.e. charitably] attending them thinks the womans life in great danger'.[31] John Cary, a surgeon of Trowbridge (Wiltshire), was even more charitable, recounting how Manoh England had been badly mangled in an industrial accident such that his cure required 'long continued attention ... the attendance and trouble were very great'. Not wishing to charge the parish for such intervention, he rather asked the vestry of Bradford-on-Avon to consider an allowance for the parents, who had to provide ongoing care.[32] Evidence for an ingrained charitable imperative comes from the records of doctors as well as the poor law. The Lancashire medical man Richard Loxham appears never to have offered free treatment, but he did adopt sliding scales of charges for patients according to his perception of their ability to pay. Moreover, he allowed debts to run on, in some cases for

decades, without interest and accepted part or full payment in kind as well as cash.[33] The early nineteenth-century shoemaker poet Robert Hird of Bedale (North Yorkshire) put the generosity of his local practitioner – Dr Campbell – to lyric:

> The poor he quickly did attend,
> When ever he'd their call,
> And med'cine sent, if they did mend,
> He'd oft no pay at all
>
> Or did he ever one distress,
> For he'd sympathy,
> For poverty and helplessness:
> Such traits are rare to see.
>
> 'Twas with a smile, that he met you,
> And did obeisance make,
> Both rich and poor received his bow
> To all he was awake.[34]

Such examples point once again to a substantial underbelly of additional doctoring for the sick poor outside the framework of formal medical welfare.

For some doctors, and as a third motivation, the issue of payment was subsumed to a sense of their professional imperative to preserve life in extremis. Their intervention in this sense was more than charity. When Robert Kerrison MD assembled a list of correspondence about 'Medical and surgical attendance on the parochial poor' from provincial doctors for the *Transactions of the Associated Apothecaries & Surgeons of England and Wales*, the difficulty of obtaining an order (and thus reimbursement) for urgent treatment was an encompassing complaint. One doctor from Skipton (Yorkshire) 'Recommends it to be legal for another person (not an overseer) to give such order in case of emergency', and he was one of many correspondents who argued for a standard table of fees for doctoring in extremis.[35] Doctors acting in such situations sometimes sought the moral high ground, as was the case with Dr Kenrick of Broughton (Wiltshire), who amputated the leg of Alice Rogers so as to save her life. He assured the overseer 'he wd take it off gratis' but requested reimbursement for the journeys and medicine.[36] In other cases, however, doctors assumed an absolute right

to act, as for instance with Joseph Hooper of Bath, whose bill of five guineas for operating on a Bradford-on-Avon pauper called Morris was refused, 'but as the case was one of life and death not allowing time for my giving notice to my Parish authority, I shall upon that plea sue you for the Payment as I am assured of its recovery by my attorney'.[37] Even before attempts in the 1830s and 1840s to construct doctors as a class of public servants, those engaged with the poor law elaborated a *de facto* professional duty rationale for their independent actions.[38] William Spacey of Halifax (West Yorkshire), writing in 1801, exemplifies this process. Noting that he had treated the pauper Allen Day 'quietly' (i.e. free of charge) in the four months from February to May as an act 'of charity lying within my professional and public duty', he now asked officials to grant Day an allowance to help with his recuperation. He was sure that the 'Gentlemen would, could they but see him [Allen Day] be called out of humanity to follow my own quiet example'.[39]

It is difficult to codify the multiple snapshots and mixture of direct and implied references to the seeking and provision of independent medical care and thus to provide a systematic chronological or spatial overview. Nonetheless, the sense of a large-scale shadow medical economy of makeshifts which mimicked the therapeutic actions of the parish is clear. The sick poor felt that they had a right to turn to doctors independently of the poor law, and they acted in this regard on a considerable scale, particularly after 1800. On the opposite side of this equation, doctors, nurses and apothecaries joined with and gave credibility to the shadow medical economy, creating for parochial officials a considerable moral and economic dilemma. Sometimes – and particularly where there was an assumption that parishes would simply pick up large retrospective bills for shadowing treatment – resistance could be strong and sustained. Yet what is striking in the data is both the frequency with which vestries re-stated a position that paupers and providers were required to seek authorisation for prior or additional treatment and their inaction when rules were broken. As we have observed in Chapter 3, such inaction rapidly turned into custom.

The complementary economy

At the same time as the dependent poor applied for and obtained medical welfare from the parish, they were accessing complementary

forms of treatment. Institutional care falls into this category and has been explored in Chapter 8. Three other medical welfare avenues – family care, medical charity and self-dosing – also, however, require particular attention if we are to understand the meaning of parish provision. First, the idea that families must have been responsible for a considerable amount of informal care and treatment is implicitly accepted, though less often proven, by historians of welfare, the family and medicine.[40] The diaries, account books and autobiographies that inform this view are rarely available for the labouring and dependent poor.[41] Nonetheless, some 3,200 pauper and advocate letters imply, detail or explain family care during sickness, across a spectrum from nursing, errands and advocacy, through provision of food and acquisition of medicines, to securing institutional care or medical devices. Familial support might also extend to seeking herbal medicines and other domestically prepared or administered remedies of the sort encountered as part of parochial provision in Chapter 6.

More broadly, kinship support seems to have shaped the complementary economy and its relationship to parochial medical welfare in three ways. Firstly, the data is redolent with explicit or implied examples of care simply being given, something we discover almost by accident. Hence, the draft 1801 census return for Binfield (Berkshire) suggests that the insane Mary Cooper was cared for by her stepmother after her father died; the aged widower William Gibbs was under the care of his sister Elizabeth Cutler; the blind Fran Gildin drew support from two lodgers, a granddaughter and two servants; and the decrepit widow Williams was cared for by her two granddaughters aged thirteen and seven respectively.[42] There is no evidence that any of these caring relationships came at a cost to the parish. Nor ultimately did the support offered by Henry Cooper, whose wife had 'through a nervous Fever, become Insane'. Then resident in Peckham lunatic asylum, 'she is not considered well enough to be removed', but Cooper was unable to meet the full costs of her sojourn there immediately. His letter to St Clement Danes (London) was emphatic and emphasised with underlining: Cooper was 'not desiring for her to be passed over to her parish' but rather he wished to agree a payment plan underwritten by the parish, and 'Should death, or recovery, take place before the deficiencies are made up, I will pay 5s per week till the whole Debt is cleared.'[43] Meanwhile, support between brothers and sisters (and

their in-law counterparts) appears to have been particularly important in terms of both the provision of advocacy and more tangible help at times of sickness, something that chimes strongly with recent attempts to re-situate the importance of sibling relationships in middling and other families.[44] An emblematic example is Jane Thorpe, resident in Stamford (Lincolnshire) workhouse, who was discharged with one of her children 'to nurse her sister'.[45] While ultimately this sort of unheralded support cannot be quantified, the sense of both vestry data and the corpus of correspondence is of its core importance.

At the other end of the experiential spectrum, the nature of the complementary economy and its relationship to parochial welfare was shaped by the absence of kin or (much more often) by the resources of a wider kinship group simply running out. The situation is exemplified in the correspondence of Joseph Richards of Colleycroft, who, when asking for an allowance on 20 April 1828, noted that 'we are very much distressed in consequence of our age and infirmities which no doubt you must well know for I am 73 and my wife 65 and my 2 girls which is the chiefest of our dependence for living is very ill & has been for sometime which makes our own case still worse'.[46] This elision of increasing need and the sudden or gradual falling-off of kinship support is a commonplace in the data. Nor was it confined to the decline associated with old age. The 'Pore Afflicted lad' that James Stiles, writing from London to Bampton (Oxfordshire) on 4 February 1818, had been obliged to 'maintain Many years and Cannot dow it any longer' was actually his grandson.[47] There is also much evidence that care might extend to a wider group than that involving immediate lateral and vertical kin. Thus when John Calvert wrote from Alston (Lancashire) on the subject of the chronically sick William Burland, he observed that 'Had it not been for me he must have taken hurt.' Calvert had, he assured the overseer of Greystoke (Westmorland) 'found him with ~~victuals~~ logins and part victuals ever since he came into this part of the Country, which I can ill afford to do as I have a large family of my own to support'. The crossing out in this letter points simultaneously to a desire for accuracy in case of inspection or further enquiry (see Chapter 3) and a struggle for Calvert himself to adequately encompass the nature of his support for Burland. Lest the overseer confuse his approach with advocacy from a neighbour, Calvert reminded him that 'the man is not to be lost, he is only a distant relation of mine, but he

has no one to do anything for him, nevertheless, I would do anything for him that lies in my power'.[48] While references to failing and absent kinship could be a useful rhetorical device for the sick poor and their advocates, a more positive reading can be supported: one in which kinship groups, often little better off than their sick relatives, complemented support or prevented dependence for as long as they could.

It is perhaps unsurprising against this backdrop that a final group of paupers, advocates, families and officials sought to blur the boundaries between parochial medical welfare and complementary kinship support by forming partnerships. Richard Eastwood, living with his daughter in Bolton (Lancashire), was in April 1825 to be 'found on a Sick Bed and speechless, It is not very likely he can continue much longer one person [presumably the daughter] is continually in attendance on him'.[49] Equally, officials might supplement family care for sick children. Charles Blades of Braceborough (Lincolnshire) had his insane granddaughter delivered to him 'to take care of her (her grandfather having been accustomed to the care of insane persons)'. Resisting a suggestion that she be placed in an asylum, he 'did not apprehend any danger would arise to his daughter or any other person, as at present she was by no means violent, and that he could take good care of her, if allowed 5s per week', which was duly granted.[50] In other work, I have argued that industrial parishes in particular actively went out of their way to foster a complementary economy by subsidising the co-residence of aged and decaying paupers with their children, but the evidence from pauper letters is that individuals, parishes and families operated more widely in a negotiative space where the systematic fusion of parochial and kinship resources underpinned a complementary medical economy of makeshifts.[51] Once again, then, parochial medical welfare formed only a subset of the resources attainable by the sick poor.

Medically related charity was a second potential part of the complementary economy. Some was organised, consistent and long-term, as for instance with the voluntary hospitals, lying-in charities and specialist institutions encountered in Chapter 8.[52] Parishes themselves sometimes blurred the dividing line between this sort of charity and medical welfare, as for instance in Oundle, where the vestry ordered (in a short-lived venture) on 13 January 1831 that 'the subscription to Peterborough Dispensary be discontinued, Mr Wildash [proxy for Watts Russell] stating that Mr Watts Russell subscribed to it which

would most probably afford means of procuring the admission of any
parish patient that might be required'.[53] Nonetheless, and despite an
early nineteenth-century renewal of the philanthropic imperative,[54] a
singular feature of the range of formal charity in my parishes is that so
little of it dealt directly with the medical needs of paupers. This echoes
Alannah Tomkins's argument that charity offered for the poor 'benefits
which did not exactly or even approximately match their needs'.[55] No
doubt for this reason, an implicit though rarely elaborated assumption of the secondary literature is that individual, *ad hoc*, charity was
a key response to sickness in most localities. Sources reflecting on the
middling sorts are indeed replete with examples of such charity running across a spectrum from the provision of sustaining resources and
nursing, through advocacy and to the purchase of medicines. James
Newton, rector of Nuneham Courtenay (Oxfordshire), was a visitor
of the sick and periodically 'order'd of them Victuals' from his own
pocket.[56] At the other end of the country, James Dawson of Troutbeck
(Cumberland) gave £12 per year to the sick poor from 1813 to 1839,
mainly in the form of food and clothing.[57] The Ampthill (Bedfordshire)
diarist Elizabeth Brown also reflected frequently on her own personal
charity. Her diary entry for 9 February 1779 noted that she had:

> In the evening visited a young woman who is sick and destitute of any
> near relations to administer comfort at these times, being also in strait
> circumstances ... Have many times remarked that nothing can induce
> so much to a desire of administering to the necessities of the poor as to
> visit them in their cottages and to behold their many wants.[58]

And visiting could turn into much more active involvement in the
remediation of sickness. The vicar of North Creake (Norfolk), having
visited the nineteen-year-old Henry Fowle and found him extremely
sick, had 'a mind to try the virtue of vervain: came home to look in the
physic books'. Put off by what he read, the vicar resorted to alternative
remedies brewed in his kitchen including infusion of hemlock, cream
of tartar, julep and his own patent 'elder ointment'.[59] This was one of
eighteen medical cases joined by the vicar, not one of which involved
poor law officials.

It is the *ad hoc* charitable activities of 'friends' and neighbours,
however, which loom particularly large in my data. W.B., writing from
Leicester to Market Harborough, noted that 'Mr Wilson had only one

penny left last night till relieved by a Neighbour [but] ... the only friend he seems to have here has gone as far as she can afford to do.'[60] Barbara Ingham, 'now lying ill at Dent (Westmorland) and in a very poor state', lived with her sister but was 'maintained by her friends', and Nanny Ormerod 'a short time ago got her bed and since that time has been unable to leave her bed and must have been removed had she not been relieved by some ladies'.[61] While charity extended to women is notably visible in the sources, the gender dimension is less important in understanding the nature of *ad hoc* support than questions of life-cycle (old people were more likely to note such support than younger applicants for medical welfare) and the severity of sickness. Within this broad framework, 'friends' often wrote directly to officials when their own charity had been exhausted. John Mitchel, encountered at the outset of Chapter 8, wrote to the vestry clerk of Rotherfield Greys (Oxfordshire) on 23 February 1818 to note that Mary Harris's daughter had three weeks previously 'lost the use of her Limbs, & has been confined to her bed ever since'. He had been requested by Harris to apply for medical relief, and in the meantime Mitchel had 'given her such assistance as I could spare'.[62] The analogue of such support can be seen in cases such as that of Hannah Blothridge, who on 7 May 1829 was 'now very ill and stands in need of your assistance' and for whom her epistolary advocate noted that 'she have no friends as can assist her'.[63] This language of active or absent friendship, and the wider individual charity that it denotes, are deeply inscribed into the correspondence used in this analysis and, if anything, become more common over the period considered here.

Evidence for a third strand of the complementary economy – self-treatment – also becomes more frequent from the later eighteenth century. Quack, folk and herbal remedies were a focus of Chapter 6 and are explored at greater length below. Another aspect of this strand was the taking of waters. We have grown accustomed to thinking of water therapy (a catch-all title that includes everything from mineral springs, through sea and freshwater bathing, to holy wells) as the preserve of the rich and middling.[64] In practice, however, there is considerable evidence that the poor also turned to water treatment of their own accord before, during or after treatment provided by the Old Poor Law. Diarists provide outline evidence of the accessibility of such cures. Dr Richard Pockocke's tours through England in the mid- and

late eighteenth century, for instance, are punctuated with information on medicinal springs. He draws a distinction between Ilkley, where 'There is here a famous alum spring, which is of great use in drying up both scrophulous and also old sores, where the constitution is strong enough to bear it', and more minor springs such as Bormhill Grange near Lake Derwent (Cumberland), where 'there is a salt spring which is much frequented by the common people, as a purging water'.[65] Similar sites for the 'common people' were noted in places as far afield as Ormskirk on the one hand and Padstow on the other. In Cullingworth (Nottinghamshire) he observed a mineral spring that 'rises out of the coal mines, and was not drunk, unless to kill worms'.[66] Access to water of various types was increasingly funded as a form of parochial medical welfare, but instances in which officials contributed to the costs of freshwater and sea visits rather than underwriting the entire venture were still in 1834 the representative mode of parochial engagement with this curative strand. There is also, however, considerable evidence in the corpus of correspondence that the sick poor sought the waters independently and without asking for parochial resources. Jonathan Sweet's sojourn in Harrogate, for instance, comes to our attention only because he broke his leg while getting into the water and was required to approach the overseer of Calverley for surgical aid.[67]

Any attempt to quantify and codify this variegated picture of familial and neighbourhood support, formal and personal charity and self-help founders on patchy sources capable of multiple readings. Even for the best-documented parishes in the underlying sample we can obtain only a partial snapshot of the complementary medical economy. It is thus difficult to discern whether parishes with lower aggregate spending on medical welfare or more focus on cash payments acted as they did simply because the complementary medical economy was more robust in the locality. Nor is it possible to discern with certainty whether the unquestionable increase in references to the complementary economy across the parochial sample from the 1800s reflects a genuine increase in its scope and depth – a reflection and embodiment of the increasingly medicalised lives of the poor – or simply a reaction to increasing medical needs unmet by parishes. We are on clearer ground in relation to familial care, references to which increase markedly in pauper letters, overseer correspondence and vestry minutes from the early 1800s. While Mary Fissell and others have argued that those with least

kinship support were most likely to become dependent on the parish and in medical institutions, in the parochial sample underpinning this study there was no systematic relationship at individual level between receipt of medical welfare and the ostensible, claimed or traced extent of kinship. Indeed, the tendency for parishes to seek partnership with families to achieve care of the sick and aged poor often meant that those garnering the highest per capita levels of welfare benefits were equally those tied most firmly into local kinship networks.[68]

The substitute economy

These are important observations, but they must be set against a backdrop in which most sick paupers were engaged at some point (and arguably more frequently than in all other welfare avenues) in a substitute medical economy of makeshifts. Patient case histories such as those taken by William Stutter at the Suffolk General Hospital in the 1830s confirm the perspective of Chapter 2 that the sick poor laboured under serious medical conditions for many years without approaching either the poor law or medical institutions.[69] One of the obvious components of this substitute medical economy of makeshifts was planned self-help. Indeed, welfare historians have sometimes drawn a negative link between the 'generosity' and scope of welfare payments and the spatial distribution of the 925,000 friendly society members active in the early nineteenth century.[70] True or not, the evidence that 'club' membership was an important part of the substitute medical economy is marked. In Lancashire the Garstang Friendly Society paid variable allowances ranging between 4s and 9s per week by the 1810s.[71] At the same date the Bampton (Oxfordshire) Friendly Society paid 5s weekly benefit and allowances of up to £6 for funerals.[72] There is also strong evidence of popular support for local friendly societies. Robert Hird visited them in his magisterial poem with the following words:

Clubs had become a common scheme,
In all the country round:
Against old age, or sickness keen,
And benefit they found.

In case of death they had a sum,
For husband and for wife,

And this was pleasant to look on,
In health and strength through life.

Five shillings they had in the week,
When sick and laid off work,
For one whole year, if they'd no trick,
In idleness to lurk;

Longer than this, they'd half a crown,
And might a little do,
And when to old age they had come,
Were pensioners life through.

But no relief was from the box,
Which rose from mens' bad ways,
The doctor viewed the sick folks,
And gave account always.[73]

We can of course overstate the strength of entitlement to benefits and of the organisations which paid them.[74] The recently bereaved Mary Ann Pearson, for instance, wrote from Finsbury (London) to Beverley (East Yorkshire) on 15 April 1834 to request relief during her sickness. Noting that her husband 'was in no society', she added that 'the one he was in for ten years in Beverley broke up, leaving the family destitute in his final illness and death'.[75] Yet parochial officials valued such insurance sufficiently to collect friendly society membership certificates as an indemnification against medical welfare claims.[76] Moreover, twenty-eight parishes blurred the boundaries between the poor law and self-help by paying the membership subscriptions of paupers.[77] Officials also involved themselves in disputes over entitlement to benefits, as did the newly formed Stamford Board of Guardians in November 1837 when the Ketton Friendly Society refused to pay benefits to the widow of Thomas Freeman, who had taken his own life.[78] How far the benefits paid kept the sick away from medical relief is difficult to discern with any precision. Periodic surveys of the poor by vestries sometimes recorded people surviving on a combination of club and parochial benefits. On the other hand, contracts between friendly societies and doctors usually specified comprehensive treatment, and the comparative lack of disputes between paupers and officials over entitlement when in receipt of 'club money' suggests some gap between the two welfare systems.

The benefit for parishes of a well-operated society is best exemplified by the case of Mary Purday, for whom Thomas Webster wrote from Bedford Row (London) on 29 September 1808. Purday 'was attacked about 2 months since with a paralytic stroke'. She had been supported by a daughter who was now suffering from fainting fits and was unable to maintain the mother. Webster noted that 'The Daughter belongs to a Sick Club and is a present on the books I do not therefore mention her case to solicit parochial relief' merely to highlight the need for medical welfare for her mother.[79] There is thus no obvious sense in which parishes with high friendly society membership paid lower per capita medical welfare costs, though they may have had fewer potential claimants.[80]

The analogue of self-help in the substitute economy was paternalism. While some employers turned out their employees at the first sign of sickness, there are balancing perspectives. The earliest substantial parochial letter sets (for Cricklade in Wiltshire, Oxford and Lancaster, all between the 1750s and 1780s) provide abundant evidence of employers supporting sick and injured employees by paying for doctors, food or allowances in cash. Such support can be seen even more clearly in the larger corpus for the post-1800 period. Most of them sought no reimbursement for their actions. John Chapman Jnr wrote from Northampton to Market Harborough on 6 April 1828 on the subject of his employee George Peabody, who was now better after a long fever. He added, 'I believe those Powders we had from the Chymists has been of great service.'[81] Similarly, William Moore wrote from Bath to Bradford-on-Avon on 11 April 1834 in the case of his employee John Hurt, who was under the charitable care of the Bath eye doctor Mr Spender. Noting that he intended to retain Hurt when his eyes were cured, Moore told the overseer: 'I have relieved him several times by subscription and other ways which I should not have been done had I not considered him deserving of relief.'[82] Other employers made claims on settlement parishes for employees but had not intended to do so at the outset of the illness. Thus John Easby wrote to Tilehurst on 21 March 1825 to say that he had parted from Mary Nibbs his servant, who 'lived with us a month but turned out to be subject to fits and was laid up with one here. The Doctors Bill was 2/6 and expences occurring from persons to sit up with her &c above 7/- more.' Easby eventually sought reimbursement from the parish, but the fact is that he relieved Nibbs not knowing that such a claim was possible. He was, as he

admitted, alerted to the fact only by 'an advertisement in the Reading Mercury for all demands upon Tylehurst parish being sent to you'.[83] A small subset of employers sought immediate reimbursement by parishes. William Plaister of George Lane, Oxford, was 'not doubting' that the parish of Witney would be 'paying all necessary expences' when his employee John Prestage was 'down with the Small Pox and as he was taken ill at my House I was under the necessity of taken care of him'.[84] Even among this group, however, such demands were usually accompanied by advocacy for ongoing support of the paupers themselves. In any case, far more representative was the 'humane Liberality' extended to the sick labourer William Gilpin by his employer at Strickland Roger (Westmorland) in 1835.[85]

Other aspects of the substitute medical economy of makeshifts are harder to analyse systematically, though no less important. Many welfare and medical historians assume that the poor, even the dependent poor, must have turned to quack remedies both because parishes themselves did and because without their demand there could have been no market.[86] Indirect evidence that itinerant providers had a presence throughout the period covered by this study is plentiful. Rosetta Trainer, for instance, was killed in Hungerford on 29 April 1783 when she was trampled by two horses 'drawing a carriage or stage belonging to a travelling mountebank', while Daniel Farroe, 'a traveller and itinerant vendor of quack medicines', was found dead in Devizes on 8 September 1783.[87] Meanwhile, in Shellingford (Berkshire) the overseer in 1814 paid for himself and another man to go and 'suppress a mountebank'.[88] Yet it was the proliferation of fixed, knowable outlets on the one hand and mail order on the other that transformed the quack trade. It is not hard to imagine the poor responding to an advertisement such as that by a Lancashire bookseller:

> Sold by Thomas [crossed out and 'Jane' substituted] Butter Bookseller near St Martins Lane in Exton where (besides books and stationary wares of all sorts) is sold the best mathematical and sea instruments, seven sorts of physical medicines, as Dr Daffy's Elixir Satuti, Stoughton's Elixir Stomachium, Spriti of scurvy grass, golden and plain … by wholesale or retail.[89]

Such vendors sold remedies and some of their constituent ingredients in quantities which ranged from full bottles to tiny 'measures'. If we add

to this picture the proliferation of druggists in the nineteenth-century medical market,[90] many of whom produced their own patent remedies and sold them by the pennyworth, the potential role of the quack remedy in the substitute medical economy of makeshifts is clear.

Finding evidence of actual usage by the dependent poor is more difficult, and much of the literature has focused disproportionately on the mid- to late nineteenth century.[91] Court cases (and newspaper reporting of them) periodically deal directly with deaths occasioned by quacks and more commonly provide witness evidence of their activities in the very poorest districts.[92] Coronial records provide more focused evidence, with children in particular often recorded as being killed by individual ingredients or composite medicines purchased, stored and administered by their parents independent of doctors or the poor law. Thus later eighteenth-century Wiltshire coroners recorded overdosing by mercury (in one case sold by 'an unskilful quack'), 'physic powder from an empiric', white hellebore (given 'from a dreadful mistake of an apothecary's servant'), 'deadly poison mixed with sulphur and treacle' instead of cream of tartar, syrup of poppy, spurge laurel (as an abortifant), Daffy's Elixir, Evans's Spirit of Comfrey and various patent pills.[93] From the 1820s onwards the *Nottingham Journal* and *Nottingham Mercury* reported coronial inquests across the whole county. As Bernard Heathcote points out when using this data, for sickness among children parents might turn to Dalby's Carminative or Godfrey's Cordial, which were 'readily obtained from grocers, corner shopkeepers and chemists'. Such 'medicines' were implicated in more than 100 traceable Nottinghamshire deaths. Nor were the preparations of druggists any safer: The mother of Alan Witham, a pauper of Sutton-in-Ashfield, went to Mr Littlewodd the druggist and asked his assistant 'to supply her with a mixture of syrup of rhubarb, syrup of violets, paregoric and honey'. The assistant accidentally included laudanum instead of paregoric and the child died.[94] The fact that Mrs Witham had sought to dose her own child and had specified the exact mixture she needed is significant to this overview of the substitute medical economy.

Doctors themselves periodically railed against unqualified medical men, and while one must be cautious in interpreting such complaints Kerrison's 1821 survey of provincial doctors is replete with testimony on the following: 'Many unqualified persons'; 'instances of mischief done by a farrier and a bonesetter'; 'qualifications not attended to';

'business ill done'; 'an impudent quack ... was a barber, then innkeeper and now farmer'; 'abuses in that part of the country by pretenders'; 'the necessity of excluding unqualified persons'; and 'mischief of practicing quacks'. Detailed case notes on 'Bad practice in midwifery and surgery' in the *Nottingham Journal* develop this theme and provide evidence of the tendency of the very poor to seek the services of bonesetters, midwives, druggists, apothecaries, truss makers and herbalists.[95] Yet direct evidence of the dependent poor consuming quack remedies is rare: Thomas Earl's wife was 'taken in the night in the Same Complaint that we thought She Ould have died but She took Some Dafies and She is a Little Recovered'.[96] She was one of only thirty-eight paupers in the entire pauper letter corpus who were noted as taking such remedies, though many more examples are probably disguised by ubiquitous references to the acquisition of 'medicines'. This label must also have included laudanum if the example of John Sawyer of Rugeley (who was 'very Ill in bed he wants more Lodonom and cant have any at Mr Bamford's on your acct'[97]) is representative. More broadly, a sense of the expectation that the sick poor ought to be able to acquire drugs in their own right is provided by cases such as that of Samuel Smith writing from Lancaster on 16 December 1823. Beset with his 'old cum-plaint' and noting he had received free advice from Dr Turnwell, he wished the overseers to know that 'the Drugest Charges very high for his drugs so that I dow not know how to get them'.[98]

For those not inclined or, like Smith, too poor to buy from the quack, 'folk remedies' provided an alternative. Moore and McLean suggest that folk medicine represents an open system rooted in the community and responsive to individual need, whereas formal medicine is closed and based upon fixed and universal assumptions. In turn, they argue, 'formal medicine treated those who could best afford it' such that it was 'the poor and uneducated that utilised folk medicine as a direct result of their impoverished circumstances'.[99] Most commentators are more circumspect, being informed by an implicit sense that the very poorest must necessarily have drawn on traditional folk and herbal remedies and a range of other 'alternative' therapies rooted in older belief systems. Indeed, the assumption that poor people inevitably drew on alternative therapies is so strong that the poor in general, and the dependent poor in particular, have little more than a walk-on part in most histories of such medical provision, even as its longevity well into the nineteenth

century in the persona of amateur botanists, cunning folk and 'fringe' practitioners has been increasingly well established.[100] This situation is in large part explained by the lack and fragility of sources, from which the current study is not immune. There are, however, some 171 references to broadly conceived alternative remedies across the sample, including the wife of John Miller of Oundle, who in 1816 'made money in an improper way – telling fortunes' to those labouring with sickness – and was 'put in workhouse' for her troubles.[101] Examples like these are the ultimate embodiment of a sense from the underlying data that the sick poor sought, and felt they had a right or even a duty to seek, remedies for their sickness which were beyond or in addition to the stock responses of parishes themselves.

Life-cycle strategies

These schematic representations of the data are useful. Yet it is the wider question of how the sick poor put together (simultaneously and sequentially) the different aspects of the medical economy of makeshifts and how this melded with simply doing nothing that is important for our understanding of the patchwork of experiences of sickness and poverty and the meanings of medical welfare. While the strength, duration and cost of engagement by the sick poor with the parochial authorities varied according to life-cycle stage, gender and place, on balance Chapter 4 suggested that more paupers had more of their poverty 'medicalised' by the 1830s than had been the case in the 1750s. At the same time, it is clear that many illnesses went unreported to or untreated by the poor law. This, the increase in the scale and longevity of sickness traced in Chapter 2 and the existence of the tri-partite medical economy of makeshifts explored here mean that it does not inevitably follow that parochial medical welfare played a progressively larger part in the life-cycles of the sick poor. The sorts of records that give definitive perspective on these issues are sparse. Patient case histories associated with admittance to medical institutions begin to proliferate only at the end of the period considered by this study.[102] It is, however, possible to garner at least a broad sense of medical life-cycles from other sources. The brief autobiography of the Suffolk poet Ann Candler, encountered already in this study, paints a picture of a woman drawn low by a miscreant husband and her own

poor decision-making. Ongoing acts of personal charity by friends and local patrons obviated the harshest consequences of her situation – she was 'by industry and the frequent donations of kind friends protected from want'[103] – keeping her out of the clutches of the Old Poor Law. Her friends rallied round particularly at times of illness, and Candler would be

> guilty of the highest ingratitude were I not to remember, with veneration and respect, the late M__e R-ss-ll, esq. who almost entirely supported me, and the two children, during an illness of eleven weeks, which afflicted me in consequence of the perturbation of mind I had laboured under upon my husband's departure [to the army].[104]

A disastrous foray into London left her destitute, and on her return to Suffolk she was once again thrown upon the charity of her friends – including for instance their provision of 'an ample supply of whatever she thought might be most useful and acceptable to me'[105] at the time of Candler's confinement – to avoid the poor law. Eventually, however, a six-month illness for her husband followed by his absconding left her a long-term resident of the house of industry, where 'all my prospects of comfort ended'.[106] Even here, however, 'friends' sent or brought resources in cash and kind, particularly at times of illness, in order to improve her lot. One gets little sense of specific medical treatments or of Candler's interaction with doctors and other medical people. Nonetheless, her story of periodic illness-driven dependence upon the poor law interspersed with rather longer spells of informal charitable support, particularly at times of sickness, chimes with other stories that comprise the very warp of this study.

Another aspect of her story – a sense that the medical economy of makeshifts for the aged could be rapidly denuded, generating a more complete overlap between illness and parochial medical welfare – is perhaps not unexpected. On the other hand, a second and more robust source of life-cycle perspective – the letters of out-parish paupers who wrote five or more narratives – suggests a more complex picture, one peppered with medical charity, simply doing nothing, purchasing care and mutual or familial nursing. Table 9.1, drawing on a complete analysis of these letter sets, presents some exemplar medical economies. William King was, as we have seen, writing from London to Braintree in the early 1830s. While his exact age is unclear, he claimed on multiple

Table 9.1 Examples of the medical economy of makeshifts

Year	Name, number of letters sent			
	Phillip James (15)	Thomas Earl (11)	William King (15)	Elizabeth Roberts (22)
1827				SIS, MC, PC
1828			SIS, SD, PR	PC, MC, MFC
1829			MC, SIS, PR, MFC	PR, PC, MC, SIS, IC
1830			MC, SIS, PR	SIS, PR, SD, MC
1831			SIS, PR	SD, SIS, MC
1832	SIS,	PR	MC, SIS, PR	PR
1833	SIS, MC	SIS, MC, MFC, IC, PR	MC, PC, PR	PR, PC, MFC, SD
1834	MC, SIS, PR, IC, PC, MFC	PR, MFC, SD, SIS	PR, MFC, SIS	SIS, IC, PC
1835	IC, SIS	PR, PC, MC, IC		SIS, PR, IC
1836	IC, SIS, PR			SIS, MC, MFC

Notes: The numbers of letters include those sent by paupers and on their behalf.
IC: institutional care; MC: medical charity (from doctors, friends or others); MFC: mutual or familial care; PC: purchased care (including nursing, medicines, etc.); PR: parochial relief (achieved rather than requested); SD: self-dosing; SIS: suffering in silence.
Sources: Phillip James: King, Nutt and Tomkins, *Narratives of the Poor*, pp. 272–83; Thomas Earl: Hurley, *Bradford on Avon*, p. 14–19; William King: Sokoll, *Essex Pauper Letters*, pp. 111–50; Elizabeth Roberts: RPC.

occasions to be old and bowed down. Suffering in silence was a constant feature of his reaction to personal or familial illness, but the centrality of parochial relief (and to a much lesser extent medical charity) for his medical economy is clear. Thomas Earl, writing from Southampton to Bradford-on-Avon, was characterised by two overseers as 'getting old'. While his medical economy was slightly more diverse than that of King, particularly in what turned out to be a final set of illnesses in 1835, the centrality of parochial medical welfare is still clear. Phillip James (writing from Leicester to Uttoxeter) and Elizabeth Roberts (writing from Birmingham to Rothersthorpe) were at very different

life-cycle stages. Roberts was thirty-four at the commencement of her extensive correspondence and had several young children. The age of Phillip James is harder to gauge, but he likewise had young children. For both of these paupers suffering in silence was a common response to illness, but the diversity of their medical economies is also striking. Of course, it is possible to construct, classify and present numerous life-cycle typologies, but the broad thrust of the reconstruction exercise is that very few paupers at any life-cycle stage confronted illness with a mixture simply of inaction and parochial support. While parochial medical welfare could be absolutely central to some paupers over a very long period or at certain times (such as the final illness before death), for many writers the engagement with the parish in the face of ongoing illness was at best episodic.

Pauper letter writers at earlier stages of the life cycle tend to provide less detail around which to reconstruct the medical economy of makeshifts, in part as a function of the fact that they more often applied for remedy of one-off sickness events rather than ongoing allowances requiring more justification. Backward-looking patient case records taken at institutions afford a richer canvas as well as removing the analytical distinction between the in- and out-parish poor. It is not always easy in such records to distinguish the cases of paupers from those of the labouring poor more generally. Nonetheless, these records have the distinct advantage that they tend to over-represent those – children, young adults and those under forty-five generally – whose voices and histories we hear intermittently in pauper letters or vestry minutes.[107] William Stutter's casebook covers the years 1839–41 but the histories that he took sometimes stretch back decades into the period covered by this study.[108] In the very broadest sense the singular observation of the case histories is that most people suffered prodigiously before they sought formal medical help. Esther Isaacson (aged nineteen) was admitted in October 1839 after having been 'taken six months ago with pain and numbness of left foot' spreading to her back and pelvis. Despite 'constant pain and giddiness' and 'repeated copious attacks of epistaxis', she had 'been able to remain in service till within a week'.[109] The eighteen-year-old Susan Sharpe had 'been out of health a year and a half', and Kezia Atkins (aged twenty) had 'enjoyed good health till about twelve months ago'.[110] Relatively few patients claimed to have experienced good health right up until their admittance, something

consistent with the perspectives offered in Chapter 2. There are considerable synergies between the case histories and pauper letters: Susan
Plumbe (aged nineteen) had been confined to her bed for six months
with a heart problem two years before her admittance and nursed by
her family, a familiar scenario to that described by Frances Soundy,
with whose letters this chapter opened.[111] Case histories also record
various engagements with doctors, unspecified medical attendants and
self-dosing: George Channel (aged sixteen) had been for one week
'under medical treatment'; Sarah Ford (aged eighteen) had previously
been blistered, as had Sarah Bryant (aged twenty-five); Frances Baker
had previously been bled for her tuberculosis; and Thomas Scott (aged
nineteen) had previously seen poultices and 'stimulating liniments'
applied to his foot.[112] Whether such interventions were paid for by
families, individuals or parochial authorities or were done charitably is
unclear, but the idea that there was a considerable degree of latent sickness and impairment in the patient population of the Suffolk General
Hospital is, as Chapter 2 might have led us to expect, overwhelming.[113]

A final source confirms the sense that even the dependent poor were
enmeshed into a complex medical economy of makeshifts. Richard
Cobbold, the rector of Wortham (Suffolk), constructed, as we have
already seen in this study, biographies of many of his parishioners after
he came to the parish in 1824. These remarkable seventy-eight case histories provide a compelling picture of age-related decay for the majority
of the population, but also of a community in which ongoing sickness
and impairment were the norm. Cases like that of William Cotton, who
until advanced old age 'never knew what a bed of sickness was', were
in the distinct minority.[114] Mirroring many of the observations already
made in this chapter, particularly in the pauper letters explored for
Table 9.1, responses to sickness were diverse. Inaction was common
as was the extensive provision of familial nursing between parents and
children, brothers and sisters, and (surprisingly common) grandpar-
ents and grandchildren. The extraordinary number of invalids – Judy
Fuller 'took to her bed at the sudden loss of one of her daughters, and
kept it for sixteen years' attended by a daughter, while Ann Taylor 'lay
in bed' for thirty years, for instance[115] – created a need for large-scale
familial and neighbourhood nursing outside the poor law. Such care
melded seamlessly into charity, as with Susan Woods, who took in the
deaf and dumb Frances Howlett when her parents (whom Wood had

nursed) died.[116] And more generally the case histories are redolent with examples of sickness-related philanthropy, on a spectrum from informal charity provided by the vicar himself – Cobbold paid for a man to sit with the deranged James Harbour for two weeks[117] – to disguised support offered in the form of odd jobs to keep the crippled, aged or mentally impaired away from parochial relief. In common with the dependent poor elsewhere, those in Wortham summoned doctors and sought complementary therapies. And the histories provide more abundant evidence than one can find elsewhere of self-dosing. Thus Noah Fake 'at times had to drink half a pint of turpentine to allay his agonies' while Sarah Goddard was 'her own doctor' and confronted illness with a twenty-four-hour starvation regime. Maria Jolly was 'cured by that far-famed food called 'Revelanta', while the rector himself also dispensed remedies, curing Norah Nichols with a pint of gin and hot water.[118] Against this backdrop, engagement with parochial welfare was generally episodic and disproportionately concentrated towards the end of life and in the cases of sudden rather than chronic illness. People like Samuel Copping, 'afflicted with two very large carbuncles on the back of his neck and could work no longer', who received parochial relief for many years, were relatively uncommon, and much suffering was not captured by the poor law.[119] There appears to have been no single path towards such parochial relief, not least because individual charity often made up for absent or dying kin, but Cobbold's observation in relation to Robert Gooderham – 'long illness and old age together empty the purse of a poor man'[120] – is compelling.

Conclusion

The extent and depth of the medical economy of makeshifts undoubtedly influenced who applied for medical welfare, the nature of their claims and the duration of relief. Reconstructing this medical economy across space and time and discerning whether a richer makeshift economy led to higher or lower parochial medical bills would be a considerable undertaking outside places like Wortham. One can observe, however, that there was no inevitable relationship between indicators such as urban status and the outlines or even depth of the medical economy of makeshifts. Reading the pauper letter sets for London parishes against the pauper biographies constructed for rural

Wortham yields few striking differences in approaches to illness or the propensity to seek parochial aid. Moreover, and as we have seen earlier in the chapter, at the same time as spending on medical welfare was increasing across the country, so different arms of the medical economy of makeshifts (individual charity, self-dosing and alternative therapies) were also affording more opportunity for the dependent poor. It is difficult to escape the conclusion that poverty was increasingly a medicalised phenomenon in either a formal or an informal sense. In this framework, however, it is clear that parochial authorities did deal with a sub-group of paupers. The strategy of pauper letter writers generalising a particular event or need into a case for ongoing entitlement increased noticeably over time and begins to suggest that the aged poor were a growing part of this sub-group. Those with impairments and those experiencing sudden, work-related sickness and accidents, probably also fall into this category. Detailed analysis of the letters of paupers writing five or more narratives confirms this perspective at the same time as it suggests that even those who took the parochial shilling were engaged in a complex supplementary medical economy. On the other hand, the Wortham case histories also suggest randomness in engagement with the parish; while it is true that old age and sustained engagement often went hand in hand, those receiving medical welfare spanned the age, gender and causative spectrum. If one is to believe Richard Cobbold, the place of parochial relief in a wider medical economy of makeshifts was as much a matter of personal character as the nature of need or the richness of available resources in the shadow and other makeshift economies.

Notes

1 BRO, D/P 91/18, letter.
2 On makeshifts, see J. Adams, 'The mixed economy for medical services in Herefordshire, c.1770–1850' (unpublished PhD thesis, University of Warwick, 2004) and E. Hurren and S. King, 'Public and private health care for the poor, 1650s to 1960s', in P. Weindling (ed.), *Healthcare in Private and Public from the Early Modern Period to 2000* (London: Routledge, 2015), pp. 15–35.
3 'Mercally' was probably not contracted to Battersea parish. It is notable that Soundy did not seek payment of his bill.

4 On this sort of partnership, see M. Gorsky, M. Powell and J. Mohan, 'British voluntary hospitals and the public sphere: Contribution and participation before the National Health Service', in S. Sturdy (ed.), *Medicine, Health and the Public Sphere in Britain 1600–2000* (London: Routledge, 2002), pp. 123–44.

5 BRO, D/P 132/18/12/7, letter.

6 Sokoll, *Essex Pauper Letters*, p. 112.

7 For the Keeling letters, see S. King, Nutt and Tomkins, *Narratives of the Poor*, pp. 219–23.

8 RPC, letter.

9 Digby, *Making a Medical Living*, p. 81.

10 In addition to material in earlier chapters, see O. Davies, 'Cunning-folk', pp. 55–73.

11 R. Moore and S. McLean, 'Introduction: Folk healing in contemporary Britain and Ireland: Revival, revitalisation or reinvention?', in R. Moore and S. McLean (eds), *Folk Healing and Health Care Practices in Britain and Ireland. Stethoscopes, Wands and Crystals* (Oxford: Berghahn, 2010), pp. 1–21, at p. 2.

12 R. Porter, *Health for Sale*.

13 These categorisations are of course artificial and overlapping. They are, nonetheless, useful shorthand for codifying disparate sources and the snapshot nature of many references to the medical economy of makeshifts.

14 LRO, DDX 386/3, vestry minutes.

15 NRO, 356p/7, vestry minutes.

16 LRO, PR 3168/5/1, vestry minutes.

17 WYRO, 15D74/10/2/10, overseers' vouchers.

18 LCRO, DE 1587/156/19, letter, 21 October 1828.

19 NRO, 261p/242/1, letter.

20 NRO, 261p/244/40, letter.

21 Hurley, *Bradford on Avon*, p. 18.

22 LRO, DDX 386/3, vestry minutes.

23 CPL, vestry minutes.

24 RPC, letter.

25 B. Heathcote, *Viewing the Lifeless Body: A Coroner and his Inquests Held in Nottinghamshire Public Houses during the Nineteenth Century 1828 to 1866* (Nottingham: Nottingham County Council, 2005), p. 26.

26 C. Lawrence, P. Lucier and C. Booth (eds), *'Take time by the forelock': The Letters of Anthony Fothergill to James Woodforde, 1789–1813* (London: Wellcome Trust, 1997), p. 84.

27 CRO, PR-5-67-61, letter and bill, 15–17 August 1835.

28 King, *A Fylde Country Practice*.

29 For a particularly good example of £100 costs for a disputed bill of 4s 6d, see Pryor vs Nicholls and others in *Jackson's Oxford Journal*, 19 July 1823.

30 LRO, DDX 386/3, vestry minutes, 3 December 1816.

31 NRO, 261p/244/3, letter.

32 Hurley, *Bradford on Avon*, p. 19.

33 LRO, DDPr/25/6, account book. See also S. King, *A Fylde Country Practice*.

34 L. Lewis (ed.), *Hird's Annals of Bedale* (Harrogate: North Yorkshire County Record Office, 1975), p. 473.

35 R. Kerrison, 'Medical and surgical attendance on the parochial poor', *Transactions of the Associated Apothecaries & Surgeons of England and Wales*, 1 (London: Burgess and Hill, 1821), 199.

36 Hurley, *Bradford on Avon*, p. 22.

37 Ibid., p. 33.

38 See R. Porter, 'The patient in England', p. 94, and M. Brown, 'Medicine, quackery', p. 256.

39 RPC, letter, 31 May 1801.

40 L. Smith, 'Reassessing the role of the family: Women's medical care in eighteenth century England', *Social History of Medicine*, 16 (2003), 327–42.

41 Though see A. Crosby, *The Family Records of Benjamin Shaw, Mechanic of Dent, Dolphinholme and Preston, 1772–1841* (Chester: Record Society of Lancashire and Cheshire, 1991). For wider context see Humphries, *Childhood and Child Labour*.

42 Eureka Partnership, *The Parish of Binfield 1801 Census* (Aylesbury: Berkshire Family History Society, 2009).

43 COWAC, B1344-31 St Clement Danes, letter, 15 December 1835.

44 See N. Miller and N. Yavneh (eds), *Sibling Relations and Gender in the Early Modern World: Sisters, Brothers and Others* (Aldershot: Ashgate, 2006).

45 A. Cole and D. Paine (eds), *Extracts from the Minutes of the Board of Guardians of Stamford Union Workhouse, 1835–41* (Lincoln: Lincolnshire Family History Society, 2010), p. 16.

46 NRO, 194p/116, letter.

47 ORO, PAR 16/5/A11/8, letter.

48 CRO, PR-5-67-34, letter, 5 August 1827.

49 LRO, PR 2391/16, letter 21, April 1825.

50 Cole and Paine (eds), *Extracts*, p. 11.

51 S. King, 'The English proto-industrial family: Old and new perspectives', *History of the Family*, 140 (2003), 1–23. Thane, *Old Age in English History*, pp. 10 and 108, argues that 'the poor law served to support rather than replace the economy of expedients' and more widely that officials did not stint on anything that might keep the aged poor as active independent members of their communities.

52 See B. Croxson, 'The foundation and evolution of the Middlesex Hospital lying-in service, 1745–86', *Social History of Medicine*, 14 (2001), 27–57.

53 NRO, 249p/164, vestry minutes.

54 See S. King, *Women, Welfare and Local Politics 1880–1920* (Brighton: Sussex Academic Press, 2010), pp. 56–87.

55 Tomkins, 'Women and poverty', p. 164. For a richly detailed illustration of the lack of medical charity see Gibson, *The Walthamstow Charities*.

56 G. Hannah, *The Deserted Village: The Diary of an Oxfordshire Rector: James Newton of Nuneham Courtenay, 1736–86* (Stroud: Alan Sutton, 1992), p. 3, 11 January 1759.

57 CURO, WDX 397/6/5, notebook of James Dawson 1813–39.

58 Anon., *Some Bedfordshire Diaries* (Streatley: Bedfordshire Historical Record Society, 1959), p. 123.

59 NRO, Sox 517/2, case notes, 10 April 1772.

60 LCRO, DE 1587/155/12, letter, 4 January 1824.

61 LRO, PR 2391/31, letter, 27 May 1831, and PR 2391/34, letter, 29 February 1832.

62 ORO, MSS D.D.Par. Rotherfield Greys c.11/7, letter.

63 ORO, MSS D.D.Par. Souldern, c.7/i/4, letter.

64 See H. Marland and J. Adams, 'Hydropathy at home: The water cure and domestic healing in mid-nineteenth-century Britain', *Bulletin of the History of Medicine*, 83 (2009), 499–529, and P. Hembry, *The English Spa, 1560–1815: A Social History* (London: Athlone, 1990).

65 J. Cartwright (ed.), *The Travels through England of Dr Richard Pococke, Successively Bishop of Meath and of Ossory, during 1750, 1751 and Later Years* (London: Camden Society, 1977), pp. 37 and 49.

66 Ibid., p. 49.

67 WYRO, BDP/17/88, overseers' accounts. For context see R. Porter (ed.), *The Medical History of Waters and Spas* (London: Wellcome Trust, 1990).

68 Fissell, *Patients, Power*.

69 Cockayne and Stow, *Stutter's Casebook*.

70 S. Cordery, *British Friendly Societies, 1750–1914* (Basingstoke: Palgrave, 2003).

71 LRO, DDX 386/3, vestry minutes.
72 Eastwood, 'The republic in the village', p. 17.
73 Lewis (ed.), *Hird's Annals of Bedale*, p. 493.
74 The central lesson of Cordery, *British Friendly Societies* is that the exist-ence of societies was often fragile or short and that a surprising number of claims were contested.
75 EYRO, PE1-702-84, letter. These weaknesses were well recognised by ratepayers: NRO, F(M), misc volumes 357, 'Some Suggestions for the Improvement of Benefit Clubs', 1824.
76 See for instance the certificates given to Abthorpe parish (Northamptonshire): NRO, ZA 1759–1809, certificates. See also Walsh, 'Poor law administration in Shropshire', p. 118.
77 On female-friendly societies see C. Topping, 'Welfare, class and gender: Non-affiliated friendly societies in Lancashire 1750–1835' (unpublished DPhil thesis, University of Oxford, 2006).
78 Cole and Paine (eds), *Extracts*, pp. 7–8.
79 COWAC, DR02-E4-1 St Mary Staines, letter.
80 Most societies also had restrictive rules on claiming for dependents and widows, which would have had consequent impact upon the poor law.
81 LCRO, DE 1587/156/10, letter.
82 Hurley, *Bradford on Avon*, p. 26.
83 BRO, D/P 132/18/12/27, letter.
84 ORO, MSS D.D. Par. Witney, c.44 c/4, letter.
85 CRO, PR -5-67-53, letter, 15 August 1835.
86 O. Davies, 'Healing charms in use in England and Wales 1700–1950', *Folk-Lore*, 107 (1996), 19–32; Curth (ed.), *From Physick*, pp. 29–47; L. Loeb, 'Doctors and patent medicines in modern Britain: Professionalism and consumerism', *Albion*, 33 (2001), 404–25; and P. Brown, 'Medicines advertised in eighteenth-century Bath newspapers', *Medical History*, 20 (1976), 152–68.
87 Hunnisett, *Wiltshire Coroners' Bills*, pp. 84 and 86. On later 'tours' see O. Davies, 'Cunning-folk', 55–73. See also Stead, *The Diary of a Quack Doctor*.
88 BRO, D/P 109/12/2, overseers' accounts.
89 BALS, ZZ/238/1/175. See also R. Davies, 'Dr Richard Stoughton'.
90 On druggists, see Marland, 'The medical activities' and H. Marland, '"The Doctor's Shop": The rise of the chemist and druggist in nineteenth cen-tury manufacturing districts', in Curth (ed.), *From Physick*, pp. 79–104. See aso A. Morrison, 'Pharmacy in the 1840s: The wholesale chemists and druggists', *Pharmaceutical Historian*, 21 (1991), 3–9. O. Davies, 'Female healers', suggests that druggists were most commonly found in

areas with the fewest doctors by the mid- and late nineteenth century, but I find no evidence of this here.

91　See O. Davies, 'Female healers'.

92　O. Davies, 'Cunning-folk'.

93　Hunnisett, *Wiltshire Coroners' Bills*, pp. 59, 80, 94, 104 and 114.

94　Heathcote, *Viewing the Lifeless Body*, pp. 25 and 36.

95　Kerrison, 'Medical and surgical attendance', pp. 194–208.

96　Hurley, *Bradford on Avon*, p. 17, 8 October 1834.

97　S. King, Nutt and Tomkins, *Narratives of the Poor*, p. 224.

98　EYRO, PE1-702-22, letter.

99　R. Moore and S. McLean, 'Folk healing in a post-scientific world', in R. Moore and S. McLean (eds), *Folk Healing*, pp. 24 and 39.

100　On acupuncture see R. Bivins, *Alternative Medicine: A History* (Oxford: Oxford University Press, 2007), p. 120. M. Neve, 'Orthodoxy and fringe: Medicine in late Georgian Bristol', in Bynum and Porter (eds), *Medical Fringe*, pp. 40–55, suggests that attempts to undermine irregular providers were really a proxy attempt to close down the medical avenues explored by the poor.

101　NRO, 249p/164, letter. O. Davies, 'Cunning-folk', pp. 55–73, argues that the poorest were excluded from accessing the supernatural, but in other work such as 'Female healers', pp. 238 and 244–5, he refers extensively to examples of fortune-telling.

102　Risse and Warner, 'Reconstructing clinical activities'.

103　Candler, *Poetical Attempts*, p. 8.

104　Ibid., pp. 8–9.

105　Ibid., p. 13.

106　Ibid., p. 14.

107　For a similar perspective, see Fissell, *Patients, Power*.

108　Cockayne and Stow, *Stutter's Casebook*, p. xxvi. The average patient age was thirty-two.

109　Ibid., p. 36.

110　Ibid., pp. 39 and 41.

111　Ibid., p. 45.

112　Ibid., pp. 49, 53, 64, 71.

113　There may have been more of a melding of parochial aid, medical charity and familial care at the end of an institutional engagement. Many patients were discharged relieved but not cured, discharged themselves or became out-patients, and we know from pauper letters that this sort of liminal status often occasioned appeals to the parish.

114　Dymond (ed.), *Parson and People*, p. 92.

115　Ibid., pp. 114 and 226.

116 Ibid., p. 158.
117 Ibid., p. 146.
118 Ibid., pp. 108, 128, 160, 179.
119 Ibid., p. 86.
120 Ibid., p. 131.

10

Making sense of diversity

In late October 1816 William Lively arrived in Blockley (Worcestershire). With him he carried a note and a bill, both written by John Lucy, the superintendent of the Liverpool School for the Blind. Noting that Lively had been at the school for eight years, the letter would:

> inform you by order of the Committee that 4 years is the Comited time for Pupils to remain in the School and has he is a good Basket Maker and can make al sorts of twine & Lines, Cart Ropes &c. he will be able to maintain himself with your assistance in setting him up – he is also a tolerable Organist provided you have a vacancy for one in your Neighbourhood. During the time he has been in the School he has conducted himself to the satisfaction of the Committee and they trust you will be able to put him in a situation which will enable him to make a decent living.[1]

This brief narrative speaks to some of the more insistent themes in the story of medical welfare traced here. William had been sent to an institution far from home and at no little cost. Moreover, he had been there for eight years rather than the normal term, which was half this number. Officials in Blockley were participating in a much wider early nineteenth-century upsurge in the importance of institutional sojourns for parochial responses to what Chapter 2 argues was a rising tide of ill-health. While the initial motivation for sending Lively to Liverpool is unclear, the reputation of the school would suggest that officials saw themselves as investing in the future of a child with a lifelong physical impairment as well as potentially controlling future welfare bills. The strategy ostensibly worked: Lively had returned with a practical skill.

But independence could not be achieved without further investment by the parish in 'setting him up', an expenditure which would appear in our 'other health' category. The officials in Blockley no doubt looked with satisfaction on the case. They would perhaps have been rather less sanguine about the rest of the Lively family, who, individually and collectively, were at this point in the 1810s experiencing a decade-long series of illnesses, incapacities, madness and old-age associated decline.

The mid-1810s marked one of two transformational points for medical welfare. A first was in the decade between the late 1780s and late 1790s. While welfare historians have increasingly come to associate this period with the beginnings of a shift in the focus of welfare resources towards male household heads and larger families,[2] 42 per cent of the 117 parishes considered here saw a permanent step-change in spending on one or more categories of medical welfare. Counties like Norfolk lagged behind the trend, but even here a core of parishes experienced the decade as transformative. The mid-1810s were different in scale and complexion. From this point medical welfare as a proportion of all spending increased in a sustained fashion, and the study has argued that once we allow for source lacunae which mean that we detect only a sub-sample of all spending on sickness, the sick poor were by some distance the key client group of the Old Poor Law by the 1820s. The so-called crisis of the Old Poor Law elides with sickness and response rather than the rise of the able-bodied welfare recipient. The response itself increasingly came to be numerically dominated by the provision of cash allowances, which in most places were packaged with other forms of welfare as part of a sustained strategy to combat sickness. We have seen that while officials occasionally struggled with how to identify a 'last illness', very serious ill-health was met with comprehensive welfare packages. Two further features of this nineteenth-century upsurge in medical welfare are also striking. The first is that institutional sojourns such as that of William Lively became part of the expectational fabric of the poor law. The number and range of institutional engagements commissioned by parishes or requested by paupers increased exponentially after 1800. In part this reflected the increased number of philanthropic and specialist medical institutions founded in the early nineteenth century, as well as greater background knowledge about institutions and their potential on the part of both officials and paupers. Yet there were also attitudinal changes at parish level, particularly in counties such as

Wiltshire, and the study has argued that officials reacted to increased curative potential with an essentially humanitarian approach which, to borrow the words of an overseer from an earlier chapter, involved doing what was right, proper and fair. A second and even more compelling feature of nineteenth century medical welfare was the insistent place of doctors as a core component of both parochial response to sickness and pauper demands for remedy. Medical men extended their grip on the spending category 'medical people' even as the relative importance of spending on doctors, nurses and others fell in relative terms into the nineteenth century. Doctoring contracts – themselves a significant part of explanation for how increased doctoring was reconciled with reducing costs – came to dominate parochial arrangements with medical men, but few parishes relied upon them in isolation. Rather, officials were willing and able to consult a raft of regional, local and national doctors as well as so-called medical irregulars in glorious variety. Treatment and visits by doctors, then, became a, perhaps the, most public representation of the increasing medicalisation of poverty that we see in the last three decades of the Old Poor Law.

Yet the sick poor never gained official rights to poor relief. Like other groups, they had a right to apply for welfare at their parish of settlement, but officials had no analogous duties to accept such applications. The process of poor relief as opposed to the fact of it recorded in the accounts of the overseers of the poor afforded many opportunities for claims to be rejected, contested or modified. There are certainly breathtaking examples of parsimony. But most overseers and vestrymen found themselves caught uncomfortably, sometimes unwillingly, in a triangular balancing act involving duties to ratepayers, moral and customary duties to the poor who presented themselves and their cases, and a personal duty to ensure they were not taken in by charlatans. On the outside of this triangular set of considerations stood the magistrate, whose role as an arbiter of appeal remained conceptually important even if we have overstated its practical importance. Against this backdrop the claims of the sick poor were problematic. In vestry minutes, pauper narratives and the letters of epistolary advocates we have found evidence of an ingrained belief on the part of the sick poor that their cases would be heard and acted upon. Few asserted rights, but plenty asserted customary, moral, humanitarian and Christian duties as a way of navigating an essentially discretionary parochial welfare system. Equally, we have found evidence

that officials facilitated such agency, sharing a rhetorical and linguistic register with the sick poor and their advocates. There is no evidence that sickness could simply be invented and yoked to other causes of need, and in this sense parishes could be confident in the identity and deservingness of this sub-group of the poor. In turn, officials struggled constantly against doctors and advocates to keep hold of their right to recognise (or not recognise) sickness and to decide what package of benefits should be attached to that recognition, but the evidence is that the outcome of this struggle was not simple parsimony.

In fact the continuous engagement between parishes, paupers and advocates in all of the parishes considered here over the nature, scale and symbolism of pauper funerals suggests exactly the opposite. This matters for our understanding of the sentiment of the Old Poor Law during its crisis stage, given the growing centrality of the sick poor for the overall welfare bill. My attempts to think more widely about the essential characteristics of European welfare systems would suggest that during this crisis period England actually had multiple poor laws rather than one. While the able-bodied male poor outside places like Essex may have been inscribed into broad disciplinary or exclusionary regimes, those who could rhetoricise sickness and its consequences were clearly navigating an entitlement regime in which, *inter alia*, the governance of access to poor relief was relatively open; institutional relief (communal or charitable) was uncommon or unstable, but where it did exist it was broadly supportive; inspection and surveillance were, and were seen to be, periodic and the outcomes usually benign; officials and communities were sensitive to the material and moral symbolism of poverty; relief may not have been adequate but it was nonetheless substantial and regular; partnership with families was desirable but not a mainstay of the relief process; and above all the ingrained sentiment of those financing relief was favourable to the right of the poor to make claims on charity and community.[3] When James Cloke and John Fanwell, overseers of East Stonehouse (Devon), wrote to Longbridge Deverill (Wiltshire) on the subject of Mary Ann Holton they suggested that 'had she been one of our own the real Relief absolutely required would be as follows, and which under the painful case, hope you will view with the like feelings as ourselves being eyewitnesses of her wretchedness'.[4] In effect, then, they were confirming the very real existence of this sort of entitlement regime.

How officials enmeshed in such a regime constellated medical welfare at parochial level was partly auto-correlated with the scale and
duration of sickness, disease-specific recovery patterns, the encompassing medical economy of makeshifts and the scale and nature of
background poverty. There was also, however, a considerable degree
of discretion, and the study has done much to draw out the range and
depth of medical welfare and the colourful variety of the experiences
of the sick poor: Woodford Halse (Northamptonshire) purchased 'an
oversize coffin' for Thomas Parr in February 1804 'on account of his
deformity'; the overseer of Warham (Norfolk) copied a recipe for the
'Bite of a Mad Dog' into his 1792 account book, presumably so that
subsequent overseers would be able to commission local remedies;
William Spacey was sent to five different institutions for the cure of his
ulcerative leg by the Calverley (West Yorkshire) overseers between
1798 and 1809; the parish of Enderby (Leicestershire) contracted a
local doctor between 1810 and 1821 but also referred pauper patients
to fourteen other medical men, including practitioners in London;
and the parish of Hulme (Lancashire) apprenticed twenty-three
children with physical impairments between 1810 and 1816. Each of
these examples points to a wider sense in the data of parishes seeking to respond constructively – even 'well' – to the conditions of the
sick poor. David Eastwood's view that 'the last years of the so-called
unreformed parish system were years of vibrancy and experiment'[5]
and Vick Walsh's argument that Shropshire relief systems in the crisis
years of the Old Poor Law were 'responsive to the needs of ratepayers
and paupers' in a spirit of 'reforming vitality' have purchase in this
context.[6]

This is not, of course, to argue that all parishes all of the time had
a clear knowledge of the sick poor nor responded favourably to their
needs and demands. When John Frewen, lord of the manor of Cold
Overton (Rutland), tore down a cottage illegally built on waste ground
at Sapcote (Leicestershire):

> there was an aged sick person in the cottage at the time who either died
> or nearly died in consequence (J F T not knowing any one was inside)
> the person was a Methodist so [Joseph] Butterworth, MP, the head of
> the Methodists, took up the case & instituted a criminal prosecution
> [against Frewen] & hoped he would be hung.[7]

The fact that Frewen tore down the cottage without checking who was inside and that repute of the sick woman had not reached him or those (presumably local men) who helped him points to deep lack of concern for the sick and aged. The act itself was clearly undertaken to prevent an illegal cottager from obtaining a settlement in the parish, and points to the prioritisation of the interests of ratepayers over the poor. Isaac Curtis also felt that his interests had been subsumed to those of the parish when he wrote to the overseers of Longbridge Deverill (Wiltshire) on 25 April 1818. He noted, 'you promised Gentlemen to pay the Doctor, it is not in my power to do it, as the Money you send me was not sufficient to bury my late wife I was obliged to borrow some on Acct where I work to make up the deficiency'.[8] Yet such experiences must be contrasted with some of the familiar names from this study – William King, Frances Soundy, Edward Buckeridge, Walter Keeling – whose sickness stories, told over multiple encounters with parochial authorities, elicited continuous support from ratepayers notwithstanding their obvious irritation at receiving renewed appeals. In this sense, sickness was the totemic problem faced by officials, and its relief occasioned their most sustained responses.

The patterning of such response was more nuanced than a focus on the all-parish sample might suggest. There was a surprising lack of typological variation. Smaller rural communities and those that formed transport hubs appear to have generated a more variegated patchwork of sickness remediation than urban or industrial parishes, but many of the normative dichotomies – urban–rural and industrial–arable, for instance – have little place in the story of medical welfare. Spatial variation at county and parish level was rather more pronounced. At its broadest extent, the data suggests that the highly diversified character of medical welfare apparent in all counties in the 1750s had by the 1830s developed into two typologies. Parishes in Northamptonshire, Leicestershire, Norfolk and West Yorkshire appear to have followed policies which continued to generate meaningful diversity, albeit that the importance of cash allowances increased everywhere except Norfolk and Leicestershire. By contrast, parishes in Lancashire, Berkshire and Wiltshire generated increasingly narrow spending profiles. Of course these characterisations carry more force than perhaps they ought to do, given the problems of interpreting the underlying sources. The fact that cash allowances could be used by paupers to fund funerals,

doctors and drugs which would otherwise have been provided by the parish and thus appeared as an augmentation to different expenditure categories constitutes an important interpretational problem. There are, however, others. Not least, relatively few parishes in the sample retained workhouses for very long periods, but the turnover of such institutions at parish level gives an aggregated continuity to their role in medical welfare which may be misleading.[9] These issues notwithstanding, county-level samples exhibit their own distinctive complexions of medical welfare. Table 10.1 provides a broad summative perspective.

For paupers in Berkshire, medical welfare was increasingly tied up with cash allowances across the range from transient and tiny through to long-term and substantial. While 'being doctored' was part of the expectational culture of officials and parishes, sustained and expensive nursing care was the single most distinctive feature of medical welfare in the county. Both absolutely and in comparison to their peers in nearby Wiltshire, the sick poor in Berkshire had limited access to medical institutions, and the medical role of the workhouse all but disappeared by the mid-1820s, something that goes some way to explaining the interrupted upward course of medical welfare in the county. Contrasts with Norfolk are very strong. Here cash allowances were barely more important in 1834 than they had been in 1750, and the dominant trend was the increasing proportion of medical welfare delivered via workhouse residence. Nursing tended to be at the less intensive and expensive end of the spectrum, while officials turned at best sparingly to medical irregulars. Rather, doctors came to be the mainstay of the spending envelope on medical people, suggesting an increasing formality to the experiences of the sick poor in Norfolk. A close reading of Table 10.1 reveals equally strong divisions in the Midlands and the north and between them, confounding some of the stock perceptions of the regionality of poor law policy and practice that I myself have helped to create.

Of course, spending curves and distribution profiles for medical welfare are in themselves the product of a complex amalgam of local experiences. Even in the two areas where we see most consistency – the involvement of parishes in pauper funerals and the access of paupers to institutional sojourns by the early nineteenth century – the study has highlighted complex inter- and intra-parish variation in practice. How much parishes were willing to spend on a funeral depended in part

Table 10.1 Summary of county-level experiences

County	Complexion of medical welfare
West Yorkshire	Above average % of resources spent on medical welfare by the 1830s; medical people as a spending category falls but with an increasing focus on nursing, medical irregulars and doctors outside contracts; cash payments rise, albeit not as strongly as elsewhere, and are focused on time-limited and open-ended allowances rather than broader welfare packages; provision of medical welfare via the workhouse is small but consistent while engagement with non-workhouse institutions is significant and paupers obtain multiple institutional admissions; in-kind payments as a spending category rise but through a multiplication of *ad hoc* or regular seasonal events; funerals have a consistent place in spending, and drug and device supply forms a relatively a significant component of medical welfare, with a strong emphasis on regional and local supply.
Leicestershire	Above average % of resources spent on medical welfare by the 1830s; spending on medical people remains stable but with an increasing focus on doctors rather than nurses or medical irregulars; cash payments remain muted throughout the period and overseers seek to impose strict time or other limitations on allowances; provision of medical welfare via the workhouse is small but consistent while engagement with non-workhouse institutions is more significant but as in other parishes single-event; in-kind payments as a spending category rise, and this provision reflects a multiplication of *ad hoc* and regular seasonal events; spending on funerals and drugs and devices is significant, and Leicestershire parishes are particularly notable for their tendency to turn to national device makers.
Northamptonshire	Above average % of resources spent on medical welfare by the 1830s; broad stability in the importance of medical people as a spending category but doctors (contracted and otherwise) become more important as the importance of nursing falls off and medical irregulars remain common; the importance of cash payments rises but with a focus on transient and packaged allowances; provision of medical welfare in the workhouse remains limited but engagement with

County	Complexion of medical welfare
	other medical institutions (usually as a single event for paupers) is consistent and significant; in-kind payments are strong/rising but as a reflection of the presence and value of food, fuel, clothing and other material relief in broad care packages offered to the sick poor rather than as discrete allowances; spending on funerals is consistent, as is that on drugs and devices from the full range of local, regional and national providers.
Lancashire	Above average % of resources spent on medical welfare by the 1830s; spending on medical people dwindles and the significant concentration on doctors in and out of contract is notable; cash payments rise rapidly and officials focus on transient, time-limited and substitution payments rather than open-ended or packaged allowances; provision of medical welfare via the workhouse is small but consistent, and engagement with non-workhouse institutions episodic but multiple where it does occur; in-kind payments as a spending category decline, particularly where we strip out the support packages offered to paupers before and after attendance at an institution; funeral provision is consistently important but spending on drugs and devices is distinctively small.
Berkshire	Below average % of resources devoted to medical welfare and the upsurge in medical welfare falters in the 1820s; the importance of medical people as a spending category falls but nursing increases in importance over time at the same time as Berkshire parishes stick closely to doctoring contracts and supplement them only in limited ways; cash payments increase over time with Berkshire parishes providing a markedly holistic and open-ended set of cash benefits in comparison to those elsewhere; provision of medical welfare via the workhouse has always been small and falls off strongly as the importance of nursing increases; engagement with non-workhouse institutions is episodic and single event; in-kind payments constitute a small but stable element of medical welfare; funerals are consistently funded, and while drugs and devices constitute a relatively small element of spending Berkshire parishes turn disproportionately to national quack remedies.

Norfolk	Below average % of resources spent on medical welfare and a high concentration of parishes which do not see a significant surge in spending from the 1810s; spending on medical people is stable but doctors (contracted and others) become more important and medical irregulars have a negligible place throughout the period; cash payments remain muted (something that is partly explained by the importance of workhouses in the provision of medical welfare) but the focus is firmly on the provision of transient allowances; engagement with non-workhouse institutions is episodic and singular; in-kind payments as a spending category fall, and this becomes especially marked where we strip out the support packages offered to paupers before and after attendance at an institution or when ague was being treated; drugs and devices absorb a small proportion of medical welfare, though the provision of alcohol is marked.
Wiltshire	Above average % of resources spent on medical welfare by the 1830s and with remarkably low inter-parish variation; the importance of medical people as a spending category falls, though within this envelope doctors become more important and medical irregulars rather less so; cash payments increase over time, though with a particular focus on time-limited and substitution payments; provision of medical welfare via the workhouse is consistent, and more generally Wiltshire parishes demonstrate the strongest engagement with non-workhouse institutions as single events in pauper treatment histories; in-kind payments as a spending category fall, particularly where we strip out the support packages offered to paupers before and after attendance at an institution; spending on drugs and devices is small at the outset of the period and falls away as cash became more common, suggesting some substitution effects.

upon the existence of friendly and burial societies (the effect of which was to push up background expectations), custom, cause of death or age. In turn, how parishes responded to the undoubted upsurge in pauper demands for institutional treatment depended in part upon when parishes tended to get involved in the sickness stories of paupers, knowledge of institutions, whether a sick pauper could call upon advocacy and the personality of the officials considering their claims. Above all, however, responses were shaped by how overseers and vestrymen constructed the notion of economy and the degree to which these same men and some women understood the growing early nineteenth-century sense that the sickness of the poor could and should be subject to full remediation. It is these situational variables which underpin the rich and colourful patchwork of pauper experiences that we see played out in their letters, in their appearances before the vestries and in the correspondence of officials and advocates.

Yet we can dwell too long on infinite variety. The core lessons of this study are clear. Medical welfare became an insistent component of parochial spending from the early nineteenth century, reflecting both increasing sickness and also wider changes in parochial understanding of how duties to ratepayers and the sick should be balanced. Within this broad envelope of medical welfare the sick poor across most parishes could expect to spend more of their sickness lives under the care of doctors, to experience more institutional sojourns, to receive more of their welfare over time in the form of cash allowances and for parishes to play a consistently high profile in the process of dying and the nature of pauper funerals. Those, like William Lively, with mental and physical impairments could increasingly expect the close attention of parochial officers. Above all, the transition from frequent epidemics and crisis years in the eighteenth century to a wider palette of sickness causation in the early nineteenth century saw the sick poor increasingly receiving tailored packages of benefits rather than the more *ad hoc* relief that had been their lot in the 1750s. Crucially, these paupers were not simply subject to the will of officials; rather, and as the rich emblematic stories told in earlier chapters show, they could and did exercise considerable agency. This is not, of course, to argue that the parish came to play a more central role in the medical economy of makeshifts explored by paupers, advocates and families. Robert Sharp of South Cave (East Yorkshire), in talking of John Dunlin, noted that 'he had good friends

who took care he wanted nothing, when he was ill the overseer asked him if he wanted any thing, but he replied he had plenty of every thing and was not in want, indeed, he seemed hurt at being asked if he could be assisted'.[10] It is important in this story that the overseer knew John Dunlin was ill, testimony to a network of knowledge that we have seen time and again in this study, and that he consulted the sick man on what the parish might do. Equally, the fact that Dunlin had an alternative to parochial assistance – his 'good friends' – speaks to the existence of a much wider medical economy of makeshifts, one that Chapter 9 has characterised as increasingly extensive and vibrant, and capable of both substituting parochial provision and complementing it. In this sense, and as I have argued throughout, focusing on medical welfare identifies only a subset of the sick poor, life-cycles of sickness and the spectrum of potential remediation.

The fact that this subset of the sick poor came to draw down such a significant part of the welfare resources of parishes by the 1830s is thus significant. It suggests again that sickness was the totemic issue for officials and that discretionary policy was highly malleable at the local level in the face of an 'uneasy intersection of the demotic and the official'.[11] What was 'fair' became more expensive, more expansive and of longer duration over the period considered here. The quality as well as the scale of entitlement rose. In this sense we must refigure the sentimental architecture of the Old Poor Law. James Taylor's view that 'Paternalism not repression is the note juste' of the Old Poor Law has sustained resonance with the data deployed for this study.[12] There is little evidence, at least in the context of the sick poor, for a 'sharp curtailment of the influence of traditional benevolence',[13] and even less for 'a watershed between a traditional society based on community obligation and a modern one founded on individualism'.[14] Efforts to 'delegitimize public support for the poor' in the early nineteenth century are certainly clear, but if they had any practical effect at all it was to generate *de facto* rights for the sick poor to receive relief in myriad and increasingly expensive forms.[15] Lynn Hollen Lees may be right to state that the fact of the able-bodied poor absorbing an increasing share of the parochial welfare resources in some places triggered 'revulsion ... against the needy who were slowly pushed to the margins of their communities', but this study has argued that 'common understandings of citizenship [and we might add custom and humanitarian or moral

duty] and social rights' ensured that the same fate did not await the sick poor.[16] While officials might act slowly, partially or with the unwillingness borne of frustration, the evidence is that they did act, and on some scale.

Against this backdrop, the increasing centrality of the sick poor to parochial welfare should lead us to simultaneously question the construct of the crisis of the poor law from the 1780s as it was experienced at parish level and to understand the Old Poor Law as not one institution but a complex amalgam of several poor laws, each with a different legitimacy in the eyes of ratepayers. Doing so will cause us to look in a more positive light on the achievements and sentiments of officials. It also carries fundamental implications for our understanding of the New Poor Law. David Eastwood has suggested in relation to southern rural parishes in the 1820s that 'from the wasteland of their failed policies arose the first pillar of the modern centralising state'.[17] Yet if we accept that by the early 1830s the Old Poor Law was accelerating into the role of a proto-health service, the advent of the New Poor Law must be viewed in a much more nuanced way. A new institution never designed with the sick in mind was imposed upon a rich and substantial patchwork of support for the sick poor, one that had been growing in scale, depth, and cost for at least fifteen years. As better economic times peeled some of the more morally problematic groups away from welfare irrespective of the actions of the New Poor Law unions and their workhouses, so the core health function of the welfare system rapidly resurfaced if indeed it had ever gone away. In most places the purpose of the New Poor Law had been subverted or re-asserted by the 1840s.[18] The central authorities were to try just once more to contradict this basic reality, during the crusade against outdoor relief in the 1870s and 1880s. As Elizabeth Hurren reminds us, these efforts were again to founder on the rocks of the moral, customary, humanitiarian and Christian rights of the poor to claim medical welfare and of the analogous duties of local and regional officials to listen and act.[19]

Notes

1 GRO, P52 OV/7–1/2, letter, 28 October 1816.
2 For a comprehensive review of this argument see French, 'An irrevocable shift', and Sokoll, 'Families, wheat prices', pp. 78–106.

3 For more on welfare regimes see S. King, 'Welfare regimes', pp. 42–66.

4 Hurley, *Longbridge Deverill*, p. 10.

5 Eastwood, 'The republic', p. 25.

6 Walsh, 'Poor law administration in Shropshire', p. 130; V. Walsh, 'Old and New poor laws in Shropshire 1820–1870', *Midland History*, 2 (1974), 225–43, at p. 232.

7 SURO, FRE 1757, letter from Mary Burrough of Drigg to John Frewen of Cold Overton, 27 June 1807.

8 Hurley, *Longbridge Deverill*, pp. 5–6.

9 This is perhaps unsurprising. In 1803, of the 1,233,768 people on relief, just 86,468 were in the workhouse. R. Cowherd, 'The humanitarian reform of the English poor laws from 1782–1815', *Proceedings of the American Philosophical Society*, 104 (1960), 328–42, at p. 334.

10 Crowther and Crowther, *The Diary of Robert Sharp*, pp. 206–7.

11 Ogborn, *Spaces of Modernity*, p. 237.

12 J. Taylor, *Poverty, Migration and Settlement*, p. 51.

13 D. Baugh, 'Poverty, Protestantism and political economy: English attitudes towards the poor, 1660–1800', in S. Baxter (ed.), *England's Rise to Greatness* (Berkeley: University of California Press, 1983), p. 91.

14 Valenze, 'Charity, custom', p. 61.

15 Lees, *Solidarities of Strangers*, p. 20.

16 Lees, *Solidarities of Strangers*, pp. 111 and 20.

17 Eastwood, *Governing Rural England*, p. 167.

18 S. King, 'Rights, duties and practice'.

19 E. Hurren, *Protesting about Pauperism: Poverty, Politics and Poor Relief in Late-Victorian England, 1870–1900* (Woodbridge: Boydell, 2007).

Appendix

As Chapter 1 notes, this study brings together four datasets through which we can explore the scale, depth, nature and pauper experience of medical welfare. At its core lies quantitative data (overseers' accounts; vestry minutes; bills and vouchers; contracts, etc.) drawn from 117 communities across the counties of Berkshire, Norfolk, Wiltshire, Northamptonshire, Leicestershire, Lancashire and West Yorkshire. The counties were chosen so as to generate a sample of communities which would map onto the standard categories for understanding eighteenth- and nineteenth-century England (pastoral, arable, lowland, upland, industrial, proto-industrial, urban and small rural areas) and which might be expected to have had markedly different poor law histories or experiences of sickness. There was also an imperative not to duplicate the (largely unpublished) work of other poor law historians working at county level, including that of Judith Hills (Surrey), Mary Barker Read (Kent), Victor Walsh (Shropshire), Jonathan Reid (Derbyshire), Hilary Marland (South Yorkshire), Neil Hopkin (North Yorkshire) and Thomas Sokoll and Eric Thomas (Essex and Berkshire).

Within these county contexts, four considerations drove the choice of communities: firstly, source survival and coverage, particularly the existence of multiple poor-law-related sources that might allow extended record linkage; secondly, pre-existing datasets, for instance those relating to Calverley, Pudsey, Idle and Stanhope (West Yorkshire) collected as part of my 1994 PhD; thirdly, the need to obtain similar coverage of different sorts of community (rural, urban, industrial, isolated, well-connected; urban, urban hinterland, etc.) in each county sample; and finally, the desire to generate county samples that roughly

encompassed the same proportion of those county populations, here measured at 1801. In terms of the latter, the communities encompass an 1801 population of 169,460, varying across a spectrum from places with fifty-five people to parishes of 16,033 souls. On average parishes in Lancashire and West Yorkshire tended to have larger populations than their Midland and southern counterparts. Nonetheless, the core sample encompasses between 6 and 10 per cent of the county populations that they represent. The exception is Norfolk, where the combination of a few large urban centres and myriad tiny rural parishes means that a large numerical sample of parishes still represents a small proportion of the 1801 county population. The fact that in 1831, 15,535 parishes, townships and unions administered the poor law but 12,034 of them had to contend with the welfare of fewer than 800 people means that the very smallest parishes are likely to be under-represented in the core sample. At the other extreme, source survival and the sheer scale of the task of implementing the definition of medical welfare set out in Chapter 2 mean that the largest urban areas are also under-represented. Nonetheless, the overall sample of 117 communities includes town hinterlands and smaller urban areas, while, as earlier chapters note, other aspects of the source base such as pauper letters begin to compensate for the lack of a large urban focus.

Figure A.1 maps the location of these communities. At various points in the text, I make reference to two broad subsets of this data: the Core, Tier 1 and Tier 2 parishes which have the most complete basic operational data and thus form the central component of Chapter 4; and community groupings based upon socio-economic or locational characteristics which help to inform and problematise county-level trends in medical welfare spending. The Core parishes are those which have complete runs of accounts or where spending can otherwise be accounted (by cash books, vestry minutes, etc.). No county or typological subset is without representation in the Core set, which comprises a mixture of older-established and newer communities: Ashwell, Belgrave, Ansty, Walton, Calverley, Pudsey, Guiseley, Idle, Otley, Winfarthing, Farsley, Barnham, South Creake, Collingtree, King's Sutton, Enderby, Passenham, Pennington, Atherton, Easington, Great Shefford, Drayton, Caversham, Shelton, Stratton, Shottesham, Holme, Trowbridge, Melksham, Charlton, Upavon, Sopworth, Luckington and Chippenham.

The 117 communities are also episodically re-constellated on the basis of socio-economic variables. Classification of communities in these terms is imprecise, being based upon a reading for each place of parochial documentation such as rate lists, population size, antiquarian and other local histories and newspaper commentaries covering, for instance, the nature of the transport infrastructure. Given this approach, the classifications are more likely to be problematic at the start of the period, when supporting sources are relatively thin, than at the end, when they are not. By way of example of this classification process, my urban subset includes market towns like Chippenham, Caversham, Marlborough and Bradfield alongside growing industrial towns (Dewsbury, Trowbridge) and rapidly growing places like Wellingborough, Rothley and Reading St Mary. By contrast my broadly conceived classification of waterside communities includes Upavon, Lacock, Salhouse and Wallingford. Drawing on perspectives from the work of Byung Song, John Broad, Richard Smith, John Langton and others, I have identified from rate books, antiquarian histories, rentals and lists of vestry members a small sample of closed parishes to contrast with the more open communities found in industrial and proto-industrial areas. These include parishes such as Brington, Stoke Albany, Geddington, Englefield and Bradden. Places like Calverley, relatively closed until the early 1800s and rather more open thereafter, could equally have been added to this list and contrasted purposefully with the adjacent community of Pudsey, which was not dominated by a single landowner.

At various points in Chapters 4 to 9, I make reference to the lack of variation in spending trends or the complexion of medical welfare across the different socio-economic or locational typologies. This is not meant to imply rigorous statistical and correlation analysis. As will be clear from a reading of Chapter 2 onwards, the sources that underpin a consideration of medical welfare are problematic in terms of the way they record (or do not record) spending and the particular subset of the sick poor and their illnesses that they keep in observation. The need for record linkage both to reconstruct the nature and level of sickness and to quantify the wide definition of medical welfare outlined in Chapter 2 magnifies these source problems at the same time as it gives an erroneous precision to the categories that I employ. It is thus appropriate only to make comparisons on the broadest level, but even

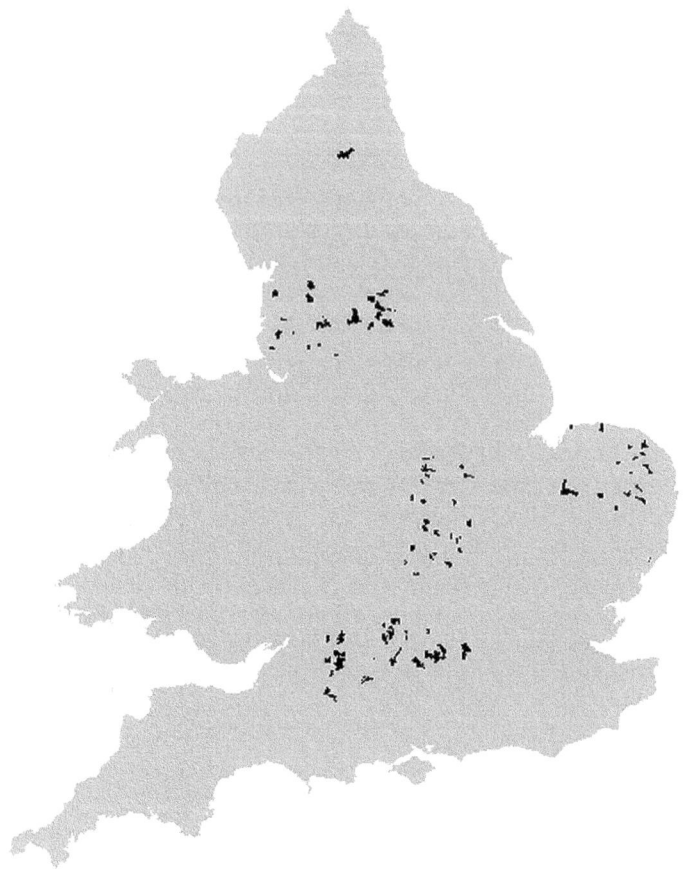

A.1 The spatial distribution of the core parochial sample

these reveal significant trends in medical welfare. If we take Figure 4.9 as an example, there are many subtle differences of trend and level in terms of the complexion of spending on medical welfare in the typological subsets, but I see only two that have real significance: the narrowing of the palette of expenditure categories over time in urban and proto-industrial communities; and the dwindling of cash allowances as a form of medical welfare in pastoral and arable communities by the

1820s. Broadly styled waterside communities had an apparently fluid approach to expenditure categories, but this may well be an artefact of the data given the low number of small communities underpinning this category.

In addition, the study episodically focuses on a second tranche of communities where operational data is more fractured. Comprising 146 parishes both within the existing county envelopes and much more widely in England, these places provide a window onto the experiences of medical welfare across a wider spatial, socio-economic and typological canvas. In particular, the sample includes both London parishes and populous places in the London hinterland, as well as definitively urban parishes in the north, Midlands and south-east. Figure A.2 locates the spatial distribution of these places. It is clear that even allowing for the existence of complementary county-level studies of the sort noted above, some areas are poorly covered. These include the far south-west, coastlines, the Scottish and Welsh borders, the northern uplands and the counties of Lincolnshire and East Yorkshire. Many of these places are also poorly served by historiographical literatures on demography, social unrest and economic infrastructure. To some extent, and as I have observed in Chapter 1, these spatial lacunae are balanced in and through a third dataset which comprises pauper letters, overseers' correspondence and letters from advocates of the poor from parochial archives across England. Because these letter sets encompass writers who may have left communities many years beforehand and had multiple migratory experiences, they tend to encompass a diverse range of communities across the English landscape.

None of these sources, as each of the substantive chapters point out, are unproblematic in terms of chronological coverage, depth, representativeness or accuracy. Gaps in overseers' accounts can be particularly galling. Many are punctured by simple summative returns of expenditure, usually reflecting periods in which the poor were farmed to a contractor at a fixed rate per head,[1] or where broad figures were transferred from other, more detailed, books and loose papers that do not survive. Hence, at Kettering St Peter and St Paul (Northamptonshire) summary overseer accounts survive for the period considered here but details of many disbursements were recorded in 'the other book now lost'.[2] Similarly, when the Halliwell (Lancashire) vestry made the following order on 28 May 1817, it was

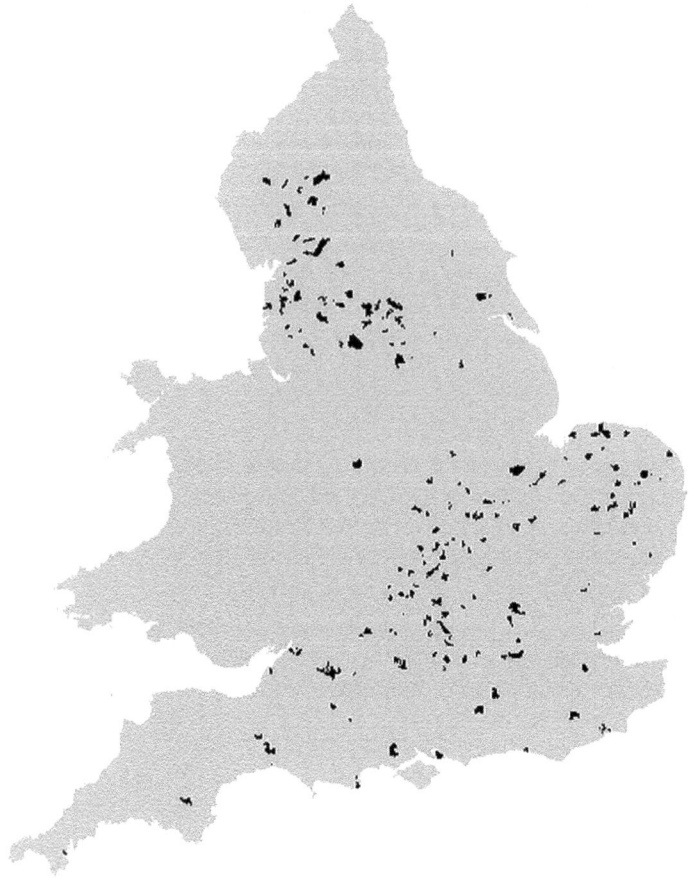

A.2 The spatial distribution of the additional samples

crystallising the fragile nature of record-keeping and decision-making in the period we are considering:

> every pauper to have a book containing what money they have received from the overseer at each time and the overseer to enter himself in their books and when at each townsmeeting each pauper to shew their books in order to see what relief they may have received and to authorise the Overseer not to pay any pauper any money if the said pauper have not brought their book for to enter the said money in as relief.[3]

The situation was no better for record-keeping in relation to the out-parish poor. An entry in the Garstang vestry minutes on 31 July 1821 resolved that the overseer must lay before the vestry all letters relating to the out-parish poor, implying that some had previously slipped through the net.[4] More widely, considering those communities in the underlying sample with overlapping overseers' accounts and vestry minutes usually reveals a disjuncture, sometimes a very considerable one, between the two sources. In some instances this disjuncture centres on the nature and scale of spending, with decisions made at the vestry modified, extended or countermanded by the overseer. Frequent injunctions by vestries that overseers must do as they were ordered testify to the fact that officials at the sharp end of decisions frequently took matters into their own hands. We see this writ large when vestries attempted to purge relief lists but overseers either failed to act or allowed re-applications once the dust had settled. As Chapters 2 and 4 suggest, then, we should be wary of ascribing the quantitative material arising out of the datasets more exactitude than actually exists. Whatever constellation of sources that we deploy, the study picks up only a subset of the sick poor, their sickness episodes and the medical welfare employed to combat such sickness. Nonetheless, this is a very substantial sample of parochial and other records, and if we understand poor relief in general and the agreement of medical welfare in particular as a process rather than an event it is possible to reconstruct the detailed experiences of the sick poor.

Notes

1 E. Murphy E., 'The metropolitan pauper farms 1722–1834', *London Journal*, 27 (2002), 1–18, at pp. 4 and 14, notes that in 1832 eighty-three from ninety-six London parishes farmed paupers and suggests that such places were 'convenient receptacles for the diverse classes of incompetent poor'.

2 NRO, 185p/103, summary book of overseers' accounts 1748–94.

3 BALS, PHA 1-3, Halliwell township books.

4 LRO, DDX 386/3, vestry minutes. This was, of course, an enduring problem in the nineteenth century, even under the New Poor Law. I am grateful to Keir Waddington for this observation.

Bibliography

Primary sources

Berkshire Record Office (BRO)

D/P 2/16/1/1–8, Abingdon correspondence 1815–25.
D/P 3/18/3, Aldermarston petitions for relief 1800–10.
D/P 7/12/1–2, Ardington overseers' accounts 1778–1831.
D/P 9/12/1–6, Ashbury overseers' accounts and vouchers.
D/P 22/12/1–5, Bradfield overseers' accounts 1771–1825.
D/P 23/12/1–9, Bray overseers' accounts and vouchers 1755–1820.
D/P 23/18/1–20, Bray workhouse documents.
D/P 26/12/1–6, Brimpton overseers' accounts and vouchers 1705–1832.
D/P 26/18/1, Brimpton letters.
D/P 27/12/1–7, Buckland overseers' accounts and vestry minutes 1693–1837.
D/P 27/28/7, List of inhabitants 1799.
D/P 29/12/1–6, Burghfield overseers' accounts 1759–1823.
D/P 29/8/1, Burghfield vestry minutes 1828–34.
D/P 41/12/1, Great Coxwell overseers' accounts 1784–1815.
D/P 41/5/1, Great Coxwell vestry minutes 1796–1922.
D/P 41/18/1, Great Coxwell miscellaneous papers 1784–1815.
D/P 45/18/4, Cumnor miscellaneous correspondence 1805–15.
D/P 48/12/1–3, Drayton overseers' accounts and poor book 1739–1836.
D/P 51/8/1–2, Enborne vestry minutes 1777–1848.
D/P 52/12/1–4, Englefield overseers' accounts 1755–1835.
D/P 52/5/1, Englefield vestry minutes 1713–85.
D/P 52/28/3, Miscellaneous papers.
D/P 53b/8/1, Little Coxwell vestry minutes 1786–1879.
D/P 53b/12/1, Little Coxwell overseers' accounts 1803–31.
D/P 70/12/1–2, Hinton Waldrist overseers' accounts 1795–1826.
D/P 71/8/1–5, Hungerford vestry and poor committee minutes.

D/P 71/12/1–17, Hungerford disbursements, workhouse accounts and bills.
D/P 71/13/7/1–47, Hungerford correspondence 1737–1838.
D/P 71/28/7, Hungerford census 1825–34.
D/P 71/28/16, Hungerford census 4 July 1831.
D/P 77/28/1–2, Kingston Bagpuize friendly society accounts 1774–1800.
D/P 78/18/4, Kintbury poorhouse minute book 1816–45.
D/P 78/12/1–11, Kintbury overseers' accounts.
D/P 91/12/1–3, Pangbourne overseers' accounts 1820–34.
D/P 91/8/1, Pangbourne vestry minutes 1820–70.
D/P 91/18/, Correspondence and vouchers.
D/P 96/8/2–5, Reading vestry minutes 1780–1859.
D/P 98/8/3 and 6, Reading St Mary vestry minutes 1760–1829.
D/P 98/12/1–227, Reading St Mary overseers' accounts and vouchers.
D/P 108/12/1–4, Great Shefford overseers' accounts and papers 1738–1835.
D/P 109/12/1–3, Shellingford overseers' accounts and vouchers 1669–1834.
D/P 118/12/1–3, Stanford-in-the Vale overseers' accounts 1733–1843.
D/P 130/8/1–2, Thatcham vestry minutes 1814–37.
D/P 130/12/1–10, Thatcham overseers' papers 1784–1836.
D/P 132/8/2–3, Tilehurst vestry minutes 1793–1844.
D/P 132/12/1–36, Tilehurst overseers' papers 1720–1835.
D/P 132/18/1–20, Tilehurst correspondence and workhouse papers.
D/P 134/8/1, Uffington vestry minutes.
D/P 134/12/2–5, Uffington overseers' accounts 1708–1825.
D/P 139/8/1, Wallingford St Peter vestry minutes.
D/P 139/12/1–7, Wallingford St Peter overseers' accounts and vouchers 1744–1835.
D/P 139/18/1–8, Wallingford St Peter correspondence and workhouse papers 1755–1847.
D/P 144/12/1–7, Warfield overseers' accounts and vestry.
D/P 162/8/1, Caversham vestry minutes 1814–22.
D/P 162/12/1–13, Caversham overseers' papers 1782–1841.
D/P 162/13/6, Vouchers and correspondence.
D/P 162/18/1–10, Vouchers, bills and notebooks.

Bolton Archives and Local Studies (BALS)
PHA 1–3, Halliwell township books 1641–1821.
ZZ/39/9, Longworth overseers' accounts.
ZZ/238/1, Memorandum book.
ZZ/250/3, Survey of the condition of the poor 1835.

Buckinghamshire Record Office (BURO)

PR 196/12/1Q-8Q, Stoke Mandeville overseers' accounts.

Cheshire Record Office (CRO)

P143/19/9/153, Undated letter, probably 1821.
PR5-67, Pauper Letters.
P120/4525/224/171, Letter.

Chorley Public Library (CPL)

Chorley Vestry Minutes 1781–1823.

City of Westminster Record Office (COWAC)

A2250, Pauper letters St Anne, Soho.
B1344, Pauper letters St Clement Danes.
B1350, Pauper letters St Clement Danes.
K418 and 437, Pauper letters Liberty of the Rolls.
DR02-E4, Parish correspondence, Staines.

Cumbria Record Office (CURO)

CPR 102-116-10, Letter, 7 February 1825.
WDX 397/6/5, Notebook of James Dawson 1813–39.
WPR 5-63 and 5-67, Greystoke parish correspondence.
WPR 70/7/3/1/31, Overseers' accounts.

Doncaster History Centre (DHC)

DD/BW/Local/58, Warmsworth Census, 9 February 1829.
PLD1/1, Memorandum book of Richard Tilburn and John Daniell, 1794–95.

Dorset Record Office (DRO)

PE/ABB/OV1/3/1, Contract, 1824.
PE/ABB/VE1/1, Abbotsbury vestry minutes 1833–35.
PE/BE/OV8/1, Beaminster correspondence 1783–1847.
PE/BER/OV9/1, Bere Regis correspondence and bills 1711–1820.
PE/BF/OV1/13/1/1–167, Correspondence 1741–1815.
PE/BF/VE1/1/1–3, Blandford vestry minutes 1731–1856.
PE/CMO/11/2, Charmouth overseers' correspondence.
PE/CMO/11/2/1–24, letters.
PE/SML/OV/1–9, Sturminster Marshall bills and letters.
PE/SW/VE1/1, Swanage vestry minutes 1788–1818.
PE/WM/OV7/3–6, Wimborne correspondence and bills.

East Yorkshire Record Office (EYRO)
PE1-702, Beverley pauper letters.

Gloucestershire Record Office (GRO)
P30 OV/7, Awre pauper letters.
P52 OV/7, Blockley parish letters.
P76 OV/3, Charlton Kings parish letters.
P78 1/OV/7, Cheltenham St Mary correspondence.
P112a OV/3, Deerhurst correspondence.
P154 OV/3, Gloucester St Nicholas letters.
P193 OV/7, Kingswood letters and bills.
P328a OV/7, Tetbury St Mary letters and bills.

Hertfordshire Archives and Local Studies (HALS)
D/P/90/18/1, Letter.

Lancashire Record Office (LRO)
DDHe 83/54, Cottage rents paid at Longton.
DDHk (Box 2), Chorley overseers' papers.
DDNW 9/8, Newton with Scales Petitions for relief 1785–95.
DDPr/25/6, Account Book.
DDX 1/6, Town book of Bispham with Norbreck.
DDX 28/51, Rules and regulations of Chatburn Friendly Society.
DDX 28/78, Clitheroe poor law accounts 1794.
DDX 28/257, Clitheroe select vestry minutes.
DDX 386/3, Garstang vestry minutes.
DDX 752, Colne overseers' accounts.
DDX 1096/1, Garstang Friendly Society books.
DDX 1822/1, Cliviger order book 1815–52.
DDX 1834/1, Duxbury overseers' accounts 1695–1820.
DDX 1852/1–5, Ulnes Walton overseers' accounts 1756–1836.
MBCh 6/1, Chorley Poor's Book 1814–35.
MBCo 7/1, Colne vestry minutes.
PR 418, 422 and 430, Bickerstaffe overseers' accounts.
PR 501, Caton vestry minutes.
PR 797–812, Kirkham overseers' accounts and papers.
PR 834, Kirkham bills and receipts.
PR 861, Clitheroe select vestry minutes 1819–29.
PR 866 and 867, Lancaster overseers' letter books.
PR 1336, Barnacre with Bonds select vestry minutes 1821–37.
PR 1349, Pauper letters.

PR 1603, Overseers' accounts.

PR 2052 and 2068, Kirkham poor law papers.

PR 2386, 2387, 2389 and 2397, Billington overseers' accounts and papers.

PR 2390/1–51 and PR 2391/2–47, Billington overseers' correspondence.

PR 2596/2–8, Bispham overseers' accounts.

PR 2853/1/2, Culcheth overseers' accounts.

PR 2853/1/5, Culcheth overseers' accounts.

PR 2935/2/7, Pilling overseers' accounts 1776–1820.

PR 2995/1/9–29, Easington overseers' accounts and vouchers 1743–99.

PR 2995/1/11–26, Easington overseers' accounts 1762–1840.

PR 2956/3/5, Pauper petitions.

PR 2995/4/2, Easington pensioners.

PR 2995/6/1, Easington pensioners.

PR 3031/8/1, Mitton vestry book.

PR 3031/10/1–5, Mitton overseers' accounts and correspondence 1764–1836.

PR 3168/5/1, Tarleton vestry minute book 1822–36.

PR 3168/5/6, Account book.

PR 3168/7/9–71, Tarleton overseers' papers 1708–1840.

PR 3243/4/1, Pilling overseers' accounts 1821–39.

Leicestershire Record Office (LCRO)

1D57/3–8 and 62, Syston overseers' accounts and bills 1761–1836.

6D43/7/3, Account book of Dr Woolaston 1757–1800.

17D64/D/1, Belgrave St Peter vestry minutes 1795–1811.

17D64/E/1–4 Belgrave St Peter overseers' accounts 1737–1834.

17D64/F/a/1–13, Supplementary overseers' accounts and bills.

17D64/F/6/1–43, Bills and letters.

23D52/16/1–21, Leicester St Michael pauper letters.

DE 64/32, Desford pauper letters.

DE 156/6, Pauper letters.

DE 157/1–4 and 34, Thurcaston overseers' accounts and bills.

DE 199/1–4, Anstey overseers' accounts, 1749–1837.

DE 199/24/1–19, Miscellaneous papers.

DE 384/43, Overseers' memorandum book.

DE 394/51, Shepshed overseers' correspondence.

DE 400/72, Overseers' correspondence.

DE 516/139, Overseers' correspondence.

DE 609/16–17, Enderby overseers' accounts and vestry minutes 1738–1836.

DE 966/20–21, Rothley overseers' accounts 1756–1826.

DE 1265/25, Cold Overton vouchers 1825–37.

DE 1369/31, Lubenham select vestry minutes 1816–35.

DE 1463/6, Town books.

DE 1587/153–170, Market Harborough letters, receipts and correspondence.

DE 1579/5–6, Normanton overseers' and churchwarden accounts 1769–1836.

DE 2132/2–5, Market Harborough overseers' accounts.

DE 2209/63–65, Hambleton overseers' accounts, rules and orders 1759–1825.

DE 2401/9–10, Sharnsford overseers' accounts and vestry minutes 1779–1837.

DE 2492/23, Billesdon constable accounts and letters 1760–1801.

DE/2559/37–69, Lutterworth overseers' accounts and bills.

DE 2575/48, Glaston correspondence book.

DE 2694/610, Vestry minutes.

DE 2704/16–18 and 23, Ravenstone overseers' accounts and vestry minutes 1756–1848.

DE 2753/11 and 14, Gilmorton overseers' accounts 1782–1836.

DE 2934/42–44, Walton overseers' accounts.

DE 3074/2, Uppingham vestry minutes.

DE 3178/7–13, Oakham letters and agreements.

DE 5199/6–8, Ashwell churchwarden and overseers' accounts 1690–1837.

DE 5962, Rothley parish records, supplementary.

DE 6348, Papers of the Winstanley family.

DE 13054/2/2, Minute books of the Leicester Infirmary, 1811.

Manchester Central Library (MCL)

L21/3/6/1–14, Workhouse and other accounts 1817–44.

L21/3/7/1–845, Bills and vouchers.

L21/3/12, Tottington survey of the poor, 1817.

L21/3/13/1–28, Tottington overseers' correspondence and bills.

L75/8/1, Newchurch overseers' accounts and bills.

L82/8/3/1–30, Goodshaw overseers' correspondence.

M10/4/2/1A-16, Blackley workhouse papers.

M10/23/1/1–3, Rusholme township ledgers 1802–28.

M10/23/2/1–6, Rusholme overseers' accounts and correspondence.

M10/23/3/1, Rusholme vestry minutes 1819–1828.

M10/808–15, Hulme letter books.

The National Archives

HO 44/51, Home Office Papers.

Norfolk Record Office (NORO)

PD 47/22, Bradfield accounts and agreements 1790–1838.

PD 48/9–11, Swafield overseers' accounts 1680–1838.

PD 50/44–53, Gissing township records.

PD 78/56–92, Winfarthing overseers' and workhouse papers.

PD 86/124–32, East Dereham overseers' accounts 1758–1823.

PD 100/88, 104–11 and 151–61, Diss overseers' papers.

PD 136/65–88, Denton overseers' accounts and vouchers 1718–1834.

PD 144/66–78, Fersfield overseers' papers.

PD 145/47–9, Scottow overseers' accounts 1759–1836.

PD 168/36–64, Thetford St Cuthbert overseers' papers.

PD 313/50–1, Methwold overseers' accounts and vouchers 1758–1833.

PD 317/92–8, Blofield parish accounts 1746–1840.

PD 330/16, West Dereham overseers' accounts 1784–1804.

PD 358/42–72, Shelton overseers' accounts and vouchers 1735–1836.

PD 385/11–16, Shotesham overseers' and workhouse papers.

PD 374/56–7, Lyng overseers' accounts 1794–1835.

PD 421/132–7, Forncett St Peter overseers' accounts 1762–1833.

PD 423, Overseers' accounts for Stratton Strawless.

PD 434/24–7, Blickling overseers' accounts and vouchers 1758–1836.

PD 502/64–81, Warham overseers' and workhouse papers.

PD 552/55–108, Wighton overseers' and workhouse papers.

PD 553/64–104, Holkham overseers' papers.

PD 612/42 and 70–73, South Creake overseers' papers.

PD 618/1, Toftrees Town Book.

PD 625/25–6, Salhouse overseers' accounts 1781–1836.

PD 629/50–52, Holme Next the Sea overseers' accounts 1721–1837.

Uncatalogued, Overseers' accounts 1800–27.

Northamptonshire Record Office (NRO)

1p/166, Abington overseers' account book 1775–1825.

1p/171/1–4, Bills for medicines 1816–20.

15p/92–95, Ashby St Leger overseers' accounts 1691–1825.

21p/105–09 and 135–37, Aynho overseers' accounts 1755–1837.

36p/19–23, Boddington overseers' papers.

43p/14–15 and G1 425, Bradden overseers' accounts and vouchers 1728–1832.

46p/60–65, Braunston overseers' accounts 1769–1814.

46p/56–58, Braunston vestry minutes.

46p/191, 1821 Braunston census.

47p/91–94, 258, 264–65, Braybrooke accounts and bills.

49p/GB4–8, Brington overseers' accounts 1777–1836.

49p/151, Bills.

58p/120–110, Castle Ashby correspondence.

92p/117–32, Crick overseers' accounts and memorandum book 1758–1835.

92p/55, Crick vestry minutes 1821–1882.

110p/258–9, 135–7, 138 and 168–70, Earl's Barton overseers' papers.

127p/77–119, Findeon overseers' accounts and papers 1753–1844.

133p/72, Select vestry minute book 1822–27.

133p/92, 102–25, Geddington accounts and vouchers.

ML 3085, 3088, 3093–4, Geddington overseers accounts.

143p/27, 59–61 and 99–109, Guilsborough overseers' papers.

185p/94 and 103, Kettering St Peter vestry minutes.

188p/13–36 and 208, King's Sutton overseers' accounts and vouchers 1757–1834.

249p/164–216, Oundle vestry minutes and correspondence.

251p/23–38 and 98–9, Great Oxendon vestry minutes and overseers' papers.

252p/244–7, 486, 411 and 131–56, Passenham accounts, letters and notebooks.

261p/220–52a and 256, Peterborough St John overseers' accounts, receipts and letters.

283p/33 and 34, Rothersthorpe vouchers and correspondence 1810–30.

284p/189–95, Rothwell Vestry minutes and vouchers 1774–1835.

302p/14–22, Stoke Albany overseers' accounts and vestry minutes 1778–1834.

325p/193 and 194, Thrapston copy letter books.

339p/40–47, Wappenham overseers' accounts 1756–1836.

350p/161–75, 270, 295, 554–79, Wellingborough overseers' accounts, vestry minutes and vouchers.

356p/7–18, Welton poor book 1773–1834.

356p/28, Welton vestry book.

361p/205, Whiston overseers' accounts 1799–1824.

372p/11/A/S, Woodford Halse overseers' accounts 1776–1830.

F(M) G 666, Reports on St Luke's Hospital, Middlesex, 1751–85.

F(M) Misc Volumes 357, 'Some Suggestions for the Improvement of Benefit Clubs', 1824.

GI 375, Volume of surgeons' accounts 1774–93.

Sox 517/2, Case notes, 10 April 1772.

ZA 1759–1809, Certificates.

Oxfordshire Record Office (ORO)

MSS. D.D. Par. Charlbury b.8/9, fol. 9, letter.

MSS. D.D. Par. Hook Norton b.12/10/9, letter.

MSS. D.D. Par. Oxford St Clements c.25, letters.

MSS. D.D. Par. Rotherfield Greys c.11/1–24, letters.
MSS D.D. Par. Souldern, c.7/i/1–7, letters.
MSS D.D. Par. Witney, c.44 c/4, letter.
PAR 16/2/A1/2, Bampton vestry minutes.
PAR 16/5/A11/8, letter.
PAR 16/5/F1/2, Bampton overseers' accounts.
PAR 207/5/A2/ 1–27, letters.
PAR 207/5/A7/1–17, letters.
PAR 236/5/A13/2/1–19, letters.
PAR Oxford St Martin 211/5/C1/1/1–48, letters.
Wooton P.C. IX/iv/1–14, letters.

Rawtenstall Library and Local Studies (RL)
RC 331.55 Lov, Apprenticeship indentures for print works.
RC 331.55 Ros, Indentures for Newchurch 1759–74.
RC 352 Raw, Overseers' accounts for Cowpe, Lenches, Newhallhey and Hall Carr.
RC 552, Higher Booths overseers' accounts.

Rothersthorpe Parish Church (RPC)
Letter collection.

Royal College of Surgeons, England (RCSE)
MS0040/1/5, Rowland Morris Fawcett miscellaneous notes.
MS Add.427, 3a, 'The Poorhouse Surgeon's Day Book' 1805–15.
MS0162, 'Westminster Hospital Remarkable Cases' 1802–18.

Somerset Record Office (SRO)
DD/WY/198, Bundle 29, blank letters.
D/P/ba.ab/13/10/1, Workhouse survey 1822.
DP Chard/13/2/14, Vouchers.
DP Chard/13/7/1, Complaints of the poor.
D/P/Chard/13/10/4, Printed leaflets.
D/P/Mls/13/2/9, Letter book 1826–35.
D/P/She/13/2/30, Shepton Mallet daily receipts and expenditure 1831–36.
D/P/Twn/9/1/1, Copy letter book 1832–33
D/P/twn/9/1/1, Vestry minutes.
DP/wor/13/10/1, Inventory.

Staffordshire Record Office (STRO)
B3891/6/100, Uttoxeter pauper letters.
D24/A/PO/2892–3106, letters.

Surrey Record Centre (SRC)
P3/5/39/9, Overseers' correspondence for the parish of Farnham.
SHER 28/8/2, Overseers' correspondence for the parish of Shere.

Sussex Record Office (SRO)
FRE 1757, Letter from Mary Burrough of Drigg to John Frewen of Cold Overton, 27 June 1807.
PAR. 400/37/12–128, Hurstpierpoint letters.

Wigan Record Office
Tr/Ath/C/2/7–33, Atherton overseers' accounts and ledgers 1743–1834.
Tr/Ath/C/7/3 and 5, Orders for relief.
Tr/Ath/C/7/17, Workhouse inventories.
Tr/Ath/C7/31, Schedule of paupers 1830–47.
Tr/Ath/C/7/59, Friendly society certificates.
Tr/Ath/C/7/61 and 65, Correspondence 1718–1841.
Tr/Ath/C/22/40–60, Vouchers.
Tr/Pe/f18, Miscellaneous papers.
Tr/Pe/p1, Pennington town book 1700–1817.
Tr/Pe/p5–9, Pennington overseers' accounts 1700–1840.
Tr/Pe/p10–14, Constables' accounts 1704–1819.
Tr/Pe/p18, Miscellaneous bills.

Wiltshire Record Office (WRO)
173/3, 27–37, Lacock overseers' papers and vestry minutes 1740–1832.
206/63–121k, Trowbridge overseers' papers.
730/324–27, Ashton Steeple friendly society.
735/32–9, Chilton Foliat overseers' accounts 1793–1839.
746/15–31, West Lavington overseers' accounts 1742–1840.
811/126–220, Chippenham overseers' papers 1742–1830.
871/62–9, 177–203, Marlborough overseers' papers.
980/22–38, Donhead with Charlton vestry minutes and vouchers 1740–1822.
1020/55–116, Longbridge Deverill overseers' papers 1753–1834.
1076/36–63, Stratford-sub-Castle St Lawrence overseers' papers.
1089/4–10, Boughton Gifford overseers' accounts and vestry minutes 1742–1829.
1097/12, Corsley accounts and vouchers 1828–1901.
1108/11, Luckington overseers' accounts 1747–1836.
1179/16–25, Corsley overseers' and workhouse accounts 1742–1800.
1186/18–20, Hardenhuish overseers' accounts 1765–1836.
1228/28–31, Sopworth overseers' papers 1685–1836.

1368/110–126, Melksham overseers' accounts 1748–1836.
1589/32–9, Malmsebury overseers' papers 1760–1836.
1719/4–32, Box overseers' accounts, vestry minutes and correspondence 1793–1829.
1757/41, Corsley bills and accounts 1776–1819.
1789/27–31, Box vestry minutes and vouchers 1797–1806.
1814/7–8, Chilton Foliat bills and letters.
1834/11–14, Upavon overseers' accounts 1729–1836.
CL/CHI/22, Bill.

West Yorkshire Record Office (WYRO)
6D74, Idle township papers 1737–1923.
15D74, Idle, Manningham and Bowling overseers' papers 1734–1837.
23D98/3/11, Guiseley poor book 1795–96.
29D93/1, Bingley township book.
33D80, Bingley and Haworth township records.
74D80, Shipley township book 1687–1846.
BDP/17/88–97, Overseers' accounts for Calverley.
BIC/8/c/8, Bowling overseers' accounts 1818–19.
BDP 29, Guiseley township papers.
BK100/1, Guiseley workhouse book 1789–98.
CP/M Mirfield township and workhouse records.
DB 3/C56, Woodmansey overseers' papers.
DB 16/C12/17, Pudsey bills 1815–17.
DB 17/C13/5, Overseers' accounts.
DB 65/c4/4, Newspaper cutting book 1815–79.
EF, Eastwood family of Stansfield.
FER, Busfield-Ferrand of Bingley papers.
FH.330, List of Sowerby benefactions 1616–1817.
Has/B:22/5, Workhouse inventories 1766–92.
HSB:1–3, 63, Sowerby overseers' accounts 1812–37.
KC 155/3, Pudsey overseers' accounts 1836–37.
KC 1023, Gomersal township records.
KC 1042, Dewsbury township records 1691–1837.
KX 296–316, Dewsbury overseers' papers.
MMC/38–42, Bingley township records.
RDP 9, Beeston township records.
RDP 17/83–8, Calverley cum Farsley overseers' papers.
RDP 43, Horsforth overseer papers.
RDP 96, Spofforth overseers' and township papers.
SpSt/11/2, Horsforth town books 1607–1767.

Sta, Stansfield papers.
Sta:217–19, Sowerby overseers' papers.
Tong/1/1–687, Bills and vouchers.
Tong/2/1–12, Tong overseers' papers.
Tong/10/1–38, Bills and vouchers.
Tong/12/a–h, Bills and vouchers
Tong/78/6, Appellant brief 1796.
Tong/Tempest family papers.
WDP 20/9/3/15, Overseers' correspondence for Sandal Magna.
WYC: 1525, Rawson papers.

Yorkshire Archaeological Society

DD12/I, The Calverley papers.
DD12/II, The Clark-Thornhill papers.

Newspapers and web resources

Jackson's Oxford Journal
Lincolnshire, Rutland and Stamford Mercury
Old Bailey Online, https://www.oldbaileyonline.org/browse.jsp?id=t1786
0222-104-defend1037&div=t17860222-104#highlight (last accessed 26 March 2017).
The Times

Printed sources

Aikin, J., *Thoughts on Hospitals* (London: Joseph Johnson, 1771).
Anon., *Administration & Operation of the Poor Laws 1833* (London: Fellowes, 1833).
Anon., *Henley-on-Thames Poor Relief 1822–1835* (Oxford: Oxfordshire Family History Society, 1987).
Anon., 'Mendicants', *Literary Speculum*, March 1822.
Anon., *The Overseers' Handbook* (1851).
Anon., *Some Bedfordshire Diaries* (Streatley: Bedfordshire Historical Record Society, 1959).
Anon., *Some Particulars of Mawnan Church and its Rectors* (Falmouth: Falmouth Printing, undated).
Barber, B. *Memorandum Book of Richard Tilburn and John Daniell: Overseers of the Poor for the Township of Doncaster* (Doncaster: Doncaster and District Family History Society, 2009).
Candler, A., *Poetical Attempts by Ann Candler, a Suffolk Cottager with a Short Narrative of her Life* (Ipswich: T. Hurst, 1803).

Cartwright, J. (ed.), *The Travels Through England of Dr Richard Pococke, Successively Bishop of Meath and of Ossory, During 1750, 1751 and Later Years* (London: Camden Society, 1977).

Cockayne, E. and N. Stow, *Stutter's Casebook. A Junior Hospital Doctor 1839–1841* (Woodbridge: Boydell, 2005).

Cole, A. and D. Paine (eds), *Extracts From the Minutes of the Board of Guardians of Stamford Union Workhouse, 1835–41* (Lincoln: Lincolnshire Family History Society, 2010).

Collins, A., *Finchley Vestry Minutes 1768–1840* (London: Finchley Libraries Committee, 1957).

Common Sense, 'Rights of the poor asserted', *Monthly Magazine*, 34 (1812), 231, pp. 123–7.

Cooper, A., *The Anatomy and Surgical Treatment of Abdominal Hernia* (London: Green, 1827).

Cowe, F., *Wimbledon Vestry Minutes 1736, 1743–1788* (Guildford: Surrey Record Society, 1964).

Crabbe, G., *The Village: A Poem in Two Books By The Rev. George Crabbe* (London: John Carr, 1783).

Creighton, C., *A History of Epidemics in Britain: Volume 2 from the Extinction of the Plague to the Present Time* (Cambridge: Cambridge University Press, 2014 repr.).

Crosby, A., *The Family Records of Benjamin Shaw, Mechanic of Dent, Dolphinholme and Preston, 1772–1841* (Chester: Record Society of Lancashire and Cheshire, 1991).

Crowther, J. and P. Crowther, *The Diary of Robert Sharp of South Cave: Life in a Yorkshire Village 1812–1837* (Oxford: Oxford University Press, 1997).

Dymond, D. (ed.), *Parson and People in a Suffolk Village: Richard Cobbold's Wortham 1824–77* (Ipswich: Wortham History Group, 2007).

Eden, F. M., *The State of the Poor: Or, an History of the Labouring Classes in England, from the Conquest to the Present*, 3 vols (Cambridge: Cambridge University Press, 2011).

Eureka Partnership, *The Parish of Binfield 1801 Census* (Aylesbury: Berkshire Family History Society, 2009).

Firth, J., *Highways and Byways in Leicestershire* (London: Macmillan, 1926).

Gibson, L., *The Walthamstow Charities. Caring for the Poor 1500–2000* (Chichester: Phillimore, 2000).

Gilbert, T. (1777), *Report from the Committee Appointed to Inspect and Consider the Returns Made by the Overseers of the Poor, in Pursuance of Act of Last Session: Together with Abstracts of the Said Returns Relating to 16 Geo III, c.40* (London: Butterfield, 1777).

Hannah, G., *The Deserted Village. The Diary of an Oxfordshire Rector: James Newton of Nuneham Courtenay, 1736–86* (Stroud: Alan Sutton, 1992).

Heathcote, B., *Viewing the Lifeless Body: A Coroner and His Inquests Held in Nottinghamshire Public Houses During the Nineteenth Century 1828 to 1866* (Nottingham: Nottingham County Council, 2005).

Hinton, F., 'Notes on the records and accounts of the overseers of the poor of Chippenham, 1691–1805', *Wiltshire Archaeological and Natural History Magazine*, CLIX (1933), 312–35.

Hodgkin, T., *On the Mode of Selecting Medical Men for Professional Attendance on the Poor of a Parish or District* (Lindfield: The Hunterian Society, 1836).

Hulbert, J., *Farming the Sick Poor and other Observations on the Necessity of Establishing a Different System of Affording Medical Relief to the Sick Poor, than by the Practice of Contracting with Medical Men or the Farming of Parishes* (London: Longman, 1827).

Hunnisett, R., *Wiltshire Coroners' Bills, 1752–1796* (Devizes: Wiltshire Record Society, 1981).

Hurley, B., *Bradford on Avon Applications for Relief From Out of Town Strays* (Devizes: Wiltshire Family History Society, 2004).

Hurley, B., *Longbridge Deverill Poor 1816–1821 and 1825–1835* (Devizes: Wiltshire Family History Society, 2005).

Hurley, B., *Cricklade Absent Poor and Warrants for Reputed Fathers 1787–1837* (Devizes: Wiltshire Family History Society, 2005).

Hutchinson, A., 'To the churchwardens and overseers of the poor, in and near London', *Gentleman's Magazine* (1824), 413–15.

Jekyll, G., *Old West Surrey: Some Notes and Memories* (Chichester: Phillimore, 1999).

Kerrison, R., 'Medical and surgical attendance on the parochial poor', *Transactions of the Associated Apothecaries & Surgeons of England and Wales*, 1 (London: Burgess and Hill, 1821), 154–216.

Kilvington, F. and S. Flood, 'Diary of Thomas Newcome Rector of Shenley 1822–1849', in J. Knight and S. Flood (eds), *Two Nineteenth Century Hertfordshire Diaries* (St Albans: Hertfordshire Record Society, 2002).

Lawrence, C., P. Lucier and C. Booth (eds), *'Take time by the forelock': The Letters of Anthony Fothergill to James Woodforde, 1789–1813* (London: Wellcome Trust, 1997).

Lewis, L. (ed.), *Hird's Annals of Bedale* (Harrogate: North Yorkshire County Record Office, 1975).

Lightning, R., *Ealing and the Poor: The Poor Law, the Workhouses and Poor Relief From 1722 to 1800* (Ealing: Ealing Local History Society, 1966).

Peat, A. (ed.), *The Most Dismal Times: William Rowbottom's Diary 1787–1799* (Oldham: Oldham City Council, 1996).

Peyton, S., *Kettering Vestry Minutes A.D. 1797–1853* (Northampton: Northamptonshire Record Society, 1933).

Report of the Metropolitan Commissioners in Lunacy to the Lord Chancellor 1844 (London: Bradbury and Evans, 1844).

Simmons, J. (ed.), *Letters from England: Robert Southey* (Stroud: Alan Sutton, 1984).

Smith, L., 'Elegy', *London Review*, 22 (1792), 382.

Snell, K. (ed.), *The Whistler at the Plough* (London: Merlin Press, 1989).

Spurrell, M. (ed.), *The Brightwell Parish Diaries* (Oxford: Oxfordshire Record Society, 1998).

Stead, J., *The Diary of a Quack Doctor: Being the Last Diary of John Swift, Aurist, of Newsome, Huddersfield, 1784–1851* (Huddersfield: Huddersfield Local History Society, 2002).

Stern, P., *Memorials of Leeds* (Leeds: Chadwick, 1828).

Sturges Bourne, W., *Report from His Majesty's Commissioners for Inquiring into the Administration and Practical Operation of the Poor Laws*, vol. 1 (London: B. Fellowes, 1834).

Walker, G., *Gatherings from Graveyards* (London: Longman, 1839).

Warren, P., *Extracts from the Accounts of the Overseers of the Poor, 1807 to 1820: For the Parish of Methwold in the County of Norfolk* (Norwich: Privately Published, 1958).

Secondary sources

Ackroyd, P., *Blake* (London: Vintage, 1999).

Andrew, D., *Philanthropy and Police: London Charity in the Eighteenth Century* (Princeton: Princeton University Press, 1989).

Andrew, D., 'To the charitable and humane: Appeals for assistance in the eighteenth-century press', in A. Cunningham and J. Innes (eds), *Charity, Philanthropy and Reform from the 1690s to 1850* (Basingstoke: Macmillan, 1998), pp. 87–107.

Andrews, J., '"Hardly a hospital, but a charity for pauper lunatics?" Therapeutics at Bethlem in the 17th and 18th centuries', in J. Barry and C. Jones (eds), *Medicine and Charity before the Welfare State* (London: Routledge, 1991), pp. 63–81.

Ashby, A., *One Hundred Years of Poor Law Administration in a Warwickshire Village* (Oxford: Oxford University Press, 1926).

Bailey, J., '"Think Wot a Mother Must Feel": Parenting in English pauper letters c.1760–1834', *Family and Community History*, 13 (2010), 5–19.

Bailey, J., *Parenting in England, 1760–1830: Emotion, Identity, and Generation* (Oxford: Oxford University Press, 2012).

Bannet, E. *British and American Letter Manuals, 1680–1810* (London: Pickering and Chatto, 2008).

Barker, H., 'Medical advertising and trust in late Georgian England', *Urban History*, 36 (2009), 376–98.

Bartlett, P., 'The asylum, the workhouse and the voice of the insane poor in 19th century England', *International Journal of Law and Psychiatry*, 21 (1998), 421–32.

Baugh, D., 'The cost of poor relief in south east England 1790–1834', *Economic History Review*, 28 (1975), 50–68.

Baugh, D., 'Poverty, Protestantism and political economy: English attitudes towards the poor, 1660–1800', in S. Baxter (ed.), *England's Rise to Greatness* (Berkeley: University of California Press, 1983), pp. 63–108.

Bennett, M., 'Inoculation of the poor against smallpox in eighteenth century England', in A. Scott. (ed.), *Experiences of Poverty in Late Medieval and Early Modern England and France* (Farnham: Ashgate, 2012), pp. 207–38.

Berry, A., 'Community sponsorship and the hospital patient in late eighteenth-century England', in P. Horden and R. Smith (eds), *The Locus of Care: Families, Communities, Institutions, and the Provision of Welfare Since Antiquity* (London: Routledge, 1988), pp. 126–52.

Bivins, R., *Alternative Medicine: A History* (Oxford: Oxford University Press, 2007).

Borsay, A., *Medicine and Charity in Georgian Bath; A Social History of the General Infirmary* (Aldershot: Ashgate, 1999).

Borsay, A., 'An example of political arithmetic: The evaluation of spa therapy at the Georgian Bath Infirmary, 1742–1830', *Medical History*, 45 (2000), 149–72.

Borsay, A., *Disability and Social Policy in Britain since 1750: A History of Exclusion* (Basingstoke: Palgrave, 2005).

Borsay, A., 'Disciplining disabled bodies: The development of orthopaedic medicine in Britain c.1800–1939', in D. Turner and K. Stagg (eds), *Social Histories of Disability and Deformity* (London: Routledge, 2006), pp. 97–116.

Borsay, A., 'Nursing, 1700–1830: Families, communities, institutions', in A. Borsay and B. Hunter (eds), *Nursing and Midwifery in Britain since 1700* (Basingstoke: Palgrave, 2012), pp. 23–45.

Borsay, A., and B. Hunter, 'Nursing and midwifery: Historical approaches', in A. Borsay and B. Hunter (eds), *Nursing and Midwifery in Britain since 1700* (Basingstoke: Palgrave, 2012), pp. 1–22.

Boulton, J., 'Welfare systems and the parish nurse in early modern London, 1650–1725', *Family and Community History*, 10 (2007), 127–52.

Boulton, J., '"The charity of our life and healthful years"? Approches to

inter-vivos giving to the poor in the Metropolis 1600–1720', in P. Jones and S. King (eds), *Obligation, Entitlement and Dispute under the English Poor Laws* (Newcastle: Cambridge Scholars Press, 2015), pp. 20–52.

Boulton, J., and L. Schwarz, '"The comforts of a private fireside": The workhouse, the elderly and the poor law in Georgian Westminster: St Martin-in-the-fields, 1725–1824', in J. McEwan and P. Sharpe (eds), *Accommodating Poverty: The Housing and Living Arrangements of the English Poor, c.1600–1850* (Basingstoke: Palgrave, 2011), pp. 221–45.

Boulton, J., and L. Schwarz, 'The medicalisation of a parish workhouse in Georgian Westminster: St Martin in the Fields, 1725–1824', *Family and Community History*, 17 (2014), 122–40.

Bound-Alberti, F., 'Emotions in the early modern medical tradition', in F. Bound-Alberti (ed.), *Medicine, Emotion and Disease, 1700–1950* (Basingstoke: Palgrave, 2006), pp. 1–21.

Bourke, J., *The Story of Pain: From Prayer to Painkillers* (Oxford: Oxford University Press, 2014).

Boyer, G., *An Economic History of the English Poor Law 1750–1850* (Cambridge: Cambridge University Press, 2008).

Braidwood, S., *Black Poor and White Philanthropists: London's Black and the Foundation of the Sierra Leone Settlement 1786–1791* (Liverpool: Liverpool University Press, 1994).

Broad, J., 'Parish economies of welfare 1650–1834', *Historical Journal*, 42 (1999), 985–1006.

Broadbridge, S., 'The Old Poor Law in the parish of Stone', *North Staffordshire Journal of Field Studies*, 13 (1973), 11–25.

Brown, M., 'Medicine, quackery, and the free market: The 'war' against Morison's pills and the construction of the medical profession, c.1830–c.1850', in M. Jenner and P. Wallis (eds), *Medicine and the Market in England and its Colonies, c.1450–1850* (Basingstoke: Palgrave, 2007), pp. 238–61.

Brown, M., 'From foetid air to filth: The cultural transformation of British epidemiological thought, ca. 1780–1848', *Bulletin of the History of Medicine*, 82 (2008), 515–44.

Brown, P., 'Medicines advertised in eighteenth-century Bath newspapers', *Medical History*, 20 (1976), 152–68.

Brundage, A., *The English Poor Laws 1700–1930* (Basingstoke: Macmillan, 2002).

Brunton, D., *The Politics of Vaccination. Practice and Policy in England, Wales, Ireland and Scotland, 1800–1874* (Rochester: University of Rochester Press, 2008).

Burrell, S. and G. Gill, 'The Liverpool cholera epidemic of 1832 and anatomical dissection – medical mistrust and civil unrest', *Journal of the History of Medicine and Allied Sciences*, 60 (2005), 478–98.

Bushaway, B., 'Things said or sung a thousand times: Customary society and oral culture in rural England, 1700–1900', in A. Fox and D. Woolf (eds), *The Spoken Word: Oral Culture in Britain 1500–1850* (Manchester: Manchester University Press, 2002), pp. 256–83.

Bynum, W., 'Treating the wages of sin: Venereal disease and specialism in eighteenth-century Britain', in W. Bynum and R. Porter (eds), *Medical Fringe and Medical Orthodoxy, 1750–1850* (London: Wellcome Trust, 1987), pp. 5–28.

Bynum, W., *Science and the Practice of Medicine in the Nineteenth Century* (Cambridge: Cambridge University Press, 1994).

Carter, L., 'Nineteenth-century treatments for rabies as reported in the *Lancet*', *Medical History*, 26 (1982), 67–78.

Charlesworth, L., *Welfare's Forgotten Past: A Socio-Legal History of the Poor Law* (London: Routledge, 2009).

Charon, R., *Narrative Medicine: Honoring the Stories of Illness* (Oxford: Oxford University Press, 2006).

Cherry, S., *Mental Health Care in Modern England: The Norfolk Lunatic Asylum, St Andrew's Hospital c.1810–1998* (Woodbridge: Boydell, 2003).

Cherry, S., 'General practitioners, hospitals and medical services in rural England: The East Anglian region, 1800–1948', in J. Barona and S. Cherry (eds), *Health and Medicine in Rural Europe (1850–1945)* (Valencia: Seminari d'Estudis sobre la Ciència, 2005), pp. 17–41.

Cliff, A., P. Haggett and M. Smallman-Raynor, *Measles: An Historical Geography of a Major Human Viral Disease from Global Expansion to Local Retreat, 1840–1990* (Oxford: Blackwell, 1993).

Condrau, F., and M. Worboys, 'Epidemics and infections in nineteenth-century Britain', *Social History of Medicine*, 22 (2007), 147–59.

Connors, R., 'Parliament and poverty in mid-eighteenth century England', *Parliamentary History*, 21 (2002), 207–31.

Cooter, R., 'Bones of contention? Orthodox medicine and the mystery of the bone-setter's craft', in W. Bynum and R. Porter (eds), *Medical Fringe and Medical Orthodoxy, 1750–1850* (London: Wellcome Trust, 1987), pp. 158–73.

Cordery, S., *British Friendly Societies, 1750–1914* (Basingstoke: Palgrave, 2003).

Corlett, H., '"No small uncertainty": Eye treatments in eighteenth-century England France', *Medical History*, 42 (1998), 217–34.

Cousins, M., *Poor Relief in Ireland, 1851–1914* (Bern: Peter Lang, 2011).

Cowherd, R., 'The humanitarian reform of the English poor laws from 1782–1815', *Proceedings of the American Philosophical Society*, 104 (1960), 328–42.

Cox, C., H. Marland and S. York, 'Itineraries and experiences of insanity: Irish migration and the management of mental illness in nineteenth-century Lancashire', in C. Cox and H. Marland (eds), *Migration, Health and Ethnicity in the Modern World* (Basingstoke: Palgrave, 2013), pp. 36–60.

Crook, T., and M. Esbester (eds), *Governing Risks in Modern Britain: Danger, Safety and Accidents c.1800–2000* (Basingstoke: Palgrave, 2016).

Crossman, V., *Poverty and the Poor Law in Ireland 1850–1914* (Liverpool: Liverpool University Press, 2013).

Crossman, V., and P. Gray (eds), *Poverty and Welfare in Ireland, 1838–1948* (Dublin: Irish Academic Press, 2011).

Crowther, M., *The Workhouse System 1834–1929* (London: Batsford, 1981).

Crowther, M., 'Paupers or patients? Obstacles to professionalization in the poor law medical service before 1914', *Journal of the History of Medicine and Allied Sciences*, 39 (1984), 33–54.

Crowther, M., 'Health care and poor relief in provincial England', in O. Grell, A. Cunningham and R. Jütte (eds), *Health Care and Poor Relief in 18th and 19th Century Northern Europe* (London: Routledge, 2002), pp. 203–19.

Croxson, B., 'The foundation and evolution of the Middlesex Hospital Lying-in service, 1745–86', *Social History of Medicine*, 14 (2001), 27–57.

Curth, L. (ed.), *From Physick to Pharmacology: Five Hundred Years of British Drug Retailing* (Aldershot: Ashgate, 2006).

Daunton, M., *Progress and Poverty: An Economic and Social History of Britain 1700–1850* (Oxford: Oxford University Press, 1995).

Davies, O., 'Healing charms in use in England and Wales 1700–1950', *Folk-Lore*, 107 (1996), 19–32.

Davies, O., 'Cunning-folk in the medical market-place during the nineteenth century', *Medical History*, 43 (1999), 55–73.

Davies, O., 'Female healers in nineteenth-century England', in N. Goose (ed.), *Women's Work in Industrial England: Regional and Local Perspectives* (Hatfield: Local Population Studies, 2007), pp. 229–31.

Davies, R., 'Dr Richard Stoughton and his great cordial elixir', *Pharmaceutical Journal*, 240 (1988), 377–87.

Dekker, R., *Autobiographical Writing in its Social Context since the Middle Ages* (Hilversum: Veloren, 2002).

Digby, A, *Making a Medical Living: Doctors and Patients in the English Market for Medicine* (Cambridge: Cambridge University Press, 1994).

Dobson, M., *Contours of Death and Disease in Early Modern England*, 2nd edn (Cambridge: Cambridge University Press, 2010).

Duncan, C., et al, 'Whooping cough epidemics in London, 1701–1812: Infection dynamics, seasonal forcing and the effects of malnutrition',

Proceedings of the Royal Society of London, Series B, Biological Sciences, 263 (1996), 445–50.

Duncan, C., S. Duncan and S. Scott, 'The dynamics of scarlet fever epidemics in England and Wales in the 19th century', *Epidemiology and Infection*, 117 (1996), 493–99.

Duncan, S., S. Scott, and C. Duncan, 'The dynamics of smallpox epidemics in Britain, 1550–1800', *Demography*, 30 (1993), 405–23.

Duncan, S., S. Scott and C. Duncan, 'Smallpox epidemics in cities in Britain', *Journal of Interdisciplinary History*, 25 (1994), 255–71.

Dunkley, P., *The Crisis of the Old Poor Law in England 1795–1834: An Interpretive Essay* (New York: Garland, 1982).

Eastwood, D., 'The republic in the village: Parish and poor at Bampton 1780–1834', *Journal of Regional and Local Studies*, 12 (1992), 17 28.

Eastwood, D., *Governing Rural England: Tradition and Transformation in Local Government 1780–1840* (Oxford: Clarendon Press, 1994).

Eastwood, D., 'Rethinking the debates on the poor law in early nineteenth-century England', *Utilitas*, 6 (1994), 97–116.

Eastwood, D., *Government and Community in the English Provinces 1700–1870* (Basingstoke: Macmillan, 1997).

Elliott, P., 'Medical institutions, scientific culture and urban improvement in late Georgian England: The politics of the Derbyshire General Infirmary', in J. Reinarz (ed.), *Medicine and Society in the Midlands, 1750–1950* (Birmingham: Midland History Publications, 2007), pp. 27–46.

Eriksen, A., 'Cure or protection? The meaning of smallpox inoculation, ca.1750–1775', *Medical History*, 57 (2013), 516–36.

Esser, R., '"They obey all magistrates and all good lawes ... and we thinke our cittie happie to enjoye them": Migrants and urban stability in early modern English towns', *Urban History*, 34 (2007), 64–75.

Etkin, N., *Edible Medicines: An Ethnopharmacology of Food* (Tucson: University of Arizona Press, 2006).

Evans, T., *'Unfortunate objects': Lone Mothers in Eighteenth-Century London* (Basingstoke: Palgrave, 2005).

Feinstein, C., 'Pessimism perpetuated: Real wages and the standard of living in Britain during and after the Industrial Revolution', *Journal of Economic History*, 58 (1998), 625–58.

Feldman, D., 'Migrants, immigrants and welfare from the Old Poor Law to the welfare state', *Transactions of the Royal Historical Society*, 13 (2003), 79–104.

Fissell, M., 'The disappearance of the patient narrative and the invention of hospital medicine', in R. French and A. Wear (eds), *British Medicine in an Age of Reform* (London: Routledge, 1991), pp. 92–109.

Fissell, M., *Patients, Power, and the Poor in Eighteenth-Century Bristol* (Cambridge: Cambridge University Press, 2002).

Fitzmaurice, S., 'Politeness and modal meaning in the construction of humiliative discourse in an early-eighteenth century network of patron-client relationships', *English Language and Linguistics*, 6 (2002), 239–65.

Flinn, M., 'Medical services under the new poor law', in D. Fraser (ed.), *The New Poor Law in the Nineteenth Century* (Basingstoke: Macmillan, 1976), pp. 45–66.

Forbes, H., 'The professionalization of dentistry in the United Kingdom', *Medical History*, 29 (1985), 169–81.

Frank, A., *The Wounded Storyteller: Body, Illness and Ethics* (Chicago: Chicago University Press, 1995).

French, H., and J. Barry, 'Identity and agency in English society, 1500–1800: An introduction', in H. French and J. Barry (eds), *Identity and Agency in England, 1500–1800* (Basingstoke: Macmillan, 2004), pp. 1–37.

French, H., 'How dependent were the "dependent poor"? Poor relief and the life-course in Terling, Essex, 1762–1834', *Continuity and Change*, 30 (2015), 193–222.

French, H., 'An irrevocable shift: Detailing the dynamics of rural poverty in southern England, 1762–1834: A case study', *Economic History Review*, 68 (2015), 769–805.

Gagnier, R., *Subjectivities: A History of Self-Representation in Britain, 1832–1920* (Oxford: Oxford University Press, 1991).

Gerber, D., *Authors of their Lives: The Personal Correspondence of British Immigrants* (New York: New York University Press, 2006).

Gestrich, A., E. Hurren and S. King, 'Narratives of poverty and sickness in Europe 1780–1938: Sources, methods and experiences', in A. Gestrich, E. Hurren and S. King (eds), *Poverty and Sickness in Modern Europe: Narratives of the Sick Poor* (London: Continuum, 2012), pp. 1–34.

Gestrich, A., E. Hurren and S. King (eds), *Poverty and Sickness in Modern Europe: Narratives of the Sick Poor* (London: Continuum, 2012).

Gittings, C., *Death, Burial and the Individual in Early Modern England* (London: Croom Helm, 1998).

Gorsky, M., 'The growth and distribution of English friendly societies in the early nineteenth century', *Economic History Review*, 51 (1998), 489–511.

Gorsky, M., 'Friendly society health insurance in nineteenth-century England', in M. Gorsky and S. Sheard (eds), *Financing Medicine: The British Experience since 1750* (London: Routledge, 2006), pp. 147–64.

Gorsky, M., M. Powell and J. Mohan, 'British voluntary hospitals and the public sphere: Contribution and participation before the National Health

Service', in S. Sturdy (ed.), *Medicine, Health and the Public Sphere in Britain 1600–2000* (London: Routledge, 2002), pp. 123–44.

Gorsky, M., and S. Sheard, 'Introduction', in M. Gorsky and S. Sheard (eds), *Financing Medicine: The British Experience Since 1750* (London: Routledge, 2006), pp. 1–20.

Green, D., 'Pauper protests: Power and resistance in early nineteenth-century London workhouses', *Social History*, 31 (2006), 137–59.

Green, D., 'Icons of the new system: Workhouse construction and relief practices in London under the Old and New Poor Law', *London Journal*, 34 (2009), 264–84.

Green, D., *Pauper Capital: London and the Poor Law, 1790–1870* (Farnham: Ashgate 2010).

Hallett, C., 'Nursing, 1830–1920: Forging a profession', in in A. Borsay and B. Hunter (eds), *Nursing and Midwifery in Britain since 1700* (Basingstoke: Palgrave, 2012), pp. 46–73.

Hampson, E., *The Treatment of Poverty in Cambridgeshire, 1597–1834* (Cambridge: Cambridge University Press, 1934).

Hanley, J., 'The public's reaction to public health: Petitions submitted to parliament, 1847–1848', *Social History of Medicine*, 15 (2002), 393–411.

Harding, V., 'Burial on the margin: Distance and discrimination in early modern London', in M. Cox (ed.), *Grave Concerns: Death and Burial in England, 1700–1850* (York: Council for British Archaeology, 1998), pp. 54–64.

Harding, V., *The Dead and the Living in Paris and London 1500–1670* (Cambridge: Cambridge University Press, 2002).

Hardy, A., '"Death is the cure of all diseases": Using the General Register Office cause of death statistics for 1837–1920', *Social History of Medicine*, 7 (1994), 472–92.

Hargreaves, A., 'Dentistry in the British Isles', in C. Hillam (ed.), *Dental Practice in Europe at the end of the Eighteenth Century* (Amsterdam: Rodopi, 2003), pp. 171–282.

Harris, B., 'Morbidity and mortality during the health transition: A comment on James C. Riley, "Why sickness and death rates do not move parallel to one another over time"', *Social History of Medicine*, 12 (1999), 125–31.

Harris, B., *The Origins of the British Welfare State: Social Welfare in England and Wales, 1800–1945* (Basingstoke: Palgrave, 2004).

Harris, B., M. Gorsky, A.-M. Guntupalli and A. Hinde, 'Long-term changes in sickness and health: Further evidence from the Hampshire Friendly Society', *Economic History Review*, 65 (2012), 719–45.

Hastings, R., *Poverty and the Poor Law in the North Riding of Yorkshire 1780–1837* (York: Borthwick Institute, 1982).

Haycock, D. and P. Wallis, *Quackery and Commerce in Seventeenth-Century London: The Proprietary Medicine Business of Anthony Daffy* (London: Wellcome Trust, 2005).

Healey, J., 'The development of poor relief in Lancashire, c.1598–1680', *Historical Journal*, 53 (2010), 567–72.

Helfand, W., 'Samuel Solomon and the cordial balm of Gilead', *Pharmacy in History*, 31 (1989), 151–59.

Helmstadter, C. and J. Godden, *Nursing before Nightingale, 1815–1899* (Farnham: Ashgate, 2011).

Hembry, P., *The English Spa, 1560–1815: A Social History* (London: Athlone, 1990).

Hilaire-Pérez, L., and C. Rabier, 'Self-machinery? Steel trusses and the management of ruptures in eighteenth-century Europe', *Technology and Culture*, 53 (2013), 460–502.

Himmelfarb, G., *The Idea of Poverty: England in the Early Industrial Age* (London: Knopf, 1983).

Hindle, S., 'Power, poor relief and social relations in Holland Fen c.1600–1800', *Historical Journal*, 41 (1998), 67–96.

Hindle, S., 'Civility, honesty and the identification of the deserving poor in seventeenth century England', in H. French and J. Barry (eds), *Identity and Agency in England, 1500–1800* (Basingstoke: Macmillan, 2004), pp. 38–59.

Hindle, S., '"Good, godly and charitable uses": Endowed charity and the relief of poverty in rural England, c.1555–1750', in A. Goldgar and R. Frost (eds), *Institutional Culture in Early Modern Society* (Leiden: Brill, 2004), pp. 164–88.

Hindle, S., *On the Parish? The Micro Politics of Poor Relief in Rural England 1550–1750* (Oxford: Clarendon Press, 2004).

Hindle, S., 'Destitution, liminality and belonging: The church porch and the politics of settlement in English rural communities, c.1590–1660', in C. Dyer (ed.), *The Self-Contained Village? The Social History of Rural Communities, 1250–1900* (Hatfield: Hertfordshire University Press, 2006), pp. 46–71.

Hinnells, J., and R. Porter (eds), *Religion, Health and Suffering* (London: Kegan Paul, 1999).

Hodgkinson, R., *The Origins of the National Health Service: The Medical Services of the New Poor Law 1834–1871* (London: Croom Helm, 1967).

Hodgkiss, A., *From Lesion to Metaphor: Chronic Pain in British, French and German Medical Writings, 1800–1914* (Amsterdam: Rodopi, 2000).

Holland, M., G. Gill and S. Burrell (eds), Cholera *and Conflict: 19th Century* Cholera *in Britain and its Social Consequences* (Leeds: Medical Museum Publishing, 2009).

Honeyman, K., *Child Workers in England, 1780–1820: Parish Apprentices and the Making of the Early Industrial Labour Force* (Aldershot: Ashgate, 2007).

Hopkin, D., 'Storytelling, fairytales and autobiography: Some observations on eighteenth and nineteenth century French soldiers' and sailors' memoirs', *Social History*, 29 (2004), 186–98.

Horrell, S., J. Humphries and H.-J. Voth, 'Destined for deprivation: Human capital formation and intergenerational poverty in nineteenth-century England', *Explorations in Economic History*, 38 (2001), 339–65.

Houlbrooke, R., *Death, Religion and the Family in England, 1480–1750* (Oxford: Oxford University Press, 1998).

How, J., *Epistolary Spaces: English Letter Writing from the Foundation of the Post Office and Richardson's Clarissa* (Farnham: Ashgate, 2003).

Hughes, F., 'Was lunacy and idiocy a rural or an urban condition? A compari son of two county asylum services 1845–1900', *Local Historian*, 44 (2014), 301–11.

Humphries, J., *Childhood and Child Labour in the British Industrial Revolution* (Cambridge: Cambridge University Press, 2010).

Hurren, E., *Dying for Victorian Medicine: English Anatomy and its Trade in the Dead Poor, c.1834–1929* (Basingstoke: Palgrave, 2011).

Hurren, E., *Protesting about Pauperism: Poverty, Politics and Poor Relief in Late-Victorian England, 1870–1900* (Woodbridge: Boydell, 2007).

Hurren, E., and S. King, 'Begging for a burial: Death and the poor law in eighteenth and nineteenth century England', *Social History*, 30 (2005), 321–41.

Hurren, E., and S. King, 'Public and private health care for the poor, 1650s to 1960s', in P. Weindling (ed.), *Healthcare in Private and Public from the Early Modern Period to 2000* (London: Routledge, 2015), pp. 15–35.

Ingram, A. and L. Weatherall Dickson (eds), *Popular Culture*, vol. 4 of L. Weatherall Dickson and A. Ingram (eds), *Depression and Melancholy, 1660–1800* (London: Pickering and Chatto, 2012).

Innes, J., 'The local acts of a national parliament: Parliament's role in sanctioning local action in eighteenth-century Britain', *Parliamentary History*, 17 (1998), 23–47.

Innes, J., 'State, church and volunterism in European welfare 1690–1850', in A. Cunningham and J. Innes (eds), *Charity, Philanthropy and Reform from the 1690s to 1850* (Basingstoke: Macmillan, 1998), pp. 15–65.

Innes, J., *Inferior Politics: Social Problems and Social Policies in Eighteenth-Century Britain* (Oxford: Oxford University Press, 2009).

Innes, J., S. King and A. Winter, 'Settlement and belonging in Europe, 1500–1930s: Structures, negotiations and experiences', in S. King and A. Winter (eds), *Migration, Settlement and Belonging in Europe, 1500s-1930s* (Oxford: Berghahn, 2013), pp. 1–28.

Jones, C., 'Disability in Herefordshire, 1851–1911', *Local Population Studies*, 87 (2011), 29–44.

Jones, P., 'Widows, work and wantonness: Pauper letters and the boundaries of entitlement under the Old Poor Law', in P. Jones and S. King (eds), *Obligation, Entitlement and Dispute under the English Poor Laws* (Newcastle: Cambridge Scholars Press, 2015), pp. 139–67.

Jones, P., and S. King, 'From petition to pauper letter: The development of an epistolary form', in P. Jones and S. King (eds), *Obligation, Entitlement and Dispute under the English Poor Laws* (Newcastle: Cambridge Scholars Press, 2015), pp. 53–77.

Jupp, P., *From Dust to Ashes: Cremation and the British Way of Death* (Basingstoke: Palgrave, 2006).

Kidd, A., *State, Society and the Poor in Nineteenth Century England* (Basingstoke: Macmillan, 1999).

King, P., 'Social inequality, identity and the labouring poor in eighteenth century England', in H. French and J. Barry (eds), *Identity and Agency in England, 1500–1800* (Basingstoke: Macmillan, 2004), pp. 60–87.

King, P., *Crime and Law in England 1750–1840: Remaking Justice from the Margins* (Cambridge: Cambridge University Press, 2006).

King, P., 'The rights of the poor and the role of the law: The impact of pauper appeals to the summary courts 1750–1834', in P. Jones and S. King (eds), *Obligation, Entitlement and Dispute under the English Poor Laws* (Newcastle: Cambridge Scholars Press, 2015), pp. 235–62.

King, S., 'Reconstructing lives: The poor, the poor law and welfare in rural industrial communities', *Social History*, 22 (1997), 318–38.

King, S., *Poverty and Welfare in England 1700–1850: A Regional Perspective* (Manchester: Manchester University Press, 2000).

King, S., *A Fylde Country Practice: Medicine and Society in Lancashire 1760–1840* (Lancaster: Centre for Northwest Regional Studies, 2001).

King, S., 'Re-clothing the English poor 1750–1840', *Textile History*, 33 (2002), 37–47.

King, S., 'The English proto-industrial family: Old and new perspectives', *History of the Family*, 140 (2003), 1–23.

King, S., '"It is impossible for our vestry to judge his case into perfection from here": Managing the distance dimensions of poor relief, 1800–40', *Rural History*, 16 (2005), 161–89.

King, S., '"Stop this overwhelming torment of destiny": Negotiating financial aid at times of sickness under the English Old Poor Law, 1800–1840', *Bulletin of the History of Medicine*, 79 (2005), 228–60.

King, S., 'Pauvreté et assistance: La politique locale de la mortalité dans l'Angleterre des XVIII et XIX siècles', *Annales*, 61 (2006), 31–62.

King, S., 'Pauper letters as a source', *Family and Community History*, 10 (2007), 167–70.

King, S., 'Regional patterns in the experiences and treatment of the sick poor, 1800–40: Rights, obligations and duties in the rhetoric of paupers', *Family and Community History*, 10 (2007), 61–75.

King, S., 'Friendship, kinship and belonging in the letters of urban paupers 1800–1840', *Historical Social Research*, 33 (2008), 249–77.

King, S., '"The particular claims of a woman and a mother": Gender, belonging and rights to medical relief in England 1800–1840s', in A. Andresen, T. Grønle, W. Hubbard, T. Rymin, and S. Skålevåg (eds), *Citizens, Courtrooms, Crossings* (Bergen: Bergen University Press, 2008), pp. 21–38.

King, S., '"I fear you will think me too presumtuous in my demands but necessity has no law": Clothing in English pauper letters 1800–1834', *International Review of Social History*, 54 (2009), 207–36.

King, S., *Women, Welfare and Local Politics 1880–1920* (Brighton: Sussex Academic Press, 2010).

King, S., 'Negotiating the law of poor relief in England 1800–1840', *History*, 96 (2011), 410–35.

King, S., '"In these you may trust": Numerical information, accounting practices and the poor law, c.1790 to 1840', in T. Crook and G. O'Hara (eds), *Statistics and the Public Sphere: Numbers and the People in Modern Britain, c.1750–2000* (London: Routledge, 2011), pp. 51–66.

King, S., 'Welfare regimes and welfare regions in Britain and Europe, c.1750–1860', *Journal of Modern European History*, 9 (2011), 42–66.

King, S., 'Poverty, medicine and the workhouse in the eighteenth and nineteenth centuries: An afterword', in J. Reinarz and L. Schwarz (eds), *Medicine and the Workhouse* (Rochester: University of Rochester Press, 2013), pp. 228–51.

King, S., 'Nursing under the Old Poor Law in midland and eastern England 1780–1834', *Journal of the History of Medicine and Allied Sciences*, 69 (2014), 1–35.

King, S., 'Constructing the disabled child in England, 1800–1860', *Family and Community History*, 18 (2015), 56–89.

King, S., 'English pauper letters, 1790s–1830s', *Groniek*, 204–5 (2015), 305–16.

King, S., 'Rights, duties and practice in the transition between the Old and New Poor Laws 1820–1860s', in P. Jones and S. King (eds), *Obligation, Entitlement and Dispute under the English Poor Laws* (Newcastle: Cambridge Scholars Press, 2015), pp. 263–91.

King, S., and P. Jones, 'Testifying for the poor: Epistolary advocates and the negotiation of parochial relief in England, 1800–1834', *Journal of Social History*, 49 (2016), 351–82.

King, S, T. Nutt and A. Tomkins, *Narratives of the Poor in Eighteenth Century Britain* (London: Pickering and Chatto, 2006).

King, S., and A. Stringer, "'I have once more taken the Leberty to say as you well know": The development of rhetoric in the letters of the English, Welsh and Scottish sick and poor 1780s–1830s', in A. Gestrich, E. Hurren and S. King (eds), *Poverty and Sickness in Modern Europe: Narratives of the Sick Poor, 1780–1938* (London: Continuum, 2012), pp. 69–92.

King, S., and A. Tomkins (eds), *The Poor in England 1700–1850: An Economy of Makeshifts* (Manchester: Manchester University Press, 2003).

Land, I., 'Bread and arsenic: Citizenship from the bottom up in Georgian London', *Journal of Social History*, 45 (2005), 89–110.

Landers, J., *Death and the Metropolis: Studies in the Demographic History of London, 1670–1830* (Cambridge: Cambridge University Press, 1993).

Lane, J., 'The medical practitioners of provincial England in 1783', *Medical History*, 28 (1984), 353–71.

Lane, J., "'The doctor scolds me": The diaries and correspondence of patients in eighteenth century England', in R. Porter (ed.), *Patients and Practitioners: Lay Perceptions of Medicine in Pre-Industrial Society* (Cambridge: Polity Press, 1985), pp. 205–48.

Lane, J., 'Eighteenth century medical practice: A Case study of Bradford Wilmer, surgeon of Coventry, 1737–1813', *Social History of Medicine*, 3 (1990), 369–86.

Lane, J., *A Social History of Medicine: Health, Healing and Disease in England 1750–1950* (London: Routledge, 2001).

Langton, J., 'The geography of poor relief in rural Oxfordshire, 1775–1832', in P. Jones and S. King (eds), *Obligation, Entitlement and Dispute under the English Poor Laws* (Newcastle: Cambridge Scholars Press, 2015), pp. 193–234.

Laqueur, T., 'Bodies, death and pauper funerals', *Representations*, 1 (1983), 109–31.

Lees, L. H., *The Solidarities of Strangers: The English Poor Laws and the People 1700–1948* (Cambridge: Cambridge University Press, 1998).

Lemmings, D., 'Introduction', in D. Lemmings (ed.), *The British and their Laws in the Eighteenth Century* (Woodbridge: Boydell, 2005), pp. 1–17.

Leong, E., and S. Pennell, 'Recipe collections and the currency of medical knowledge in the early modern medical marketplace', in in M. Jenner and P. Wallis (eds), *Medicine and the Market in England and its Colonies, c.1450–1850* (Basingstoke: Palgrave, 2007), pp. 133–52.

Levene, A., *Childcare, Health, and Mortality at the London Foundling Hospital, 1741–1800: 'Left to the mercy of the world'* (Manchester: Manchester University Press, 2007).

Levene, A., 'Children, childhood and the workhouse: St Marylebone, 1769–1781', *London Journal*, 33 (2008), 41–59.

Levene, A., 'Parish apprenticeship and the Old Poor Law in London', *Economic History Review*, 63 (2010), 915–41.

Levene, A., *The Childhood of the Poor: Welfare in Eighteenth Century London* (Basingstoke: Palgrave, 2012).

Lilly, R., *An Account of Rural Medical Practice from the 18th Century Onwards in Long Bucky, Northamptonshire* (Dunton Bassett: Volcano, 1993).

Lindert, P., *Growing Public: Social Spending and Economic Growth since the Eighteenth Century* (Cambridge: Cambridge University Press, 2004).

Litten, J., *The English Way of Death: The Common Funeral since 1450* (London: Robert Hale, 1991).

Litten, J., 'The English funeral 1700–1850', in M. Cox (ed.), *Grave Concerns: Death and Burial in England, 1700–1850* (York: Council for British Archaeology, 1998), pp. 1–23.

Lloyd, S., *Charity and Poverty in England, c.1680–1820: Wild and Visionary Schemes* (Manchester: Manchester University Press, 2009).

Loeb, L., 'Doctors and patent medicines in modern Britain: Professionalism and consumerism', *Albion*, 33 (2001), 404–25.

Lord, E., '"Weighed in the balance and found wanting": Female friendly societies, self-help and economic virtue in the east Midlands in the eighteenth and nineteenth centuries', *Midland History*, 22 (1997), 100–12.

Loudon, I., 'The origins and growth of the dispensary movement in England', *Bulletin of the History of Medicine*, 16 (1981), 322–42.

Loudon, I., 'The nature of provincial medical practice in eighteenth-century England', *Medical History*, 29 (1985), 1–32.

Loudon, I., *Medical Care and the General Practitioner 1750–1850* (Oxford: Clarendon Press, 1986).

Loudon, I., 'The vile race of quacks with which this country is infested', in W. Bynum and R. Porter (eds), *Medical Fringe and Medical Orthodoxy, 1750–1850* (London: Wellcome Trust, 1987), pp. 106–28.

Loudon, I., 'Medical practitioners 1750–1850 and the period of medical reform in Britain', in A. Wear (ed.), *Medicine in Society: Historical Essays* (Cambridge: Cambridge University Press, 1992), pp. 353–71.

Lyle, M., 'Regionality in the late Old Poor Law: The treatment of chargeable bastards from Rural Queries', *Agricultural History Review*, 53 (2013), 141–57.

Lyons, M., 'Writing upwards: How the weak wrote to the powerful', *Journal of Social History*, 48 (2015), 311–36.

Lyons, M. (ed.), *Ordinary Writings, Personal Narratives: Writing Practice in 19th and early 20th Century Europe* (Frankfurt: Peter Lang, 2007).

Mackay, L., 'A culture of poverty? The St. Martin's in the Fields workhouse 1817', *Journal of Interdisciplinary History*, 26 (1995), 209–32.

Maehle, A.-H., *Drugs on Trial: Experimental Pharmacology and Therapeutic Innovation in the Eighteenth Century* (Amsterdam: Rodopi, 1999).

Marland, H., *Medicine and Society in Wakefield and Huddersfield 1780–1870* (Cambridge: Cambridge University Press, 1987).

Marland, H., 'The medical activities of mid-nineteenth century chemists and druggists, with special reference to Wakefield and Huddersfield', *Medical History*, 31 (1987), 415–39.

Marland, H., '"The Doctor's Shop": The rise of the chemist and druggist in nineteenth century manufacturing districts', in L. Curth (ed.), *From Physick to Pharmacology: Five Hundred Years of British Drug Retailing* (Aldershot: Ashgate, 2006), 79–104.

Marland, H., and J. Adams, 'Hydropathy at home: The water cure and domestic healing in mid-nineteenth-century Britain', *Bulletin of the History of Medicine*, 83 (2009), 499–529.

Marshall, D., *The English Poor in the Eighteenth Century* (London: Longman, 1926).

Martin, J., 'The rich, the poor and the migrant in eighteenth century Stratford-on-Avon', *Local Population Studies*, 20 (1978), 28–48.

Mathisen, A., 'Mineral waters, electricity, and hemlock: Devising therapeutics for children in eighteenth-century institutions', *Medical History*, 57 (2013), 28–44.

Melling, J., B. Forsythe and R. Adair, 'Families, communities and the legal regulation of lunacy in Victorian England: Assessments of crime, violence and welfare in admissions to the Devon asylum, 1845–1914', in P. Bartlett and D. Wright (eds), *Outside the Walls of the Asylum: The History of Care in the Community 1750–2000* (London: Athlone, 1999), pp. 153–80.

Métayer, C., *Au tombeau des secrets: Les écrivains publics du Paris populaire, cimetière des Saints-Innocents XVIe–XVIIIe siècle* (Paris: Albin Michel, 2000).

Miller, E., 'Variations in the official prevalence and disposal of the insane in England under the poor law, 1850–1900', *History of Psychiatry*, 18 (2007), 25–38.

Miller, E., 'English pauper lunatics in the era of the old poor law', *History of Psychiatry*, 23 (2012), 318–28.

Miller, N., and N. Yavneh (eds), *Sibling Relations and Gender in the Early Modern World. Sisters, Brothers and Others* (Aldershot: Ashgate, 2006).

Mitchison, R., *Coping with Destitution: Poverty and Relief in Western Europe* (Toronto: University of Toronto Press, 1991).

Mooney, G., 'Shifting sex differentials in mortality during urban epidemiological transition: The case of Victorian London', *International Journal of Population Geography*, 8 (2002), 17–47.

Mooney, G., 'Infectious diseases and epidemiologic transition in Victorian Britain? Definitely', *Social History of Medicine*, 20 (2007), 595–606.

Mooney, G., 'Diagnostic spaces: Workhouse, hospital, and home in mid-Victorian London', *Social Science History*, 33 (2009), 357–90.

Moore, R., and S. McLean, 'Folk healing in a post-scientific world', in R. Moore and S. McLean (eds), *Folk Healing and Health Care Practices in Britain and Ireland: Stethoscopes, Wands and Crystals* (Oxford: Berghahn, 2010), pp. 22–54.

Moore, R., and S. McLean, 'Introduction: Folk healing in contemporary Britain and Ireland: Revival, revitalisation or reinvention?', in R. Moore and S. McLean (eds), *Folk Healing and Health Care Practices in Britain and Ireland: Stethoscopes, Wands and Crystals* (Oxford: Berghahn, 2010), pp. 1–21.

Morgan, G., and P. Rushton, 'The magistrate, the community and the maintenance of an orderly society in eighteenth century England', *Historical Research*, 76 (2003), 54–77.

Morgan, J., 'The burial question in Leeds in the eighteenth and nineteenth centuries', in R. Houlbrooke (ed.), *Death, Ritual and Bereavement* (London: Routledge, 1989), pp. 95–104.

Morgan, P., 'Service of the truth: Quaker poor relief in Staffordshire to the mid-eighteenth century', in P. Morgan and A. Phillips (eds), *Staffordshire Histories* (Keele: Staffordshire Record Society, 1999), pp. 157–76.

Morley, S., *Oxfordshire Friendly Societies, 1750–1918* (Oxford: Oxfordshire Record Society, 2011).

Morrison, A., 'Pharmacy in the 1840s: The wholesale chemists and druggists', *Pharmaceutical Historian*, 21 (1991), 3–9.

Muldrew, C., and S. King, 'Cash, wages and the economy of makeshifts in England, 1650–1800', in P. Scholliers and L. Schwarz (eds), *Experiencing Wages: Social and Cultural Aspects of Wage Forms in Europe since 1500* (Oxford: Berghahn, 2003), pp. 155–82.

Muldrew, C., *Food, Energy and the Creation of Industriousness: Work and Material Culture in Agrarian England 1550–1780* (Cambridge: Cambridge University Press, 2011).

Murphy, E., 'The metropolitan pauper farms 1722–1834', *London Journal*, 27 (2002), 1–18.

Murphy, M., *Cambridge Newspapers and Opinion 1780–1850* (Cambridge: Oleander Press, 1977).

Myers, N., 'Servant, sailor, soldier, tailor, beggarman: Black survival in white society 1780–1830', *Immigrants and Minorities*, 12 (1993), 47–74.

Neuman, M., *The Speenhamland County: Poverty and the Poor Laws in Berkshire 1782–1834* (New York: Garland, 1982).

Neve, M., 'Orthodoxy and fringe: Medicine in late Georgian Bristol', in W. Bynum and R. Porter (eds), *Medical Fringe and Medical Orthodoxy, 1750–1850* (London: Wellcome Trust, 1987), pp. 40–55.

O'Day, R., *The Professions in Early Modern England, 1450–1800: Servants of the Commonweal* (London: Longman; 2000).

Ogborn, M., *Spaces of Modernity: London Geographies 1680–1780* (London: Guilford Press, 1998).

Ottaway, S., *The Decline of Life: Old Age in Eighteenth-Century England* (Cambridge: Cambridge University Press, 2004).

Oxley, G., *Poor Relief in England and Wales 1601–1834* (London: David and Charles, 1974).

Parry-Jones, W., *The Trade in Lunacy: A Study of Private Madhouses in England in the Eighteenth and Nineteenth Centuries* (London: Routledge, 1972).

Pelling, M., 'Thoroughly resented? Older women and the medical role in early modern England', in L. Hunter and S. Hutton (eds), *Women, Science and Medicine 1500–1700* (Stroud: Sutton, 1997), pp. 63–87.

Pemberton, N., and M. Worboys, *Mad Dogs and Englishmen: Rabies in Britain, 1830–2000* (Basingstoke: Palgrave, 2007).

Phillips, G., *The Blind in British Society: Charity, State and Community, c.1780–1930* (Aldershot: Ashgate, 2004).

Pickstone, J., 'Dearth, dirt and fever epidemics: Rewriting the history of British "public health", 1780–1850', in T. Ranger and P. Slack (eds), *Epidemics and Ideas: Essays on the Historical Perception on Pestilence* (Cambridge: Cambridge University Press, 1992), pp. 125–48.

Poland, S., and A. Pedersen, 'Reading between the lines: Interpreting silences in qualitative research', *Qualitative Enquiry*, 4 (1998), 293–312.

Pooley, C. and J. Turnbull, *Migration and Mobility in Britain since the Eighteenth-Century* (London: UCL Press, 1998).

Porter, D., 'Health care and the construction of citizenship in civil societies in the era of the enlightenment and industrialisation', in O. Grell, A. Cunningham and R. Jütte (eds), *Health Care and Poor Relief in 18th and 19th Century Northern Europe* (London: Routledge, 2002), pp. 15–37.

Porter, D., and R. Porter, *Patients Progress: Doctors and Doctoring in Eighteenth Century England* (Cambridge: Polity, 1989).

Porter, R., 'Lay medical knowledge in the eighteenth century: The evidence of the *Gentleman's Magazine*', *Medical History*, 29 (1985), 138–68.

Porter, R., *Health for Sale: Quackery in England, 1660–1850* (Manchester: Manchester University Press, 1989).

Porter, R., 'Expressing yourself ill: The language of sickness in Georgian England', in P. Burke and R. Porter (eds), *Language, Self and Society: A Social History of Language* (Cambridge: Polity, 1991), pp. 276–99.

Porter, R., 'Medical journalism in Britain to 1800', in W. Bynum, L Stephen and R. Porter (eds), *Medical Journals and Medical Knowledge: Historical Essays* (London: Routledge, 1992), pp. 6–29.

Porter, R., 'The patient in England 1660–1800', in A. Wear (ed.), *Medicine in Society: Historical Essays* (Cambridge: Cambridge University Press, 1992), pp. 91–118.

Porter, R., 'Spreading medical enlightenment: The popularization of medicine in Georgian England, and its paradoxes', in R. Porter (ed.), *The Popularization of Medicine 1650–1850* (London: Routledge, 1992), pp. 215–31.

Porter, R., 'Introduction', in R. Porter (ed.), *Rewriting the Self: Histories from the Renaissance to the Present* (London: Routledge, 1997), 1–13.

Porter, R., *Quacks: Fakers and Charlatans in English Medicine* (Stroud: Sutton Publishing, 2000).

Porter, R., *Bodies Politic: Disease, Death and Doctors in Britain, 1650–1900* (London: Reaktion, 2003).

Porter, R. (ed.), *Patients and Practitioners: Lay Perceptions of Medicine in Pre-Industrial Society* (Cambridge: Polity Press, 1985).

Porter, R. (ed.), *The Medical History of Waters and Spas* (London: Wellcome Trust, 1990).

Porter, R., and D. Porter, *In Sickness and in Health: The British Experience 1650–1850* (London: Fourth Estate, 1988).

Poynter, J., *Society and Pauperism: English Ideas on Poor Relief, 1795–1834* (Toronto: University of Toronto Press, 1969).

Price, K., *Medical Negligence in Victorian Britain: The Crisis of Care under the English Poor Law 1834–1900* (Basingstoke: Palgrave, 2015).

Razzell, P., *The Conquest of Smallpox: The Impact of Inoculation on Smallpox Mortality in Eighteenth Century Britain* (Firle: Caliban Books, 1977).

Razzell, P. and C. Spence, 'The history of infant, child and adult mortality in London, 1550–1850', *London Journal*, 32 (2007), 272–91.

Reay, B., *Micro-Histories: Demography, Society, and Culture in Rural England, 1800–1930* (Cambridge: Cambridge University Press, 1996).

Redford, A., *The History of Local Government in Manchester*, vol. 1: *Manor and Township* (London: Longman, 1939).

Reinarz, J., 'Introduction', in J. Reinarz (ed.), *Medicine and Society in the Midlands, 1750–1950* (Birmingham: Midland History Publications, 2007).

Reinarz, J., *Healthcare in Birmingham: A History of the Birmingham Teaching Hospitals, 1779–1939* (Woodbridge: Boydell, 2009).

Reinarz, J., and L. Schwarz (eds), *Medicine and the Workhouse* (Rochester: University of Rochester Press, 2013).

Reinarz, J., and R. Wynter, 'The spirit of medicine: The use of alcohol in nineteenth-century medical practice', in S. Schmid and B. Schmidt-Haberkamp

(eds), *Drink in the Eighteenth and Nineteenth Centuries* (London: Pickering and Chatto, 2014), pp. 127–39.

Reiser, S., *Medicine and the Reign of Technology* (Cambridge: Cambridge University Press, 1978).

Richards, N., 'Dentistry in England in the 1840s: The first indications of a movement towards professionalization', *Medical History*, 12 (1968), 137–52.

Richardson, R., *Death, Dissection and the Destitute* (London: Phoenix Press, 2001).

Riley, J., *Sickness, Recovery and Death: A History and Forecast of Ill-Health* (Basingstoke: Macmillan, 1989).

Riley, J., *Sick Not Dead: The Health of British Workingmen during the Mortality Decline* (Baltimore: Johns Hopkins University Press, 1997).

Riley, J., 'Why sickness and death rates do not move parallel to one another over time', *Social History of Medicine*, 12 (1999), 101–24.

Risse, G., and J. Warner, 'Reconstructing clinical activities: Patient records in medical history', *Social History of Medicine*, 5 (1992), 183–206.

Rose, M., 'Social policy and business: Parish apprenticeship and the early factory system 1780–1834', *Business History*, 31 (1989), 5–32.

Rosenberg, C., and J. Golden (eds), *Framing Disease: Studies in Cultural History* (New York: Rutgers University Press, 1992).

Rugg, J., 'A new burial form and its meanings: Cemetery establishment in the first half of the 19th century', in M. Cox (ed.), *Grave Concerns: Death and Burial in England, 1700–1850* (York: Council for British Archaeology, 1998), pp. 44–53.

Rugg, J., 'From reason to regulation, 1760–1850', in P. Jupp and C. Gittings (eds), *Death in England: An Illustrated History* (Manchester: Manchester University Press, 1999), pp. 202–29.

Rugg, J., 'Constructing the grave: Competing burial ideals in nineteenth century England', *Social History*, 38 (2013), 328–45.

Ruggles, S., 'Marriage, migration and mortality: Correcting sources of bias in English family reconstitutions', *Population Studies*, 46 (1992), 507–22.

Ruggles, S., 'The limitations of English family reconstitution: *English Population History from Family Reconstitution 1580–1837*', *Continuity and Change*, 14 (1999), 105–30.

Rushton, P., 'Lunatics and idiots: Mental disability, the community and the poor law in north-east England, 1600–1800', *Medical History*, 32 (1988), 34–50.

Rusnock, A., 'Catching cowpox: The early spread of smallpox vaccination, 1798–1810', *Bulletin of the History of Medicine*, 83 (2009), 17–36.

Rusnock, A., and V. Dietz, 'Defining women's sickness and work: female friendly societies in England, 1780–1830', *Journal of Women's History*, 24 (2012), 60–85.

Schor, E., *Bearing the Dead: The British Culture of Mourning from the Enlightenment to Victoria* (Princeton: Princeton University Press, 1994).

Schweber, L., *Disciplining Statistics: Demography and Vital Statistics in France and England, 1830–1885* (Durham, NC: Duke University Press, 2006).

Scull, A., *The Most Solitary of Afflictions: Madness and Society in Britain 1700–1900* (New Haven: Yale University Press, 1993).

Secord, A., 'Science in the pub: Artisan botanists in early nineteenth century Lancashire', *History of Science*, 32 (1994), 269–315.

Sharpe, P., 'Survival strategies and stories: Poor widows and widowers in early industrial England', in S. Cavallo and L. Warner (eds), *Widowhood in Medieval and Early Modern Europe* (London: Longman, 1999), pp. 220–39.

Sharpe, P., *Population and Society in an East Devon Parish: Reproducing Colyton, 1540–1840* (Exeter: Exeter University Press, 2002).

Sharpe, P., 'Parish women: Maternity and the limitations of Maiden Settlement in England 1662–1834', in P. Jones and S. King (eds), *Obligation, Entitlement and Dispute under the English Poor Laws* (Newcastle: Cambridge Scholars Press, 2015), pp. 168–92.

Shave, S., 'The welfare of the vulnerable in the late 18th and early 19th centuries: Gilbert's Act of 1782', *History in Focus*, 14 (2008), 14.

Shave, S., 'The dependent poor? (Re)constructing individual lives "on the parish" in rural Dorset 1800–1832', *Rural History*, 20 (2009), 67–98.

Shave, S., 'The impact of Sturges Bourne's poor law reforms in rural England', *Historical Journal*, 56 (2013), 399–429.

Shepard, A., 'Poverty, labour and the language of social description in early modern England', *Past and Present*, 201 (2008), 51–95.

Shuttleton, D., *Smallpox and the Literary Imagination 1660–1820* (Cambridge: Cambridge University Press, 2007).

Siena, K., *Venereal Disease, Hospitals and the Urban Poor: London's 'Foul Wards' 1600–1800* (Rochester: University of Rochester Press, 2004).

Siena, K., 'Hospitals for the excluded or convalescent homes? Workhouses, medicalization and the poor law in long eighteenth-century London and pre-confederation Toronto', *Canadian Bulletin of Medical History*, 27 (2010), 5–25.

Siena, K., 'Contagion, exclusion, and the unique medical world of the eighteenth-century workhouse: London infirmaries in their widest relief', in J. Reinarz and L. Schwarz (eds), *Medicine and the Workhouse* (Rochester: University of Rochester Press, 2013), pp. 19–39.

Slack, P., *Poverty and Policy in Tudor and Stuart England* (London: Longman 1988).

Smith, C., 'Parsimony, power, and prescriptive legislation: The politics of pauper lunacy in Northamptonshire, 1845–1876', *Bulletin of the History of Medicine*, 81 (2007), 359–85.

Smith, C., 'Living with insanity: Narratives of poverty, pauperism and sickness in asylum records 1840–1876', in A. Gestrich, E. Hurren and S. King (eds), *Poverty and Sickness in Modern Europe: Narratives of the Sick Poor, 1780–1938* (London: Continuum, 2012), pp. 117–41.

Smith, G., 'Prescribing the rules of health: Self-help and advice in late eighteenth-century England', in R. Porter (ed.), *Patients and Practitioners: Lay Perceptions of Medicine in Pre-Industrial Society* (Cambridge: Polity Press, 1985), pp. 249–82.

Smith, L., 'Reassessing the role of the family: Women's medical care in eighteenth century England', *Social History of Medicine*, 16 (2003), 327–42.

Smith, L., *'Cure, Comfort and Safe Custody': Public Lunatic Asylums in Early Nineteenth-Century England* (Leicester: Leicester University Press, 1999).

Smith, L., *Lunatic Hospitals in Georgian England 1750–1830* (London: Routledge, 2007).

Smith, L., '"The keeper must himself be kept": Visitation and the lunatic asylum in England, 1750–1850', in G. Mooney and J. Reinarz (eds), *Permeable Walls: Historical Perspectives on Hospital and Asylum Visiting* (Amsterdam: Rodopi, 2009), pp. 199–222.

Smith, R., 'Charity, self-interest and welfare: Reflections from demographic and family history', in M. Daunton (ed.), *Charity, Self-Interest and Welfare in the English Past* (London: UCL Press, 1996), pp. 36–41.

Smith, R., 'Ageing and well-being in early modern England: Pension trends and gender preference under the English Old Poor Law 1650–1800', in P. Johnson and P. Thane (eds), *Old Age from Antiquity to Postmodernity* (London: Routledge, 1998), pp. 64–95.

Snell, K., *Annals of the Labouring Poor: Social Change and Agrarian England, 1660–1900* (Cambridge: Cambridge University Press, 1985).

Snell, K., 'Gravestones, belonging and local attachment in England, 1700–2000', *Past and Present*, 134 (2003), 47–73.

Snell, K., *Parish and Belonging: Community, Identity and Welfare in England and Wales 1700–1950* (Cambridge: Cambridge University Press, 2006).

Snell, K., 'Belonging and community: Understandings of "home" and "friends" among the English poor, 1750–1850', *Economic History Review*, 65 (2011), 1–25.

Sokoll, T., 'Old age in poverty: The record of Essex pauper letters, 1780–1834', in T. Hitchcock, P. King and P. Sharpe (eds), *Chronicling Poverty: The Voices and Strategies of the English Poor, 1640–1840* (Basingstoke: Macmillan, 1997), pp. 127–54.

Sokoll, T., 'Negotiating a living: Essex pauper letters from London, 1800–1834', *International Review of Social History Supplement*, 8 (2000), 19–46.

Sokoll, T., *Essex Pauper Letters 1731–1837* (Oxford: Oxford University Press, 2001).

Sokoll, T., 'Writing for relief: Rhetoric in English pauper letters 1800–1834', in A. Gestrich, S. King and L. Raphael (eds), *Being Poor in Modern Europe: Historical Perspectives 1800–1940* (Bern: Peter Lang, 2006), pp. 91–112.

Sokoll, T., 'Families, wheat prices and the allowance cycle: Poverty and poor relief in the agricultural community of Ardleigh, 1794–1801', in P. Jones and S. King (eds), *Obligation, Entitlement and Dispute under the English Poor Laws* (Newcastle: Cambridge Scholars Press, 2015), pp. 78–106.

Song, B., 'Parish typology and the operation of the poor law in early nineteenth century Oxfordshire', *Agricultural History Review*, 50 (2002), 203–24.

Sorge-English, L., *Stays and Body Image in London: The Staymaking trade, 1680–1810* (London: Pickering and Chatto, 2011).

South, S., 'Smallpox inoculation campaigns in eighteenth-century Southampton, Salisbury and Winchester', *Local Historian*, 43 (2013), 122–37.

Stanley, P., *For Fear of Pain: British Surgery, 1790–1850* (Amsterdam: Rodopi, 2003).

Stapleton, B., 'Inherited poverty and life-cycle poverty: Odiham, Hampshire, 1650–1850', *Social History*, 18 (1993), 339–55.

Stolberg, M., *Experiencing Illness and the Sick Body in Early Modern Europe* (Basingstoke: Palgrave, 2011).

Strange, J.-M., 'Death and dying: Old themes and new directions', *Journal of Contemporary History*, 35 (2000), 491–9.

Strange, J.-M., *Death, Grief and Poverty in Britain, 1870–1914* (Cambridge: Cambridge University Press, 2005).

Suzuki, A., *Madness at Home: The Psychiatrist, the Patient and the Family in England, 1820–1860* (Los Angeles: University of California Press, 2006).

Taylor, G., *The Problem of Poverty 1660–1834* (London: Longman, 1969).

Taylor, J., 'The unreformed workhouse 1776–1834', in E. Martin (ed.), *Comparative Developments in Social Welfare* (London: George Allen and Unwin, 1972), pp. 57–84.

Taylor, J., *Poverty, Migration and Settlement in the Industrial Revolution: Sojourners' Narratives* (Palo Alto: Stanford University Press, 1989).

Taylor, J., 'Voices in the crowd: The Kirkby Lonsdale township letters, 1809–1836', in T. Hitchcock, P. King and P. Sharpe (eds), *Chronicling Poverty: The Voices and Strategies of the English Poor, 1640–1840* (Basingstoke: Macmillan, 1997), pp. 109–26.

Thane, P., *Old Age in English History: Past Experiences, Present Issues* (Oxford: Oxford University Press, 2000).

Thomas, E., 'The Old Poor Law and medicine', *Medical History*, 24 (1980), 1–19.

Thomson, D., 'Welfare and the historians', in L. Bonfield, R. Smith and K. Wrightson (eds), *The World We Have Gained: Histories of Population and Social Structure* (Oxford: Basil Blackwell, 1986), pp. 355–78.

Tilly, C., 'The rise of the public meeting in Great Britain, 1758–1834', *Social Science History*, 34 (2010), 291–9.

Timmermann, K., and J. Anderson, 'Devices, designs and the history of technology in medicine', in J. Anderson and K. Timmermann (eds), *Devices and Designs: Medical Technologies in Historical Perspective* (Basingstoke: Palgrave, 2006), pp. 1–16.

Tomkins, A., 'Paupers and the infirmary in mid-eighteenth century Shrewsbury', *Medical History*, 43 (1999), 208–27.

Tomkins, A., 'Women and poverty', in H. Barker and E. Chalus (eds), *Women's History: Britain 1700–1850* (London: Routledge, 2005), pp. 152–73.

Tomkins, A., *The Experience of Urban Poverty, 1723–82: Parish, Charity and Credit* (Manchester: Manchester University Press, 2006).

Tomkins, A., '"The excellent example of the working class": Medical welfare, contributory funding and the North Staffordshire Infirmary from 1815', *Social History of Medicine*, 21 (2008), 13–30.

Tomkins, A., 'Demography and the midwives: Deliveries and their denouements in north Shropshire, 1781–1803', *Continuity and Change*, 25 (2010), 199–232.

Tomkins, A., 'Retirement from the noise and hurry of the world: The experience of almshouse life', in J. McEwan and P. Sharpe (eds), *Accommodating Poverty: The Housing and Living Arrangements of the English Poor, c.1600–1850* (Basingstoke: Palgrave, 2011), pp. 263–83.

Tomkins, A., '"Labouring on a bed of sickness": The material and rhetorical deployment of ill-health in male pauper letters', in A. Gestrich, E. Hurren and S. King (eds), *Poverty and Sickness in Modern Europe: Narratives of the Sick Poor* (London: Continuum, 2012), pp. 51–68.

Tomkins, A., 'Workhouse medical care from working-class autobiographies, 1750–1834', in J. Reinarz and L. Schwarz (eds), *Medicine and the Workhouse* (Rochester: University of Rochester Press, 2013), pp. 86–102.

Tomkins, A., 'Poverty, kinship support and the case of Ellen Parker, 1818–1827', in P. Jones and S. King (eds), *Obligation, Entitlement and Dispute under the English Poor Laws* (Newcastle: Cambridge Scholars Press, 2015), pp. 107–38.

Topham, J., 'Publishing "popular science" in early nineteenth-century Britain', in A. Fyfe and B. Lightman (eds), *Science in the Marketplace* (Chicago: University of Chicago Press, 2007), pp. 135–68.

Turner, D., *Disability in Eighteenth-Century England: Imagining Physical Impairment* (London: Routledge, 2012).

Turner, D., and A. Withey, 'Technologies of the body: Polite consumption and the correction of deformity in eighteenth-century England', *History*, 99 (2014), 775–96.

Valenze, D., 'Charity, custom and humanity: Changing attitudes to the poor in eighteenth century England', in J. Garnett and C. Matthew (eds), *Revival and Religion since 1700: Essays for John Walsh* (London: Hambledon, 1993), pp. 59–78.

van Voss, L.-H., 'Introduction', in L.-H. van Voss (ed.), *Petitions in Social History* (Cambridge: Cambridge University Press, 2001), pp. 1–10.

van Voss, L.-H. (ed.), *Petitions in Social History* (Cambridge: Cambridge University Press, 2001).

Waddington, K., *Charity and the London Hospitals 1850–98* (Woodbridge: Boydell, 2000).

Wall, R., 'Families in crisis and the English poor law as exemplified by the relief programme in the Essex parish of Ardleigh 1795–7', in E. Ochiai (ed.), *The Logic of Female Succession: Rethinking Patriarchy and Patrinlineality in Global and Historical Perspective* (Kyoto: International Research Centre for Japanese Studies, 2002), pp. 101–27.

Wallis, P., 'Exotic drugs and English medicine: England's drug trade, c.1550– c. 1800', *Social History of Medicine*, 25 (2012), 20–46.

Walsh, V., 'Old and New poor laws in Shropshire 1820–1870', *Midland History*, 2 (1974), 225–43.

Weatherall, M., 'Making medicine scientific: Empiricism, rationality, and quackery in mid-Victorian Britain', *Social History of Medicine*, 9 (1996), 175–94.

Webb, S., and B. Webb, *English Poor Law History Part I: The Old Poor Law* (London: Cass, 1963).

West, J., *The Taylors of Lancashire: Bonesetters and Doctors 1750–1890* (Worsley: Privately Published, 1977).

Wheeler, M., *Heaven, Hell and the Victorians* (Cambridge: Cambridge University Press, 1994).

Whyman, S., *The Pen and the People: English Letter Writers 1660–1800* (Oxford: Oxford University Press, 2009).

Wild, W., *Medicine-by-Post: The Changing Voice of Illness in Eighteenth-Century British Consultation Letters and Literature* (Amsterdam: Rodopi, 2006).

Williams, G., *Angel of Death: The Story of Smallpox* (Basingstoke: Palgrave, 2011).

Williams, N., 'The reporting and classification of causes of death in mid-nineteenth-century England: The example of Sheffield', *Historical Methods*, 29 (1996), 58–71.

Williams, P., 'Religion, respectability and the origins of the modern nurse', in R. French and A. Wear (eds), *British Medicine in an Age of Reform* (London: Routledge, 1991), pp. 234–47.

Williams, S., 'Malthus, marriage and poor law allowances revisited: A Bedfordshire case study, 1770–1834', *Agricultural History Review*, 52 (2004), 56–82.

Williams, S., 'Caring for the sick poor: Poor law nurses in Bedfordshire c.1770–1834', in P. Lane, N. Raven and K. Snell (eds), *Women, Work and Wages in England 1600–1850* (Woodbridge: Boydell and Brewer, 2004), pp. 141–69.

Williams, S., 'Practitioners' income and provision for the poor: Parish doctors in the late eighteenth and early nineteenth centuries', *Social History of Medicine*, 18 (2005), 159–86.

Williams, S., 'The experience of pregnancy and childbirth for unmarried mothers in London, 1760–1866', *Women's History Review*, 20 (2011), 67–86.

Williams, S., *Poverty, Gender and Life-Cycle Under the English Poor Law 1760–1834* (Woodbridge: Boydell, 2011).

Williamson, S., *The Vaccination Controversy: The Rise, Reign and Fall of Compulsory Vaccination for Smallpox* (Liverpool: Liverpool University Press, 2007).

Wilson, A., *The Making of Man-Midwifery: Childbirth in England 1660–1770* (Harvard: Harvard University Press, 1995).

Wilson, A., 'The Birmingham General Hospital and its public, 1765–69', in S. Sturdy (ed.), *Medicine, Health and the Public Sphere in Britain 1600–2000* (London: Routledge, 2002), pp. 83–116.

Woods, R., *The Demography of Victorian England and Wales* (Cambridge: Cambridge University Press, 2000).

Woods, R., and A. Hinde, 'Mortality in Victorian England: Models and patterns', *Journal of Interdisciplinary History*, 18 (1987), 27–54.

Woods, R., N. Williams and C. Galley, 'Differential mortality patterns among infants and other young children: The experience of England and Wales in the nineteenth century', in C. Corsini and P. Viazzo (eds), *The Decline of Infant and Childhood Mortality: The European Experience 1750–1990* (The Hague: Martinus Nijhoff, 1997), pp. 57–72.

Woodward, J., *To Do the Sick No Harm: A Study of the British Voluntary Hospital System to 1875* (London: Routledge and Kegan Paul, 1974).

Wright, D., *Mental Disability in Victorian England: The Earlswood Asylum 1847–1901* (Oxford: Oxford University Press, 2001).

Wrigley, E., 'The effect of migration on the estimation of marriage age in family reconstruction studies', *Population Studies*, 48 (1994), 81–97.

Wrigley, E., R. Davies, J. Oeppen and R. Schofield, *English Population History from Family Reconstitution, 1580–1837* (Cambridge: Cambridge University Press, 1997).

Wyman, A., 'The surgeoness: The female practitioner of surgery 1400–1800', *Medical History*, 28 (1984), 22–41.

Unpublished works

Adams, J., 'The mixed economy for medical services in Herefordshire, c.1770–1850' (unpublished PhD thesis, University of Warwick, 2004).

Hill, J., 'Poverty, unrest and response in Surrey, 1815–1834' (unpublished PhD thesis, University of Roehampton, 2006).

Hitchcock, T., 'The English workhouse: A study in institutional poor relief in selected counties, 1696–1750' (unpublished DPhil thesis, University of Oxford, 1985).

Hopkin, N., 'The Old and New Poor Law in East Yorkshire, 1760–1850' (unpublished MPhil thesis, University of Leeds, 1968).

Neuman, E., 'The Old Poor Law in Kent 1606–1834' (unpublished PhD thesis, University of Kent, 1979).

Philipson, T., 'The sick poor and the quest for medical relief in Oxfordshire ca 1750–1834' (unpublished PhD thesis, Oxford Brookes University, 2009).

Ramsbottom, M., 'Christopher Waddington's peers: A study of the workings of the poor law in townships of the Fylde of Lancashire 1803 to 1865' (unpublished PhD thesis, Oxford Brookes University, 2011).

Taylor, S., 'Aspects of the socio-demographic history of seven Berkshire parishes in the eighteenth century' (unpublished PhD thesis, University of London, 1987).

Thomas, E., 'The treatment of poverty in Berkshire, Essex and Oxfordshire 1723–1840' (unpublished PhD thesis, University of London, 1971).

Topping, C., 'Welfare, class and gender: Non-affiliated friendly societies in Lancashire 1750–1835' (unpublished DPhil thesis, University of Oxford, 2006).

Walsh, V., 'Poor Law administration in Shropshire, 1820–1855' (unpublished PhD thesis, University of Pennsylvania, 1970).

Index

Page numbers in italics refer to figures, tables or other images

CW01508606